Chemotherapy in Emotional Disorders

CHEMOTHERAPY IN EMOTIONAL DISORDERS

The Psychotherapeutic Use of Somatic Treatments

FREDERIC F. FLACH, M.D., F.A.P.A.

Assistant Professor of Clinical Psychiatry,
Cornell University Medical College, New York;
Assistant Attending Psychiatrist,
Payne Whitney Psychiatric Clinic of The New York Hospital,
and St. Vincent's Hospital, New York

PETER F. REGAN, III, M.D., F.A.P.A.

Professor and Head of the Department of Psychiatry,
The J. Hillis Miller Health Center,
University of Florida College of Medicine,
Gainesville, Florida

THE BLAKISTON DIVISION

McGraw-Hill Book Company, Inc.

NEW YORK   TORONTO   LONDON

128991

*Dedicated to our wives, Patricia and
Laurette, and to our teachers, among
them Oskar Diethelm in particular*

FOREWORD

During the last 25 years we have witnessed a most impressive and hitherto unprecedented advance in that phase of medicine which deals with mental and emotional illness. The progress that has been achieved, however, has been so rapid, and the increase in both the scope and complexity of the whole field so great, that it has become essential to undertake a systematic organization of the new data in order to make it possible to apply in practice the knowledge that has been acquired.

From a clinical point of view this need for more adequate organization of the new material has been made particularly necessary because of two special features in this progress. The first of these is the introduction of a large number of new methods of treatment, especially in the area of somatic therapy. The second one is the knowledge that has been gained in regard to the importance of emotional factors in the causation of somatic illness and the development of the concept of psychosomatic medicine.

In regard to the former, it has become quite obvious that many of the new methods are primarily symptomatic in nature and, in the treatment of a number of these illnesses, may result in only temporary relief. This means that their usefulness can be vastly enhanced when combined with other methods, either in the same category or of the group included under the general term of psychotherapy. At the same time, the knowledge gained of the importance and significance of emotional and social stress in the development of somatic illness has attracted the attention of members of the medical profession in general and has made it necessary for them to acquire experience in using these new methods in the treatment of problems encountered in general practice. A systematic discussion of the entire range of these new methods of treatment, their indications and contraindications, as well as their relationships to the more time-honored psychotherapeutic procedures and the manner in which both can be combined in the total treatment of the patient, is not only timely, but also universally useful. It can be applied in the specialized area of psychiatry, as well as in the practice of general medicine.

The present book fulfills this need in a most satisfactory manner. The authors approach this problem with the advantage of a thorough knowledge of dynamic psychopathology and sophisticated, but also realistic, experience in psychotherapy, as well as practical experience in the use of the somatic therapies, both shock and pharmaceutical. They are also quite aware of the benefits that can be obtained from both, either separately or in combination, as well as of the caution that must be considered in using all of them. The material is presented in an orderly fashion, the style is lucid and avoids the pitfalls of being either too technical or oversimplified and of talking down to their readers. It should command a broad representation of readers in the field of psychiatry and in the general practice of medicine.

WILLIAM MALAMUD, M.D.
Professional and Research Director,
The National Association for Mental Health, Inc.

PREFACE

The development of psychopharmacologic agents has profoundly influenced psychiatric thought and practice. With the help of these agents, many patients have been able to resume productive, satisfying lives, and a dramatic realignment of treatment attitudes has taken place in the United States. This realignment of attitudes and the ease with which the many physical agents may be used have made a profound impact on research and treatment. New impetus has been given to investigations into biochemical and metabolic aspects of psychopathologic disorders. Simultaneously, prescriptions for the new drugs have multiplied at an almost unbelievable rate.

As with any rapid change, this research and therapeutic progress has created a host of unanswered questions and inviting challenges. These developments point up the fact that psychiatry can no longer continue as a house divided against itself. Instead, the time has come when it is crucial that psychodynamic and physiological concepts be unified in a fashion that will combine the complementary assets of each.

How may the physician integrate these somatic and psychologic therapeutic approaches in a meaningful way? When confronted with a particular patient, how can he decide whether or not to employ a somatic agent? If he elects to use a somatic agent, which one will he select in order to achieve his desired goal?

The preparation of this book was stimulated by these questions. Although specific information about somatic therapies is provided, the book has been designed primarily to present what appears to us to be a sound, practical basis for the incorporation of these therapies into psychotherapeutic treatment programs. We have attempted to discuss major areas of interest and to present principles which would be applicable to the clinical use of somatic agents currently available and of the others which will surely be developed in the next few years. No attempt has been made to outline the therapeutic management of every conceivable clinical situation which may arise, since to do so would distract from the primary purpose of this presentation.

It will quickly become apparent to the reader that we consider psycho-therapy a fundamental, indispensable element in the treatment of all patients with psychopathologic disturbances. When somatic treatments are introduced, they are best utilized in the setting of a dynamically oriented program of therapy.

It seems important, moreover, for the physician using these somatic agents to recognize that he is not treating an illness, such as schizophrenia, but rather that he is alleviating certain factors which significantly affect the clinical state of the patient. The analogy to the use of diuretics in the management of a patient with cardiovascular disease appears appropriate. The pharmacologic elimination of excess fluid will relieve the stress to the damaged heart. Thereby the patient will be able to function at a higher level and be relieved of subjective distress. Diuretics, however, will never in themselves restore healthy tissue to the heart injured by a coronary occlusion. In like manner, the administration of chlorpromazine to an angry, suspicious, delusional, paranoid schizophrenic patient will reduce his disturbing emotions and decrease the need for his misinterpretations. He may then make a satisfactory social adjustment and be able to par-ticipate in psychotherapy. However, the drug will not change those con-scious and unconscious personality factors and environmental considera-tions which contributed to his upheaval.

In using physical treatments to achieve such specific goals within a psychotherapeutic framework, our present state of knowledge imposes certain reasonable limitations on us. Many investigators are seeking screen-ing devices that will increase the accuracy with which treatments can be prescribed. At the moment, however, the only available guides are those which can be obtained by careful study of the psychodynamic and psychopathologic factors in the patient's condition. From this information, the physician can construct a profile which, when combined with a work-ing knowledge of the somatic therapies, will help him to pinpoint the correct form of treatment for the correct patient at the correct time.

In the first section of this volume, the principles and techniques in-volved in the evaluation of patients are discussed. In the second section, the various physical treatments and their spheres of effectiveness are described in detail. In the third section, these considerations are blended to illustrate the manner in which physical treatments can be used to en-hance psychotherapeutic treatment.

Careful attention to these criteria will increase the objectivity of the physician who is responsible for creating a plan of treatment. He will be less likely to be influenced by conscious and unconscious factors within his own personality in deciding whether to recommend or to avoid somatic therapies. We hope, therefore, that this presentation may be of interest and value to the psychiatrist, the psychoanalyst, the general practitioner, and all physicians who are confronted with the responsibility of helping the emotionally ill patient.

In the preparation of this manuscript, the authors wish to acknowledge the generous and capable assistance of Dr. Joseph F. Reilly, Susan Gould, Beatrice Rittenberg, and Christina Rockefeller.

Frederic F. Flach
Peter F. Regan, III

CONTENTS

Part One

THE EVALUATION OF THE PATIENT
FOR TREATMENT

1

PRINCIPLES OF PSYCHIATRIC
TREATMENT

Before embarking on an exploration of physical treatments in psychiatry, it is necessary to define the principles upon which the discussion is based. The notions of psychiatric illness and treatment that lie behind the practical techniques must be established, and it is the purpose of this chapter to make the authors' concepts explicit. A definition of this length has become necessary because of several developments in the present field of psychiatry. These developments are signs of growth and progress, but they are currently responsible for considerable confusion in the minds of psychiatrist and nonpsychiatrist alike.

The first of these confusion-breeding developments is the recent discovery of the tranquilizing and antidepressant drugs. On all sides, one hears zealous exponents of these various medications; enthusiastic claims for one treatment or another are balanced by equally enthusiastic counterclaims, and denunciations by counterdenunciations. Anyone who attempts to study one of the "wonder drugs" will quickly find it necessary to reconcile an enormous number of contradictory statements.

At the same time that this confusion exists in the field of physical treatment, another healthy, but confusing, conflict is taking place within the broader field of psychiatry. Exponents of different physical treatments suggest that these treatments are fundamental, basic, curative measures, which deal with the roots of psychiatric illness. Other psychiatrists, however, who are more exclusively psychotherapeutic in orientation, view these claims with great misgivings. It is the rule, rather than the exception, that the individual psychiatrist tends to align himself with the somatic or the psychotherapeutic camp. The patient, therefore,

3

seldom has the opportunity to receive a combined therapeutic approach. His treatment, more often, is guided by the orthodoxy—psychotherapeutic or somatotherapeutic—of the physician whom he consults.

In the light of this situation, it is no surprise that many physicians turn away from this field in dismay or resign themselves to using physical treatments on a completely empirical basis. It is the basic premise of this volume that such dismay and empiricism is regrettable and unnecessary. Although the field of physical treatment in psychiatry is most assuredly a young one, with many facts yet to be accumulated, nevertheless it contains a strong and firmly established core of knowledge. This knowledge, if used cautiously and intelligently, can greatly increase the effectiveness with which any physician can treat psychiatric disorders. Such treatment is based on the recognition that physical and psychologic factors combine to produce the phenomena we recognize as psychiatric illness. These two factors will now be considered, beginning with the physical forces which may contribute to the illnesses.

Physical Factors in Psychiatric Illness

At the most fundamental level, it is generally recognized that processes of thought and perception cannot exist without concomitant physiologic activity in the central nervous system. Such an apparent combination is obviously logical, and it is also buttressed by extensive experimental evidence. It is well recognized that attention and inattention, sleep and wakefulness, sensory stimulation and lack of stimulation, idle thought and problem-solving thought can all produce variations in the electroencephalographic recordings of brain activity. At a clinical level, many studies indicate that distortions of the normal electroencephalographic pattern are more frequently found in the presence of behavioral abnormality, as seen in personality disorders.

It is also apparent that the sympathetic nervous system and the endocrine system may influence thinking and behavior. Funkenstein (1957) has shown the close link which exists between the types of cardiovascular and behavioral response which subjects will display in a stressful situation. The studies of Flach (1959), Grinker (Basowitz, et al., 1955), and others indicate how closely other metabolic processes, such as calcium metabolism and liver function, are interwoven with illness and behavior. Outside the laboratory, one need only consider the "myxedema madness" of hypothyroidism, the depression of hypoparathyroidism, and the dementia associated with avitaminoses to be convinced that metabolic processes can indeed produce and influence the course of psychiatric illness.

When one begins to explore how these functions arrive at such a state of disorder, one is approaching the borderland of present-day research.

The work of Magoun and others (Jasper, et al., 1958) suggests that the reticular and limbic systems occupy pivotal roles in regulating central nervous system activity, possibly through the medium of the hypothalamus. At the same time, other work makes one suspect that these processes may be initiated by aberrations in intracellular or enzyme metabolism in specific areas of the central nervous system. It must be admitted, however, that these explorations can only give tentative leads at the present time. The situation is probably best seen as one in which disorders of thinking, emotions, and behavior are certainly linked to some extent with a complex of physiologic activities. This complex of activities must extend from cortical activity in the central nervous system, on the one hand, through midbrain electrical and metabolic activity to peripheral sympathetic, hormonal, and metabolic activities. Only time, and further exploration, will give definitive answers as to how these many factors work together.

In the light of this complex background of disrupted physiology which is associated with psychiatric illness, one must ask why these disordered processes come about. Certainly few etiologic factors are known. Examples include syphilis in causing paresis, the aftereffects of encephalitis and meningitis, and the avitaminoses already referred to. For the most part, however, one must admit ignorance of why the aberrations have come about, except to say that they *may* be attributed to genetic and constitutional factors. These factors, so well illustrated in studies of body build, certainly indicate that there are a large number of patients in whom the illness can be closely linked with the genes of the individual.

In summary, therefore, it may be said that there exists a large body of evidence to substantiate the claim that psychiatric illness is linked with physiologic disorders of one sort or another. We must recognize, however, that even the most advanced research workers are in doubt as to how these physiologic disruptions can influence behavior and how they are initiated in the first place. Only in rare cases is it possible to use a specific physiologic treatment, which deals directly with the causative factors in psychiatric illness. Most physiologic treatments are symptomatic, at best. Only when the real causes become known will these treatments become more truly curative.

Psychologic Factors in Psychiatric Illness

When one approaches psychiatric illness from the standpoint of psychologic etiology, one finds the same volume and complexity of etiologic factors as were found from the physiologic approach. Most physicians are probably aware of the dynamic constellations which different psychotherapists have suggested as causative of psychiatric illness. These therapists, whose number includes such illustrious names as Sigmund

Freud, Karen Horney, Harry Stack Sullivan, Franz Alexander, and Frieda Fromm-Reichman, have placed great emphasis on the internal psychologic mechanisms which persons may use to handle their emotional problems. These mechanisms, which include such devices as repression, sublimation, substitution, and conversion, may be viewed as analogous to the detailed electroencephalographic patterns found in electrophysiologic studies of the central nervous system. The fact that such mechanisms exist is not, in itself, news; common experience indicates that they exist and that they operate in our everyday lives. The brilliance of Freud and other investigators lies in the fact that they were able to define the mechanisms adequately and to illustrate in a detailed fashion how they work and how they become distorted in the course of psychiatric illness.

In describing these psychologic mechanisms, various investigators have used different terminology and this has led to a considerable amount of confusion. It may be difficult for the uninitiated to equate the variable terminology that may be found in the volumes of Freud and Sullivan. This semantic confusion is obviously regrettable, but it is also more or less inevitable, with our present understanding of the psychologic etiology of psychiatric illnesses. Every investigator who has approached the psychologic etiology of psychiatric illness has done so with a particular frame of reference in mind, e.g., the sexual and instinctual emphasis of Freudian psychoanalysis, the emphasis on interpersonal relationships of Sullivan, or Horney's emphasis on the social situation. When these different viewpoints are recognized, it becomes clear that the different investigators are almost obliged to use different terminology, owing to the current absence of means for correlating the findings of one with the findings of the next.

Although it is currently impossible to dovetail all the findings of various investigators, it is perfectly feasible to utilize their findings in a complementary fashion. In the study of personality development during infancy, for example, the impact of the social situation may be viewed in the light of Horney's work, while at the same time the infant's instinctual urges and the influences of the intimate interpersonal relationships between him and his mother may be regarded as crucial in his development.

Departing from the study of the individual subject, a number of investigators have provided ample evidence for the impact of psychologic factors on the development of psychiatric illness in different ways. In the social sphere, the findings of Bowlby (1952) with children isolated from maternal care gave evidence of how psychologic deprivation may lead to the development of personality distortions. On different scales of social psychiatric research, studies in large cities (Rennie, et al., 1957), medium-sized cities (Hollingshead and Redlich, 1958), and small towns (Leighton, et al., 1957) illuminate a seemingly endless series of pertinent facts. Thus, these studies provide evidence that psychiatric illness differs in its timing and its nature according to the ethnic group in which it is found; there is a marked difference, for example, between schizophrenic illness among Irish populations and that among Italian populations (Opler, et al., 1956). There are also differences in the nature of psychiatric illness according to the level of social class; the awareness of illness, and the expectations of treatment, are radically different in upper-class, middle-class, and lower-class persons, for cultural, educational, and economic reasons. Finally, it has been found that the highest incidence of psychiatric illness occurs in persons and families who are involved in the process of social change. Whether moving up or down on the socio-economic ladder, mobile groups are most likely to have the highest frequency, and the greatest severity, of psychiatric illness.

When these studies are linked with the elaborate investigations of the effect of environmental stresses on the individual, the fact that psychologic factors may induce psychiatric illness becomes a virtual certainty. One need only think of the clear-cut relationships which many workers have demonstrated between life situations and such variable physiologic changes as duodenal ulcers, migraine headaches, and cardiovascular illness to recognize that these factors are indeed associated with physiologic change. Currently, there is great interest in the effects of "sensory deprivation"; persons placed in isolation will, within a matter of 6 or 8 hours, demonstrate delusions, hallucinations, and thinking difficulties which mirror the development and some of the characteristics of schizophrenic reactions. The similarity between these findings and the clinical phenomena which follow the administration of such drugs as lysergic acid diethylamide is well known.

Thus, everyday experience, together with experimental evidence from individual studies, group studies, and large-scale social investigations, indicates the fact that psychologic factors are important in the etiology of psychiatric illness. Once again, as with the physiologic factors, the details are not yet known. How much of the influence of the psychologic factors is direct, and how much is mediated through the effect of experience on the person's physiologic state, is unclear. Certainly, treatment of psychologic factors almost always modifies illness to some extent.

The Dangers of Therapeutic Exclusiveness

Even these brief surveys indicate the strength of the arguments that can be raised in favor of the fact that psychiatric illnesses have a combined cause, produced in part by both psychologic and physiologic factors. One would think that physicians, faced with this likelihood, would use a combined approach in dealing with these illnesses. Such, however, is not the case. On the contrary, physicians are apt to concentrate on one approach or another. In consequence, they guide their therapy along the specific lines with which they are familiar. It will be found, time after time, that a physician will routinely use certain drugs or certain interview techniques, regardless of the nature of the situation with which he is dealing.

This same dichotomy exists among psychiatrists, who, because of their more continuous experience with psychiatric illness, might be expected to be highly aware of the combined cause of psychiatric illnesses. The studies of Hollingshead and Redlich (1958), for example, indicate that psychiatrists tend to fall into one of two groups: the directive-organic group of therapists or the analytic-psychological group of therapists. Members of the former group tend to use the most abbreviated forms of psychotherapy, and they emphasize the use of drugs and other physical treatments in their therapeutic endeavors. Members of the latter group, conversely, avoid the use of any medications and concentrate almost solely on the use of interview psychotherapeutic techniques. This dichotomy, with its therapeutic exclusiveness, is manifested in individual practice and is also reflected in the existence of various schools, groups, academies, and societies, which intermingle only on rare occasions and which foster the exclusive use of one or the other of these two distinct approaches.

In the light of this realistic situation, Hollingshead and Redlich doubt the existence of an eclectic therapist. They point out that an eclectic therapist, if he does exist, is rare indeed. The experience of the authors tends to justify this skepticism and even to carry it one step further. The so-called eclectic therapist, when he is found, is apt to be a person who uses various forms of therapy, psychologic and physiologic, but uses them on an either-or basis. He uses these methods of therapy *without* combining them with other methods which might be complementary. The eclectic therapist may use electroconvulsive therapy in one patient and intensive psychotherapeutic interviews in another patient. It is only rarely, unfortunately, that he combines the physical and the psychologic approach in his treatment of a single patient.

This is the current pattern of therapeutic exclusiveness. For reasons linked with training or personality, most physicians tend to slip into a groove of physiologic or psychologic treatment. Those who try to use both approaches tend to do so on an either-or basis, using only one approach with any one patient. As a result, the general treatment of patients suffers. Neither a psychologic nor a physiologic approach can, at present, make a pretense of dealing with genuine causative factors. Both approaches work at symptomatic levels. Both, moreover, may influence symptoms in the other area; physiologic measures can alter psychologic symptoms, and vice versa. To eliminate one or the other of these approaches is to deprive the patient of an additional chance for benefit from treatment and is the unfortunate effect of therapeutic exclusiveness.

A Combined Therapeutic Approach

It is because of the existence of this widespread segmentation of psychiatric treatment that the present book is written. The authors firmly believe that the existence of a patient with only a physical problem or only a psychologic problem is a theoretical possibility, but a practical impossibility. Even in general paresis, for example, the treatment cannot be centered solely on the physical etiologic factors. On the contrary, the personality configuration and the specific nature of the patient's symptoms make it necessary to apply the physical treatment measures in a specific fashion; this specific treatment, moreover, must be suitable not only for the patient, but also for his family and for the social situation in which he lives. At the other end of the physiologic-psychologic scale, even the most classical of the psychoneuroses is associated with some physiologic abnormalities. One must always be aware of these and be prepared to use physical means of intervention, however mild, if such intervention can promote the effective utilization of the intensive psychotherapy which is carried out.

A combined therapeutic approach, therefore, is not one in which the physician uses *either* physical *or* psychologic treatment measures. Instead, it is one in which the use of any physical treatment depends on its validity in the psychotherapeutic situation; e.g., will the administration of chlorpromazine not only control an excitement but also aid the long-range psychotherapeutic plans? Conversely, the combined approach demands that psychotherapy be carried out with full awareness that it is not the only treatment medium, but may be speeded or aided enormously by the properly timed application of physical treatments, e.g., use of shock treatment to overcome massive resistance in the psychotherapeutic treatment of a schizophrenic patient (Hill, 1955). The two approaches, psychotherapeutic and physical, must be continually intertwined.

The Course of Personality Development

This combined therapeutic approach is based on a belief that the development of personality is influenced by both physical and psychosocial forces. When psychiatric symptoms or illnesses exist in the personality, all these forces should be considered and controlled. In the next few pages, the course of personality development will be sketched, to illustrate how the two kinds of forces relate to each other and to provide a frame of reference for later etiologic comments.

It is a generally accepted notion that an individual comes into the world with relatively fixed genetic and constitutional characteristics. These characteristics, in themselves, will alter the way in which the individual proceeds through various stages of development. At each of these stages of development, in turn, a variety of physical factors may intervene: these include accidents, infections, nutritional factors, and the indirect effect of other physical illnesses. Throughout the course of life, therefore, an individual's personality is influenced by basic inherited characteristics and by subsequent modifications.

The influence of physical factors of personality, however, is not a one-way street. Coming into the world with certain genetic characteristics, the individual is also subjected to a number of psychologic factors, intra-personal and environmental. These factors, in turn, will create their own influences on his development, accelerating or retarding the rate at which he grows to fulfill his potential. Not only will they act directly, in a psychologic fashion, but also they will greatly modify, by direct and indirect means, the physical characteristics which the individual possesses. Thus, there exists a never-ending circle of interaction, with physical and psychologic factors combining and recombining to produce different constellations of personality as the individual grows and develops.

Being subject to these factors, physical and psychologic, the individual may be seen to go through the following stages of development.

INFANCY

During this stage, which lasts from birth to approximately 15 months, the individual must learn to delineate himself from his environment. Just as he must learn to evaluate the length of his arms and legs and his physical limitations as he proceeds to walk, talk, grasp objects, and the like, so must he learn his psychologic limits. He must learn to recognize the world as existing apart from himself and to see that it does not respond magically to his wishes. The ordinary degree of delineation of self is one which allows a certain healthy relatedness to the world and which allows the individual to retain a comfortable sense of power and self-centeredness. These are healthy remnants of an egocentric world and may be seen, in adult life, in the ordinary sensitivity of the individual to the feelings of other persons, in the use of daydreams and fantasies, and in the importance which most persons attach to their own existence and ideas. Inadequate delineation of one's self may exaggerate these characteristics, as in the extreme sensitivity, personalization, and magic distortions of reality which are found in schizophrenic reactions.

EARLY CHILDHOOD

This period of life may be said to extend from age 15 months to age 35 months. Having delineated himself, the child now has to learn ways of dealing with the external reality which he has recognized. During this period of his development, therefore, he learns over-all patterns for controlling his emotions, obtaining what he wants in the world, and avoiding what he does not want. Depending on his perceptions and his situation, he acquires traits of emotionality, rigidity, habit formation, cleanliness, morality. He adopts a set of pervasive characteristics, which we see as the core features of the personality in persons with whom we deal. These characteristics are used in an across-the-board fashion; a rigid, obsessive pattern, for example, will be used by an individual, in his dealings with person after person, in shifting situations, without regard for greater or lesser appropriateness.

If the work of this state of development is not accomplished satisfactorily, one will find such later distortions as excessive rigidity, obsessive-compulsive symptomatology, the psychopathic acting out of personality disorders, and the pleasure-empty existence of the depressed patient.

LATE CHILDHOOD

This developmental period extends from age 3 to age 5. When a child enters this developmental period, he has delineated himself from the environment and has learned over-all methods of dealing with this environment. During the stage of late childhood, it is necessary for him to accomplish two objectives. The first of these is *individualization,* the ability to modify his over-all patterns in accordance with varying needs of different aspects of the environment. Having learned *over-all traits,* such as neatness and cleanliness, and having adopted *over-all mechanisms* for revealing and concealing emotions, the child must now learn how different persons and different situations will modify these over-all standards. He must learn to show more love and affection in protected situations and to guard himself in new or unfriendly situations. He must learn that different standards of behavior are maintained in the bedroom, in the dining room, in the playground, and in the kindergarten. If his development during early childhood has been excessively rigid, it will not be possible for him to modify his patterns. With normal previous development, however, it should be possible for a child to learn a realistic amount of variability and to succeed at the first objective of late childhood—individualization.

Linked with this need to modify the over-all patterns in dealing with the environment is the second part of the work to be done during the period of late childhood. This work is that of *forming identifications*. As surrounding persons come into sharper individual focus during the period of late childhood, the child will find that he is more attracted to some, less attracted to others. Gradually, he will have to adapt himself to the reality of the situation. Early in the period of late childhood, at approximately age 3, the child will wish immediately to take the place of those whom he admires. The male child, for example, will usually show jealousy of the prerogatives and pleasures of the father and will frequently wish to assert his own authority and take the father's place; these unrealistic wishes for substitution, when expressed in the sexual area, are commonly regarded as the matrix of the oedipal situation. Over the succeeding 2 years, however, the child must learn that the wishes for immediate substitution are impossible. He must see himself more and more realistically, in his physical and intellectual lack of development, and gradually change his attitude toward the person he admires. Instead of wishing immediately to replace the object of his admiration, he gradually forms an identification; i.e., he sets the person up as an ideal and bends his energies toward striving to equal the ideal by developing his own intelligence, physical power, and experience.

The complex interaction of these two processes which go on in late childhood—individualization and identification—makes this period a very significant one for later life development. Failure to individualize, of course, results in an inability to utilize one's assets in an adaptable fashion. It prevents, at the same time, mature and unhampered relationships by forcing all adult relationships into a single mold, one which was workable in early childhood but is now unworkable. Failure to individualize hampers the development of identifications. Identifications may also be hampered by activities on the part of those with whom the child is attempting to identify. An overly protective and yielding attitude, for example, may fail to bring the reality of the situation to the child's attention. The parent, for example, who attempts to "make things easy" for his child, by yielding to the unrealistic demands seen in the earlier part of late childhood, can produce in the child an unrealistically powerful sense of security. Since he is able to gratify his desires by simply wishing, he may develop a pattern of boastfulness and overambition, without having learned the need to work for the things which he desires. The result, in adult life, is frequently seen in the individual of high aims without matching ability.

An opposite type of impediment to identification may also be found. Parents who are excessively punitive and frightening, in the face of rivalry during the period of late childhood, can smother the child's attempts to assert his own independence and individuality. The child learns that expressions of independence bring only retribution and that it is easier for him to remain identified as a child than to strive for his own place in the world. This constellation is frequently seen in association with such clinical illnesses as psychoneurotic conversion reactions and psychoneurotic reactions associated with phobias and anxiety hysteria. Obviously, parents who do not fulfill their traditional roles impair the process of identification in a number of ways; the mother who dominates the household, the sadistic father, and many other types of parents and parental relationships can warp and distort the process of identification. Among other results, it is not unusual to see the development of sexual deviations, which may range from nymphomania to homosexuality.

LATENCY

This period of development extends from age 6 until 11. As a time of life, it has received little attention from psychiatric investigators, although there are many studies about educating children in this period. Apparently, it is used by most children as a time in which they devote themselves wholeheartedly to growing and learning, in order to work toward fulfilling the role which they adopted by identification. Thus, we see children of ages 7 to 11 as active, industrious, almost voracious seekers after knowledge, strength, and power. Wrapped up in their quest, it is common to find that they do not involve themselves with great strength in other emotional attachments. If strong traumatic influences intervene, however, profound damage can be done to the child's ability to work and to maintain persistence in achieving goals in later life.

PUBESCENCE AND ADOLESCENCE

This period of life extends from approximately age 12 to age 17 to 19, depending on the socioeconomic and cultural level of the individual. Roughly, it may be said to range from the time of development of the secondary sexual characteristics until that time when the person is expected to move out of the family situation and adopt his independent and mature role in society. Typically, the child is growing into physical maturity, which he usually achieves by the age of 16 or 17. He relives all the different problems of the first years of life. He must again find himself in a world, learn over-all patterns of dealing with this world, and learn individual modifications of the over-all patterns. All this work is now done, however, in a situation which is much more fraught with significance. The reason for this is simple: the child is now a near adult, almost ready to put his wishes and ambitions to the test. He now has the physical strength and intellectual power to put his hostile or loving feelings into action. They are no longer "harmless" fantasies, but thoughts which are only a hairbreath away from execution. As a result, the testing of the environment is more potent, and dangerous, than that done by the 3-year-old. The game is now "for real."

In this setting, the child must go through the painful process of separation from his family. Typically, this object is achieved through a series of steps. In young adolescence, the individual takes the first step by immersing himself in peer groups of his own sex. He develops close attachments to children of his own age, occasionally taking part in some overt homosexual activity, such as mutual masturbation. Using the security of this closely knit group, with its uniformity in clothing, amusement, and other activities, the adolescent can begin to explore heterosexual relationships. He gradually works through the stages of group dating and individual dating, using group standards as his guide.

As the group activity shifts to individual heterosexual activity, the adolescent is torn by many conflicts. His rising sexual and aggressive urges are in conflict with his dependency needs of the family, his feelings of insecurity, and frequently with his moral, ethical, and social standards. In the face of this tumultuous situation, the adolescent presents a façade of contradictions. Beneath the hard shell of rebellion and self-assurance, he is in great need of security and understanding, as he strives to harness his drives in a way that will obtain the world's approval and still give him satisfaction.

The outcome of this period of development, of course, is an individual who has more or less established his goals in life and is prepared to set out independently in pursuit of those goals. He has reconciled the varying demands of his drives, his standards, and the world. Many illnesses arise, and seeds of many more are planted, before this reconciliation is achieved. The most common illness to appear during adolescence is the schizophrenic reaction.

Schizophrenic reactions are apt to occur at any time from the age of 15 until the end of adolescence. They are commonly found in persons whose basic delineation of the world is imperfect and who collapse into illness under the stress of the conflicts that they must resolve.

Other difficulties appear in adolescence. Some adolescents cope with their problems by behavior disorders; these include shyness, extreme rebelliousness, and delinquency. In the shifting of adolescence, they have not become fixed, nor can they always be diagnosed by the standards that are applied to adult difficulties. They are, nonetheless, indicative of serious trouble and of more trouble to come in the future.

Finally, it must be remembered that adolescence is the period during which the personality is finally becoming fixed. In some situations, the "shell" of the adolescent can be frozen into a shell of conformity. Lacking support from his home or his environment, the adolescent may easily come to feel that his own feelings, opinions, and ambitions are worthless. He then is led to deny these feelings, guiding his actions and life only by external standards. Whether those standards be common or uncommon, exemplary or criminal, is irrelevant. The total externalization of standards is likely to result in an inability to satisfy one's own needs; it is this inability which, in later years, may give rise to the dynamic situations leading to paranoid illnesses.

YOUNG ADULTHOOD

This period of development ranges from the end of adolescence to the age of 40. It is the time of life when an adult is expected to complete his entry into the world and to establish himself in his permanent role of life. This period is commonly associated with marked optimism in its early years. During the third decade of life, as the individual separates himself from the family, he commonly uses mechanisms such as denial, as he projects overoptimistic goals in marriage and career. By such mechanisms as conversion, he may protect himself from the threat of facing the need for independence. Illnesses which occur during this period include those illnesses, such as psychoneuroses and schizophrenic reactions, which are associated with strains of dealing with the environment in an independent fashion.

In the fourth decade of life, during the period of gradual adjustment of goals, the early optimism fades. While the healthy individual feels sadness when he recognizes his limits, the excessively rigid tend toward overcompensation through increased obsessive-compulsive symptomatology. Alternatively, they may sink into psychoneurotic depressive reactions or psychosomatic illnesses. If environmental standards have been paramount, a paranoid illness frequently develops.

MIDDLE AGE

This period of life extends roughly from the age of 40 until the age of 60. It is during this time that an individual must recognize that he needs to be satisfied by the pleasures that he is obtaining in the social and environmental situation in which he lives. Until this period of life, persons are frequently buoyed up by hopes for the future and by their assumptions that achieving their goals in life will bring them satisfaction. Thus, the businessman will aim at being the president of his concern and the housewife at raising her children satisfactorily; both will aim at a future goal. During the time of middle life, however, one must face the fact that the future has arrived. Sometimes former goals have been achieved; sometimes they have not.

When goals are not reached, depression may ensue; it may also be found when the goals *are* reached. As the man achieves the presidency and the woman finds her children going off to be married, the previously accepted goals no longer offer a *hope* of satisfaction. If the satisfaction has not already been obtained, there is nothing to look forward to and depression appears. Middle age is the time for evaluation of one's self and for learning to obtain satisfaction from what *is* rather than from what *will be.*

In addition, the person in middle age is almost always forced to make some plans for modifying his life. This is necessary because of social situations, such as the departure of children for college and marriage, and the demands of work. It is also necessary because of physical factors, such as pulmonary or cardiac illnesses, as well as generally decreased energy and capacity. As a result of these pressures, the person in middle life may find himelf giving up many of the physical pleasures and satisfactions, and the prestige-producing activities, which he previously utilized. In devising his future, he must compensate for these losses or he will make the problem of obtaining day-by-day satisfaction even harder to solve.

The work to be done during the period of middle age, therefore, requires reevaluation of life goals and the establishment of reasonable patterns for continued satisfying life. The successful working through of this problem will produce an individual who obtains his pleasure from his daily activities and no longer needs a life in which pleasure is anticipated in the distant future. The unsuccessful resolution of this conflict commonly results in myriad physical complaints and frequently in overt depressive reactions.

OLD AGE

This period in life begins at about the age of 60 or later and continues until death. Even more than in middle age, the individual is called upon to face his limitations and to make a radical readjustment of his previous mode of living. He must be prepared to give up many of the achievement patterns of previous years and to satisfy himself with new, more restricted patterns. As the process of aging continues, he must recognize that he is no longer able to be as quick in grasp, as malleable in methodology, as incisive in thinking, and as ambitious as he was previously. Instead, he must depend more and more on experience to substitute for adaptability. He must recognize that he possesses the resources of experience and maturity which are denied to more energetic, ambitious, and adaptable youth. Successful working through of these problems can lead to activity, productivity, and satisfaction in old age. The unsuccessful working through of these problems leads to an acceleration of withdrawal and to the ineffectiveness associated with senility; it is frequently seen in the anxious, bewildered, and agitated depressions of aging persons.

Significance of Developmental Periods

It is clear, in reviewing these developmental periods, that each of them is associated with physical and environmental stresses and that the mode of passing through one developmental period will, in turn, radically affect the way in which the succeeding developmental periods are handled. At any given stage, an individual is subjected to myriad forces—physical, social, broad environmental, cultural, intrafamilial, intrapersonal. What goes wrong, and what goes right, in each of these periods may be influenced by variations of any one of these forces. When any one force is modified, in turn, there will be compensatory modifications in other forces.

It is this mutual interdependence that determines the theme which the authors will follow in succeeding chapters. It is the belief of the authors that the physician, when he is called on to deal with a patient, must view carefully every single factor which may currently influence the person's life and which may have influenced it in the past. His treatment should be a balanced treatment, utilizing every possible resource to deal with each one of the determining forces, physical, psychologic, and social.

Most especially, this holds true with regard to the use of physical treatments. With rare exceptions, there are no definitive somatic treatments available for psychologic complaints. Such treatments, therefore, must be used in the light of a thorough evaluation of the other forces which guide the individual patient. Only by doing so can somatic treatments achieve their maximum effectiveness and fulfill their role in a truly comprehensive treatment program.

2

DIAGNOSTIC CONSIDERATIONS

In dealing with the many complexities of a psychiatric illness, it is clear that the physician must be able to construct a worthwhile therapeutic plan. Such a plan, of necessity, must deal with a number of variables in the most effective fashion possible. Just this necessity has caused much difficulty in psychiatry during recent years. On the one hand, the multiplicity of factors which characterize the illness indicates that each patient, and each illness, must be considered an individual entity. When one approaches each patient in this fashion, however, one loses the benefits of accumulated experience, because the unique individual entity, as such, cannot be related to other patients and other illnesses; the physician is alone in the dark. If he adopts this viewpoint in its totality, he is exploring an unknown territory, without the benefit of his own past experience and that of others.

In order to compensate for this difficulty, various sorts of terminology can be applied to psychiatric illnesses. As soon as diagnostic considerations appear, however, one is faced with the inescapable fact that diagnoses do not reveal a sufficiently detailed story to allow for intelligent individualized treatment. A schizophrenic reaction, for example, will show wide variations in different settings, in different persons, and in different cultures; the schizophrenic reaction which appears during a landing on a South Pacific beach during World War II (Ripley and Wolf, 1951), for example, differs from a schizophrenic reaction which occurs in a 15-year-old school boy. Conversely, however, each of these schizophrenic reactions will have certain features in common. They will share certain common pathology and certain common etiologic problems.

The problem, therefore, is to join an individualized approach with a nosologic approach. To some extent, this can be accomplished by recognizing the different *levels* at which descriptive terms operate. Descriptive terms, for example, may be found at three levels: (1) diagnostic terms; (2) emotional terms; (3) symptomatic terms. At each one of these three levels, a number of commonly recognized terms may be found. Moreover, terms at these three different levels may occur in any kind of combination. Hysterical symptoms may be found in schizophrenic illnesses, in psychoneurotic illnesses, and in all other diagnostic categories. Emotions, such as anxiety and anger, may be found in association with varying symptoms and, once more, may be found in all diagnostic categories.

In addition to the diagnostic, emotional, and symptomatic characteristics which the patient may display, there are other factors, which include his physical condition, his personality configuration, and the setting in which he becomes ill. It requires no more than a brief review of the possible combinations to realize that categorizing a patient at each of these levels will produce a highly specific statement of the illness which that person manifests, within the framework of present-day nosology.

The ability to arrive at this degree of specificity in describing the illness with which a patient suffers would have a value in itself, if only to allow for duplication of results. Above and beyond this benefit, however, is the fact that, at each of the levels suggested, the specific terms convey a large amount of etiologic information. The diagnosis of a schizophrenic reaction, for example, calls to mind certain physical, emotional, intellectual, and historical factors, which most schizophrenic reactions hold in common. The existence of hysterical symptoms, likewise, calls to mind a rather specific image of personality structure and past dynamic conflicts.

Finally, the terms which are used at different levels convey information about the methods of treatment that may be used in dealing with a specific situation. As a patient is classified at each level, therefore, there is formed a multifaceted image of his illness. Every term is specific. Every term helps the physician to place the patient in proper perspective and also to understand etiologic factors and decide on the optimal treatment measures.

It is the use of these different levels of information, in this specific fashion, which is being suggested in the present section of this book. It must be remembered that the physician must never lose sight of the individuality of his patient. At the same time, he must not allow this human aspect of therapy to serve as an excuse for careless or illogical thinking. Each individual finding should be fitted into the nearest appropriate classification, at each of the several levels which will be discussed in succeeding chapters. In the process of doing so, the physician will be able more and more clearly to see the proper therapeutic course. Naturally, categories will never substitute for recognition of the individual in adequate psychotherapeutic treatment. It is possible, however, when the use of descriptive terms is approached in a multilevel fashion, to make the individual treatment much more organized and effective.

In approaching these different levels of considering a patient, two factors should be borne in mind. The first factor is that the authors will attempt, in the following chapters, to limit themselves to those descriptive terms which are obvious. Thus, when a patient is described as "angry," the reader may assume that the patient is obviously angry; it is not necessary to embark on elaborate speculations, with analyses of defenses, in order to recognize that the anger exists. Although many symptoms, emotions, and other important considerations may remain hidden and may be seen only by specialized techniques, these are not considered in the current volume. The current volume, on the contrary, is concerned with obvious, clear-cut, clinical manifestations, such as may be seen without difficulty in any physician's office.

The second consideration to be borne in mind is that the emphasis in the present volume is on dynamic *somatic* treatment in psychiatry. Physical treatment is usually treatment of the individual, as opposed to group treatment; as a result, a great deal more emphasis is placed on the diagnostic, symptomatic, and emotional characteristics of the individual concerned than upon the social and cultural setting in which he operates. This bias is unavoidable, because of the purpose of the present volume. It is wise to remember, however, that the environmental considerations may be of far more importance in the treatment of some patients than the factors to which we shall turn the major portion of our attention. This recognition should serve only to emphasize once again the need to regard physical treatments as auxiliary to the over-all course of psychotherapeutically oriented treatment.

The consideration of terms which are used at different levels will begin with those terms which are used at the diagnostic level.

PSYCHONEUROTIC REACTIONS

A psychoneurotic reaction may be regarded as an emotional illness in which unconscious conflicts produce an emotional disturbance which incapacitates the patient in his functioning in daily life. In a psychoneurotic illness, anxiety is the common emotional denominator. This anxiety may be manifested directly, in the setting of a psychoneurotic anxiety reaction, or it may be manifested indirectly, through the symptoms which produce other subdivisions of the psychoneuroses. In none of the psychoneuroses is there found any significant disruption of the normal contact with environment and reality. The patient evaluates environmental situations accurately and recognizes the existence of his own illness.

The Etiology of Psychoneurotic Reactions

At the present time, it is commonly believed that the cause of psychoneurotic reactions lies in early personality development, predominantly between the ages of 2 and 6. During this period of time, as the individual first learns over-all patterns of adjustment and then acquires individualized patterns, distortions may be produced in a number of ways. Owing to the child's faulty perception of his environment, to undue environmental stresses produced by parents, or to other factors, the child may come to have anxiety about perfectly normal drives or feelings. A rigid, compulsive family situation, for example, may create absolute condemnation of expression of emotions; the child quickly experiences anxiety whenever he feels such emotions as anger. As a child, he may try to alleviate his anxiety by constructing defense mechanisms to control the feelings which produced the threatening anxiety. This may be done during the period of early childhood by the construction of over-all obsessive-compulsive defenses; the anger or the loneliness or the need to show love is quickly suppressed by focusing attention on details, neatness, and routines, until the latter become the only outward expression of the child's emotional life. In late childhood, the child may adopt patterns of avoidance or dependency in order to avoid anxiety-producing situations, such as rivalry with parents or sibling difficulties; he may learn to use physical complaints to avoid every environmental threat. These defensive maneuvers, although perhaps appropriate in the situations of early and late childhood, become fixed with the passage of time. When the individual has grown to adulthood, however, he will be expected to take his place in the world as an independent human being, and he will therefore be called upon to respond to situations in a number of healthy and direct fashions. The problems of work adjustment, marriage, aggressiveness, and companionship will then be at odds with the individual's fixed pattern. Every day they will demand that he express his feelings and that he take some risks in pursuing his goals; his personality, however, will continue to call for concealment of these and other feelings. Depending upon the strength of the defense mechanisms, the power of the underlying feelings, and the nature of the environmental situations, a disharmonious situation may then be produced. If the power of the hidden feelings is too strong, then the defense mechanisms increase to control them. With every increase in such mechanisms as compulsions, the person becomes less able to deal with his environment and is finally incapacitated by overt illness.

This brief sketch has indicated some of the necessities that must be satisfied before an adequate diagnosis of a psychoneurotic reaction may be made. First of all, there must be the existence of anxiety or of defense mechanisms which control anxiety. Secondly, there must be a logical sequence of past personality development into which the anxiety or the anxiety defense mechanisms will fit. Thirdly, the environmental situation must be such that it would call forth the symptomatic response which is seen. Fourthly, the symptomatic response must interfere with life functions. Finally, there must be no evidence of any break with reality or the existence of another psychiatric illness. The over-all story, in short, must make sense, and the physician must be able to point to a definite etiologic pattern which has produced the illness which he sees. The diagnosis of a psychoneurosis may *not* be made merely because of the absence of indications of another illness.

Types of Psychoneurotic Reactions

Within this over-all framework, there are several syndromes and subdivisions of psychoneurotic reactions. These are as follows.

CONVERSION REACTION

This illness usually occurs in pleasant, immature persons, more frequently female, in the late teens or early twenties. Surface anxiety is usually absent, being expressed through a number of conversion symptoms, which may include such manifestations as paralyses, amnesia, and sensory difficulties, none of which have a neurologic basis. The background of the individual usually includes an early life in which the relationship with parental figures was marked by domination by the parent of the opposite sex, and the patient has had difficulty in achieving a proper heterosexual identification. The symptoms will fluctuate in accord with the demands of the environmental situation. They will usually be most severe at times of crisis, when the patient is expected to take a mature and independent heterosexual role, e.g., moving out of the home, becoming engaged, taking an aggressive position in society. At such times of crisis, the severity of the symptoms will serve to prevent action on the proposed move, and the patient will be "forced" to give up his goal. The prognosis, with treatment, is usually good.

ANXIETY HYSTERIA

This type of psychoneurotic reaction also occurs in the late teens and early twenties, in persons with personality configurations, family backgrounds, and environmental situations similar to those described under conversion reactions. In anxiety hysteria, however, anxiety is overtly present. The patient does not connect the anxiety with his personality or the environmental stresses, however. Instead it is displaced and linked to certain kinds of symbolically significant situations; the classic examples of this displacement are the various phobias. On investigation, it is almost invariably found that these phobias will produce the same degree of incapacity and secondary gain as do the conversion symptoms. The prognosis with this illness is good, though not so uniformly good as with conversion reaction.

OBSESSIVE-COMPULSIVE REACTION

This illness occurs in the late twenties and early thirties. Patients develop this illness gradually, over a period of months and years. Such persons are usually rigid, tight, and bound in. Examination of their background reveals that they come from strong, rigid, and suppressive families and that they have used defenses of neatness, denial, and compulsiveness throughout their lives. Most frequently, these defenses were quite successful in producing initial emancipation from the home, and the late teens and early twenties were marked by success, as meticulous work drew rewards from teachers in school and from early employers. By the time the patient has entered the third decade of life, however, the inability to modify his fixed and unemotional approach becomes increasingly unrewarding; he finds that he cannot enjoy relaxed emotional relationships with other persons, even his family, and that he cannot mobilize his resources in an aggressive fashion when dealing with social or work situations. Increasing dissatisfaction with the situation, however, merely produces an increase in the basic characteristics, and a vicious circle is thus established. Finally, the full-blown clinical picture supervenes. The patient carries on compulsive activity, such as checking locks or gas fixtures; his thinking becomes preoccupied with obsessive thoughts on such subjects as violence, sin, or sexuality. The obsessions and compulsions increasingly fill the patient's days, and he becomes incapacitated. There is marked anxiety associated with the illness, but this is attributed to the existence of the obsessions and compulsions. The prognosis in this illness is grave, with the possibility of complete recovery being limited. Frequently, therapeutic efforts can modify the over-all course of illness, but it is difficult, and sometimes impossible, to do so; some patients require continuous hospitalization.

DEPRESSIVE REACTIONS

In many respects, the psychoneurotic depressive reactions are similar to the obsessive-compulsive reactions. They occur in persons with much the same family backgrounds, personality characteristics, and previous history. Gradually, the basic rigidity and concealment of feelings produce the same degree of dissatisfaction. The rigidity of personality, however, is not such that it produces the flagrant obsessive and compulsive symptoms found in the previous group. Instead, after struggling with his dissatisfaction for a number of years, the patient gradually experiences increasing feelings of depression and futility. These become apparent in the late twenties and early thirties, together with severe anxiety about the origin of the problem. Prognosis for these patients is variable.

To understand the subdiagnosis of anxiety reaction, it is necessary to see the interrelationships of the preceding four groups. Conversion re-actions and anxiety hysteria, as we have seen, occur in persons whose problems of identification probably have their origin in difficulties in late childhood; these persons have difficulty as they face the problems of independence in adult life, particularly in the area of heterosexuality. Obsessive and compulsive and depressive psychoneurotic reactions, on the other hand, tend to occur in rigid, tightly organized persons, whose difficulties probably originated in early childhood; these illnesses become manifest later in life, as the patients become dissatisfied with their initially successful adaptation.

From a dynamic viewpoint, anxiety reactions may fall into either one of these two categories; they may occur early, in passive and dependent persons, or late, in rigid persons. They differ from the other groups in the fact that the outstanding symptom, instead of being a paralysis, a phobia, an obsession, or a depression, is now straightforward anxiety. The anxiety, moreover, is recognized as such and is usually thought by the patient to be due to unknown personality difficulties. In essence, the anxiety reaction is the same as the other kinds of psychoneurotic reac-tions, with the secondary symptoms stripped away. The physician must use care when he establishes the diagnosis of an anxiety reaction. He should consider the personality pattern and the dynamic background. Only then can he decide which of the two types he is dealing with and thus orient his treatment properly. The prognosis, of course, will vary with the nature of the etiologic situation.

SCHIZOPHRENIC REACTIONS

The schizophrenic reactions are a widely scattered group of illnesses, with a multitude of manifestations, but with a common base of difficulty of thought and emotion. A series of monographs would hardly do justice to the various ways in which this illness could show itself. It is of primary importance to the physician, however, to recognize (1) that schizophrenic illnesses exist at every level of severity and (2) that the diagnosis does *not* carry with it a pessimistic prognosis. On the contrary, most schizophrenic reactions which are seen are found in patients who can be treated successfully, and whose illnesses may be eliminated or greatly controlled, by adequate, psychotherapeutically oriented treatment. One of the reasons for the common nihilistic attitude about schizophrenic reactions is the fact that these reactions are too often recognized only when they are most severe and when the prognosis is therefore less hopeful. The fact, of course, is that many more schizophrenic patients are treated by physicians *without* having their illness recognized. As a result, physicians have tended to overlook the majority of the patients with a good prognosis. At the same time, of course, this oversight has resulted in depriving these persons of optimal treatment.

Basic Characteristics

There are many kinds of schizophrenic reactions, and they may be grouped into a number of clinical syndromes. Throughout all these syndromes, however, certain basic characteristics are always found. These characteristics may be considered in two categories: thinking disorders and emotional disturbances.

THINKING DISORDER

The thinking difficulty of a schizophrenic patient is a disruption of associations. His thoughts do not follow the accepted logical order of society, and, in consequence, sentences, actions, and plans appear to be vague, rambling, and confused.

This thinking difficulty may best be understood as being rooted in a personalized view of the universe. The objects, persons, and situations which the patient sees are not viewed as existing in themselves, in an independent fashion. Instead, each thing is viewed only as it relates to the patient himself. The laugh of a passer-by on the street is interpreted as a laugh *at* the patient; the physician's blue tie is interpreted as a sign of affection, because blue is the color which the patient associates with affection. Because of the personalization of the patient's world, his speech and behavior frequently seem irrational and incomprehensible. It is only when each of the highly personal links in his chain of thinking is explored, and the origin of these links is understood, that the talk and the logic of the schizophrenic person become completely sensible. They become sensible, however, only for that particular individual. The thought sequence of the schizophrenic person uses a different, personalized framework for viewing the world.

In early stages of the schizophrenic reaction, this thinking disorder is manifested by wandering speech, by blocking, and by seemingly illogical comments and conclusions, especially in important personal matters. In late stages, the disruption of associations may be exaggerated to the form of highly personalized, organized fantasies which are invested with all the meaning of reality. By such autistic thinking the patient with a hebephrenic schizophrenic reaction is able virtually to create his own world and to ignore the world in which he actually lives; in the similar fashion, the patient with a paranoid schizophrenic reaction can form delusions and hallucinations.

EMOTIONAL DISTURBANCES

The emotional disturbances of the schizophrenic patient may be summarized in the term *inappropriateness.* Looking at the world with a viewpoint different from the rest of society, the schizophrenic individual tends to show emotional responses that are different from those of other persons. Consequently, his emotional responses frequently appear bizarre. These emotional responses may be inappropriate in *kind* or in *degree.* The schizophrenic patient may show joy when he is told what appears to be unhappy news or may show sorrow in a situation that would be expected to produce happiness; his reaction will thus display inappropriateness in *kind.* If the emotion is appropriate in *kind,* it may still be inappropriate in *degree.* Instead of a moderate amount of anger at a minor inconvenience, for example, the patient with a schizophrenic reaction may go into a homicidal rage. Similarly, he may become suicidal at what appears to be a slightly discouraging situation.

As an end result of the inappropriateness in *kind* and *degree,* it is common to find that there is a flattening of affect in the late stages of schizophrenic reactions. This flattening is manifested by expressionless voice and facies and by a failure to respond emotionally to stimuli; it has poor prognostic implications. Living in a world which he sees differently from other persons and one in which his emotions are constantly being twisted in an extreme fashion, the schizophrenic patient may retreat into the marked emotional withdrawal of flatness. He lives more and more in an autistic fantasy world, with his emotional life internalized.

The Etiology of Schizophrenic Reactions

At this point, there is great interest in the subject of the origin of schizophrenic reactions. Many investigators are concentrating on physiologic factors which may be pertinent to the origin of schizophrenic reactions. Others are exploring the influence of drugs, such as lysergic acid, in mimicking some of the manifestations of schizophrenic reactions. Genetic and constitutional studies have indicated that the illness may be linked to these factors. At the same time, investigators such as Fromm-Reichmann (1950) and Hill (1955) have explored the characteristic psychopathologic patterns in schizophrenic reactions and have described some effective psychotherapeutic methods for dealing with them. Large-scale family and social studies have begun to reveal characteristic patterns of environment in ethnic, cultural, and family situations.

All these etiologic studies, however, appear to lead to a single point. That point, most frequently, is that the factors that produce the illness create an inability of the individual to delineate himself adequately from the world. Investigator after investigator finds that this difficulty has taken place in the early stages of development and that probably the crucial period for this delineation to take place is the period of infancy. The interfering elements may be physiologic or psychosocial, or some combination of both, but the end result is the same—a person who, under stress, sees the world in an excessively personalized way.

With the common findings of thinking and emotional disorder and with a common problematical origin, schizophrenic reactions may be found in a number of different syndromes. These syndromes, essentially, are nothing more than characteristic maneuvers. The patient uses such maneuvers in order to escape from the conflicts which his basic difficulties of thought and emotion create between him and the environment. The various categories of schizophrenic reactions may be viewed as follows.

SIMPLE SCHIZOPHRENIC REACTION

This is the type of schizophrenic reaction which is the earliest to appear, and it is probably the most common. The simple schizophrenic reaction usually has a gradual onset between the ages of 15 and 20. Characteristically, it is manifested by the basic signs of a schizophrenic reaction, together with marked anxiety, fear, and withdrawal from environmental activities. On the surface, the patient appears to be a shy, withdrawn, tense, anxious, clumsy, socially maladapted person. On closer examination, he reveals the thinking and emotional difficulties already described. The defense mechanism which is utilized in a simple schizophrenic reaction is withdrawal from the environment, emotionally and physically.

The course of a simple schizophrenic reaction is variable. In many instances, the illness is a mild one and can be adequately handled by gentle manipulation of the environment, by reassurance, or even by the absence of severe stresses. From this mild reaction, there is a range of illness to the very severe simple schizophrenic reactions. The latter classically follow a gradual downhill course, ending in a state of marked withdrawal and deterioration. Such a downhill course usually takes approximately 5 years; for better or worse, the simple schizophrenic person has usually stabilized into a relatively fixed pattern by the age of 25.

HEBEPHRENIC SCHIZOPHRENIC REACTION

The hebephrenic schizophrenic reaction is a less frequent syndrome. Its time of onset and initial course is parallel to that of the simple schizophrenic reaction. From the first, however, there is one significant difference. In its early stages, the hebephrenic schizophrenic reaction is usually found in a person who gives more dramatic evidence of suffering as a result of his basic thinking and emotional difficulties. This increased profoundness of suffering is reflected in the individual's own descriptions and also by the fact that the person with a hebephrenic pattern shows much more emotional turmoil and variability than does the patient with a simple schizophrenic reaction. It is not uncommon for a person with a hebephrenic schizophrenic reaction to experience episodes of joy and ecstasy intermixed with periods of severe suicidal depression and other periods of homicidal rage. The emotional turbulence is shown in bizarre and distorted fashions, with eccentricities in dress and behavior; these include such devices as new words, eccentric costumes, tassels, and peculiar living schedules.

After 3 to 4 years of such a turbulent, gradually settling course, the patient enters a state of withdrawal, which terminates in deterioration and dementia similar to the deteriorated state of the simple schizophrenic patient. The person with a hebephrenic reaction, however, shows a more bizarre final picture than does the person with a simple schizophrenic reaction. Instead of quiet withdrawal, his illness is characterized by flamboyant delusions and hallucinations; he creates a full hallucinatory and delusional world. The person with a hebephrenic schizophrenic reaction, for example, is one who experiences delusions in which he is God, Napoleon, or other figures, and who peoples an autistic hallucinatory world with persons and things which substantiate his delusions. The prognosis is poor for patients with hebephrenic schizophrenic reactions from the first. It is extremely poor once the stage of deterioration has been achieved.

Dynamically, it is possible to see a hebephrenic reaction as a step further than the simple schizophrenic reaction. In the latter, the suffering person withdrew from the realistic world. In the hebephrenic schizophrenic reaction, this withdrawal from the realistically threatening world is followed by a further withdrawal. This additional step takes the patient into a delusional world, which is a more satisfying one than the withdrawn autistic world of the simple schizophrenic. From a therapeutic viewpoint this second step makes the physicians' task much more difficult. In the simple schizophrenic reaction, the doctor's problem is to lead the patient back into the world which is threatening. With a person with a hebephrenic schizophrenic reaction, however, the doctor has the dual problem of first persuading the patient to give up a pleasant autistic world and then persuading him to enter the threatening realistic world. It may be this dynamic difficulty which explains the profound lack of success which is associated with the treatment of hebephrenic schizophrenic reactions.

CATATONIC SCHIZOPHRENIC REACTION

The catatonic schizophrenic reactions are of two types: the catatonic excitement and the catatonic stupor. Both these types of reactions tend to occur at the end of adolescence and immediately at the time when the patient is about to assume an independent role in adult life. It is common to see these reactions occurring when a person is about to leave school and obtain a job, or at the time of marriage, or at some other significant period of change in his life. Usually there have been scanty evidences of a schizophrenic reaction prior to the onset of the acute episode.

The acute episodes of catatonic excitement are characteristic. The onset is rapid over a period of several days or weeks. There is increasing psychomotor activity, commonly associated with increased strength of hostile and sexual impulses. During the short period of onset, the person changes from a somewhat shy, well-controlled individual into an assaultive, destructive, combative individual, with active delusions and hallucinations. At the peak of the catatonic excitement, it is common to find exposure, masturbation, sexual assaultiveness, homicidal rage, and speech which is filled with delusional material and incoherence. The course of the catatonic excitement is occasionally interrupted by brief periods, lasting only 3 to 4 minutes, when the patient suddenly ceases his overactivity and enters into a stuporous state. Such a sudden shift in the manifestations of the illness is frequently a worthwhile sign, distinguishing the catatonic excitement from the manic excitement. The duration of a catatonic excitement is of critical importance, and patients can die if the peak excitement lasts much longer than several days. Usually, however, the peak period will end rapidly; the complete course of the excitement will be finished within 6 months.

The catatonic stupor occurs in the setting similar to that in which the catatonic excitement is found. Once again, the onset is unexpected. A catatonic stupor, however, develops less rapidly; several weeks or months may go by before the peak of the stupor is achieved. At the end of this onset, the patient is found to be immobile, with waxy flexibility, remaining in any position in which he is placed. He fails to eat, drink, defecate, or urinate and requires nursing care for his every need. It is important to remember during this time when the patient does not respond to external stimuli in an overt fashion that he is continually aware of what is going on in the environment; in point of fact, he will be able to describe incidents and repeat conversations, in extremely fine detail, several months later. Casual words and gestures of physicians and other staff, therefore, may make a dramatic difference in the way that the patient responds to treatment. The peak of the catatonic stupor is usually long, extending from a period of several weeks to several months; there have been instances in which catatonic stupors have lasted for 20 years. Recovery is frequently spontaneous, but it may be helped by other treatments, as will be described.

The prognosis, for both catatonic excitements and catatonic stupors, is a favorable one for the first episode. This is especially so when adequate psychiatric treatment is administered. One may expect that 90 per cent of persons with these illnesses will recover to a satisfactory behavioral level and will be able to resume their life in the community. At the conclusion of one episode, however, it is common to find that some evidences of the basic thinking and emotional difficulties of a schizophrenic reaction persist. There is a great likelihood then of recurrence of the illness. With each recurrent episode of catatonic stupor or excitement, the prognosis becomes progressively worse; each time, the episode is followed by more crippling degrees of autistic thinking and inappropriate emotions.

Dynamically, the catatonic schizophrenic reaction may be viewed as another way which the schizophrenic person may use to defend himself against his difficulties with the world that surrounds him. Just as the simple schizophrenic person withdrew and the person with a hebephrenic schizophrenic reaction created a fantasy world, so does the person with a catatonic schizophrenic reaction deal with unhappy life situations. In this case, however, instead of withdrawing, the person turns on the world with hostility and attempts to destroy it. His attempts to destroy his world may go in either of two directions: the destruction may be on the physical plane, with actual assaults and physical destructiveness, as manifested in the catatonic excitements; the destruction may be on the psychologic plane, with the patient denying the existence of the world around him, as in the catatonic stupor. In each of these instances, clearly, it is up to those who conduct the patient's treatment to reconcile his difficulties with the world, in order that he will be able to accept its existence and to deal with it.

PARANOID SCHIZOPHRENIC REACTION

The paranoid schizophrenic reaction is commonly the latest of the schizophrenic reactions to appear. It usually occurs in the late twenties, with a gradual onset over a period of 3 to 4 years. The initial signs are increasing anxiety, tension, withdrawal, and disruption of a previously well-integrated life organization. Within a matter of several years, the patient demonstrates increasing suspiciousness, hostility, delusions, and hallucinations. At the peak of a paranoid schizophrenic reaction, the delusions and hallucinations are very marked and shift from day to day, as the patient deals with different situations and different persons. This shifting in the paranoid structure is sometimes viewed as a favorable sign, but it must be viewed cautiously. It is a reflection of the severity of the patient's thinking difficulty that he is able to maintain mutually incomparable delusions on successive days and maintain them with such belief and sincerity that such actions as homicide or suicide are possible. The course of a paranoid schizophrenic reaction is, very frequently, a downhill one. Over a period of several years, the paranoid ideation may become more fixed or may indeed disappear, as the patient gradually enters a state of deterioration similar to that which is found in the simple and hebephrenic schizophrenic reactions. The final status of the illness is most frequently achieved by the age of 35.

Once more, the dynamic defense utilized by the patient becomes important in treatment. One usually finds a person who has compensated for the basic schizophrenic thinking and emotional difficulties by adopting the standards of the world in a rigid and cold fashion. In late adolescence, he adopted a shell, covering his own feelings with behavior which seemed to satisfy the world's standards. As this shell failed to satisfy his inner insecurities and also interfered with his ability adequately to relate to the environment, there developed increasing dissatisfaction. When this dissatisfaction and unhappiness reached a sufficiently high threshold, the individual then turned on the standards of the environment. Whereas he had previously held the world up to himself as a guide, he now regards it as the reason for his difficulties; instead of condemning himself, he now condemns the environment. This pattern of defense dictates the need to show the individual how he can reconcile his own desires with those of the world around him and can give up the drive to impose environment standards on himself or impose his own standards on the environment.

MIXED SCHIZOPHRENIC REACTION

Just as with the psychoneurotic reactions, it is very common to find elements of all kinds of schizophrenic reactions in any one patient. Thus, it is rare to find a person who goes through a prolonged simple schizophrenic reaction who has not had some paranoid episodes. It is equally uncommon to find a person with a paranoid schizophrenic reaction who does not show some of the features of withdrawal and thinking difficulty of the simple hebephrenic schizophrenic reactions. The reactions must be viewed as a group of illnesses, with some interchangeability. When they are viewed from a dynamic standpoint, it is obvious that the person with a schizophrenic reaction has a set of basic difficulties. It would be illogical to assume that, having adopted one defense to use in handling these difficulties, the person would not be willing also to use other defenses in dealing with varying situations and problems. Thus it is, clinically, that one is commonly able to associate any individual patient *predominantly* with one type of schizophrenic reaction. This predominance, however, is not exclusive, and the predominant pattern is modified by the existence of other patterns from time to time. The variability of outcome which may result from this mixture is obvious; in general, however, the outcome will be most closely associated with the predominant pattern of the schizophrenic reaction.

PSEUDONEUROTIC SCHIZOPHRENIC REACTION

The pseudoneurotic schizophrenic reaction is a special syndrome which has been described by Hoch and Polatin (1949). In this group, the basic difficulties of a person with a simple schizophrenic reaction are present. Instead of being handled by the more typical pattern of withdrawal and seclusiveness, they are handled by a multiplicity of psychologic complaints. These psychologic complaints include anxiety, phobias, conversion phenomena, and other symptoms which are commonly associated with psychoneurotic reactions. When the patient consults a physician, he presents a façade which is predominantly a psychoneurotic one. On examination, however, it will be found that the psychoneurotic symptomatology does not make sense, in the fashion described previously under the psychoneuroses. Instead, the symptomatology is much more widespread, involving every aspect of the person's life. Moreover, examination will reveal the definite evidences of thinking difficulty and emotional difficulty which are the hallmark of the schizophrenic reaction.

The significance of this syndrome lies in the fact that it appears to have a specific prognosis. Occurring in the late teens or early twenties, these illnesses tend to be extremely difficult to treat. If treatment is successful, the outcome is usually a very good life adjustment. If treatment is unsuccessful, however, deterioration commonly ensues. Contrary to many other kinds of schizophrenic reactions, it appears that there is no mid-point between good adjustment and poor adjustment. There are very specific needs in treatment, which will be considered later.

AFFECTIVE REACTIONS

The affective reactions are primary disturbances in mood, with secondary thinking difficulty which is appropriate to the emotion.

There are two over-all types of affective reactions: manic-depressive illnesses and the depressions of middle life and old age. In each type, certain characteristic phenomena are common. In each instance, it is common to see the illness beginning after the age of 35. In both types of illness, it is common to find personality configurations which are marked by a tendency toward physical activity to a marked degree. Persons who develop affective reactions are usually successful, according to their station in life. They have followed a pattern of existence which has been marked by outgoing, cheerful, optimistic, energetic, and generally successful interpersonal relationships in their social and community life, and they have generally contributed widely and well to charitable activities and organizations. In their business life, they have usually been responsible for success and expansion of their working organization. In their home life, they have generally provided a good living situation and many material benefits for their spouses and children. Throughout all this, however, it is common to find that the patient has failed to achieve any sense of satisfaction from all the valuable work and good effort which he has produced. There is usually an emotional isolation, which the person strives to overcome by all the outward gestures which have been described.

The Etiology of the Affective Illnesses

Once again, there is evidence that physical factors are operative, especially genetic and constitutional ones. This evidence, based on family studies and studies of body types, is buttressed by the fact that the affective illnesses respond so well to physical treatments, such as electric shock. Regarding psychosocial etiology, there are many reports which have clarified, to some extent, the nature of feelings of depression, emphasizing the fact that depression is somewhat akin to a hopeless grief and that it is characterized by anger which is directed inwardly, presumably toward introjected parental figures. Recently, Cohen, et al. (1954), have described a typical family constellation for persons who develop a manic-depressive illness. This constellation is one in which the family, operating as a minority in its community, uses each individual member as a means of maintaining status and uses the child in this same fashion as soon as he begins to make the transition from infancy into childhood. At the time of this transition, instead of learning to deal with the world in ways which will yield satisfaction and avoid dissatisfaction, the infant-child learns to deal with the world out of a sense of obligation and responsibility to the family. In this fashion, he is deprived of the ability to gain personal and emotional satisfaction from his activities. Such a theme in a person's life, forced by the parental figures, does not conflict with the theoretical formulations of introjected figures, which have been suggested by others. The high ratio and familial incidence of the affective reactions, however, make one cautious in assuming that the logical psychodynamic structure is solely responsible for the clinical pictures which are presented. Certainly, it is rare that the treatment of a person with an affective illness can be exclusively either psychologic or physiologic.

Types of Affective Reactions

DEPRESSIVE REACTION

Depressive reactions in middle or late life are characterized by a typical pattern. They usually take 3 to 6 months in onset, achieve their maximum intensity for a period of another 3 to 6 months, and gradually subside over yet another 6 months. Frequently, the illness is precipitated by an outstanding event: achievement of success in business, departure of children for college, sudden deaths in the family, or severe physical illness. These events are the sort that demand from the patient a reevaluation of himself and of his goals in life. Depressions may also occur when the individual has been subjected, for a number of years, to unhappy or dismaying situations. In either instance, the early signs of depression are commonly sleeplessness, restlessness, and some hypochondriac concern. Gradually, over the course of months, symptoms increase, and to the picture are added such symptoms as early morning awakening, anorexia, weight loss which may total 40 or more pounds, constipation, loss of sexual desire, impotence, social withdrawal, poor concentration, and, finally, convictions of hopelessness and suicidal ideation. When the illness has reached this point, one sees the peak of a classical retarded depression. At this time, the patient shows slowing in his motor activities and speech and is continually preoccupied with thoughts of his own guilt, worthlessness, and hopelessness. Recovery is frequently spontaneous after a period of several months have elapsed, especially if some of the environmental pressures have been modified.

The simple retarded depression, which has been described, is found most commonly during the late fifth and through the sixth decades of life. There are two other forms of depressive reactions, which may be regarded as modifications of the simple retarded pattern. The first of these, chronologically, is the paranoid depression, which occurs during the later part of the fourth and earlier part of the fifth decade. As depression mounts, it is common to find the patient becoming increasingly suspicious and gradually delusional. The delusions are self-depreciatory and self-condemnatory in nature and support the basic hopeless attitude of the individual.

A second modification of the basic retarded depression is the anxious and agitated depression. In this clinical picture, anxiety becomes a much more prominent feature associated with the depression. This type of illness usually occurs after the sixth decade and alters the clinical picture into one of marked agitation, with the patient pacing the floor, wringing his hands, and crying desperately for help and succor.

Just as schizophrenic reactions may be seen in varying degrees of intensity, so also may the affective disorders. The patterns which have been described are frequently followed to their most severe levels, it is true. Just as frequently, however, they stop short of these levels. Depressions and excitements of mild or moderate intensity may be observed in many patients. Such patients will reveal the same descriptive and dynamic features as may be found in the more pronounced states, but to a less intense degree. Recognizing these features, the physician is then in a position to undertake proper treatment in the office.

MANIC EXCITEMENTS

Manic excitements are frequently the earliest manifestations of manic-depressive illnesses. Brief, mild manic excitements may appear as early as the late teens and twenties but are much more commonly seen for the first time in the thirties. A full-blown manic excitement usually presents a characteristic picture. Over the course of 1 or 2 weeks, the normally cheerful and optimistic individual becomes gradually more and more elated, with feelings of omnipotence and omniscience. There is increasing psychomotor activity, heightened awareness of environmental stimuli, increased appetite, decreased sleep, increased sexual desire and potency, increased irritability and anger, and, finally, delusions of grandeur and persecution. When seen at the peak of a manic excitement, the patient is hyperactive, shouting, moving continually, angry and frequently assaultive if contradicted, hyperaware of stimuli, speaking with flight of ideas, and in a predominantly euphoric and elated emotional state. A manic excitement may last as long as several weeks, but if it maintains itself at its peak intensity for more than several days, death may ensue. Recovery is usually spontaneous if the patient survives the peak of the attack.

MANIC-DEPRESSIVE REACTION

The manic-depressive reactions are frequently confusing, because of the suggestion in their name that they are associated with cyclic patterns of manic excitements and depressive reactions. On the contrary, a manic-depressive reaction with alternating spells of depression and elation is highly unusual. Much more commonly, the patient demonstrates predominantly one type of reaction, with occasional episodes of the opposite reaction. Thus, one sees recurrent depressions with an occasional manic excitement or recurrent manic excitements with occasional depression. The range for this type of illness is wide, and its diagnosis is based on the recurrent nature of the illness and on the apparent absence of precipitating factors.

The depressive episode of a manic-depressive illness is usually identical to that which has been described for depressions in middle or late life. It differs in that usually there are not the same clear-cut precipitating factors which have led to the illness. It differs, also, in the fact that recurrent episodes are common. With recurrence the prognosis for recovery becomes increasingly poor, and it is common to find patients with repeated depressions who have entered a chronic depressed state, requiring continued hospitalization, by the age of 50.

PARANOID REACTIONS

The paranoid reactions are illnesses characterized by a persistent difficulty in thinking, which is associated with emotional disturbances that are appropriate to the thought content. They may be seen as being halfway between the paranoid schizophrenic reactions, which have already been discussed, and the theoretical entity of paranoia vera. In the latter illness, one would expect to find a single distortion of thinking, a false premise upon which the individual would then build a coherent, logical delusional system. In paranoia vera, one would expect that the individual would show absolutely appropriate emotions and that his personality and behavior would be perfectly acceptable, if his basic false premise were to be accepted. In the paranoid schizophrenic reaction, at the other pole, one finds a gross disturbance of every aspect of an individual's life; he manifests the thinking and emotional difficulty of a schizophrenic reaction, his appearance, behavior, and speech are disturbed, and his delusional system shifts from day to day, often being associated with supporting hallucinatory experiences.

The paranoid reactions share some qualities of each of these two kinds of illnesses. In these reactions, the person is disturbed by a single kind of preoccupation, e.g., a belief that a spouse is being unfaithful, a belief that persons at work are hampering his success, or a belief that neighbors are conspiring to keep him out of social activities. With fairly constant belief, the person with a paranoid reaction will misinterpret activities which he observes in the environment, will form ideas of reference, and will construct delusional interpretations of what he sees. These interpretations will vary somewhat from day to day, as in the paranoid schizophrenic reactions, but will maintain a persistent general theme, as in paranoia vera. The emotional responses of the patient to his paranoid ideas will be appropriate for the nature of the ideas; e.g., if he believes that the neighbors are conspiring against him, he will be angry and critical of the neighbors, making efforts to break up their conspiracy. Thoughts, actions, and feelings will be largely appropriate in areas other than those involved directly in the delusional beliefs. There are no hallucinatory experiences in the course of paranoid reactions.

The Etiology of Paranoid Reactions

Paranoid reactions have not been closely considered from an etiologic point of view. Since they have a definite similarity to the paranoid schizophrenic reactions, it is not unlikely that there may be physiologic bases for this illness. From a psychosocial point of view, it is common to find that patients with paranoid reactions were brought up in a harsh and condemnatory environment. Especially during adolescence, they were again and again reminded of their unworthiness and of the invalidity of their own opinions and feelings. In a fashion similar to that of the paranoid schizophrenic individual, they tended to adopt a shell of conformity to the world's standards. Once again, as with the paranoid schizophrenic person, this shell did not produce adequate satisfaction in life and, gradually, illness ensued.

Clinical Picture

The clinical picture of a paranoid reaction is a typical one. The illness usually appears in the early thirties in cold, rigid, unemotional, tightly organized persons. Over a period of 2 to 3 years, the person gradually develops increasing anxiety, tension, restlessness, concentration difficulties, lack of interest in business and household activities, irritability, suspiciousness, ideas of reference, and, finally, delusions of persecution. The delusional beliefs usually center on that area of the patient's life which is producing the greatest amount of dissatisfaction, e.g., marital relationships or work relationships. In the course of acting upon the delusional beliefs, the patient's behavior is sometimes slightly inappropriate, as when the suspicious wife calls the husband's secretaries or superiors to check on supposed extramarital behavior. It is never, however, completely unreasonable. On examination, these patients display few signs of illness, except in the area of their distorted beliefs. Untreated paranoid reactions are likely to progress to a state of depression and deterioration not unlike the end state of the paranoid schizophrenic reaction. They can respond well to organized treatment, however, such as will be described.

Once again, as in schizophrenic and affective reactions, one finds a variation in the intensity of illness. Unhappy and suspicious persons in their thirties frequently seek the physician's help under the guise of physical complaints or with reference to marital or business problems. When a careful examination reveals mild or moderate signs of the descriptive and dynamic features of paranoid reactions, excellent therapeutic results may be anticipated if treatment is instituted rapidly. The earlier these reactions are treated, the better the prognosis.

PERSONALITY DISORDERS

The term *personality disorder* has come to include those conditions formerly called *psychopathic personality*. As the name implies, personality disorders differ from the illnesses described above, in that they are not linked so much to the appearance of symptoms and signs. On the contrary, personality disorders are associated with over-all disruptions of personality functioning and integration. Just as with the schizophrenic reactions, personality disorders include a multitude of syndromes, which may range from the highly sophisticated "con man" to the habitual alcoholic. Throughout all the varying manifestations of the personality disorders, however, two findings are virtually omnipresent.

The first basic characteristic of the personality disorder is the person's need for immediate gratification. Persons with personality disorders find it virtually impossible to delay the satisfaction of their physical and emotional desires. This need for immediate gratification may lead them into disastrous activity, when only a brief postponement of satisfaction would have resulted in great success. Examples of this type of activity include antisocial promiscuity on the eve of marriage, petty thievery by a businessman on the road to success, entry into a drinking bout by a salesman about to seal a major contract, "spree spending" by a thief who has just completed an otherwise successful robbery. Even when a slight postponement of the gratification will produce gratification ten times more profuse, the person with a personality disorder cannot wait for the increase. Coupled with this inability to postpone gratification is the corollary inability to benefit from past experience. No matter how often the person has found that immediate gratification has led to failure and unhappiness, he will still leap to gratify a new desire immediately.

The second basic characteristic of personality disorders is that such patients regard their difficulties as egosyntonic; i.e., the behavior that has brought the person into difficulty and has brought him to the attention of a physician will not be regarded by him as alien, or symptomatic, or needing explanation. On the contrary, his promiscuity, his alcoholism, his spree, or whatever his behavior might be will be considered by him to have been perfectly natural and logical in the situation in which he was. He will be critical of the environment and persons around him for their lack of understanding, or for forcing him into the activity which he carried out. He will not, however, experience guilt or blame himself for the difficulties in which he finds himself. By the same token, one fails to find in the person with a personality disorder feelings of depression, sadness, or guilt, except when the environment creates inescapable difficulties. He does not build up anxiety because of frustrated feelings, for the simple reason that his need for immediate gratification leads him into activities which satisfy the frustrated feelings rapidly.

The Etiology of Personality Disorders

From an etiologic point of view, we find once again that there is evidence for physiologic and for psychosocial factors. On the physiologic side, most of the evidence comes from electroencephalographic studies. These have shown that a larger percentage of persons with personality disorders, including those in prisons, tend to have abnormal EEGs than of the normal population. On the psychosocial side, the studies of Bowlby (1952) have indicated that deprivation of maternal guidance between the eighteenth and thirty-sixth months of life, for a period of not less than 6 months, will frequently result in the development of personality disorders. This finding fits in with psychoanalytic writings, which have tended to regard personality disorders as the acting out of infantile conflicts, instead of the acting out of defenses against such conflicts.

Clinical Picture

The clinical picture includes several different kinds of personality disorders. These are (1) the immature personality, (2) the passive-dependent personality, (3) the cyclothymic personality, and (4) the antisocial personality. Each of these four types of personality disorders tends to appear as the individual enters adult life. Forging his way into adulthood, he adopts patterns of dependency, immaturity, criminal aggressiveness, or unpredictable variability, depending on the personality needs which he has and the ways in which he can most easily gratify these needs. Since the individual has little awareness that his difficulties are symptomatic, he is rarely brought to the attention of a physician except when some physical illness intervenes or when legal authorities demand a psychiatric examination. After the pattern has continued for a number of years, the patient may be forced to see a physician at the behest of his family. Therapy for these persons is difficult and will be described in the last section of this book. It is well to remember, in considering personality disorders, several clinical observations. The first is that there are many persons with some tendencies toward immediate gratification who do not actually become incapacitated by this difficulty. On the contrary, they may be quite successful, outgoing, aggressive, and productive persons. The second fact worthy of consideration is that the personality disorders apparently reach their peak during the age period of 20 to 40. By the time the person reaches the age of 40, apparently, his pattern is stabilized to the point where he is often able to maintain a satisfactory adjustment for the remainder of his life.

ORGANIC REACTIONS

The basic characteristics of the organic reactions are three primary kinds of difficulty: (1) memory difficulty, (2) disturbances in orientation, and (3) emotional lability. These three characteristics are found in all the many kinds of organic reactions, from brain tumors to arteriosclerotic cardiovascular diseases. In each of these diseases, the origin of the difficulties is obvious. With destruction of cortical tissue, the person has less and less capacity to understand what is going on in the environment. Having this difficulty in understanding, he naturally shows this through inability to orient himself properly in the environment and, as time passes, inability to recollect accurately what has been happening to him. Emotional lability stems from the fact that the person cannot place things which happen to him in the proper perspective. A minor threat, therefore, can produce panic; a lighthearted word can produce excessive laughter. The usual brake on emotional manifestations, namely, recognition of what is appropriate in an over-all context, has been taken away from a person with an organic reaction.

It is well to recognize that the origin of the symptoms for organic reactions is *not* by any means completely physical. On the contrary, clinicians will easily recognize that every person with an organic reaction, no matter what the nature of the physical cause, will show specific individual manifestations, according to his own personality structure. In the face of a frontal lobe tumor, for example, some persons may enter a panic, while others may exaggerate previously present obsessive-compulsive defenses. The changes of arteriosclerotic cardiovascular disease, in aging, may bring on depressive reactions in some persons, while others are able to compensate and carry on.

For purposes of the present book, a further discussion of the organic reactions would be unprofitable. Whatever the operative physical cause, this cause must be approached in the best therapeutic way possible. At the same time, it is crucial that the personality structure of the individual be considered. Various specific uses of physical treatments, combined with psychotherapeutic approaches, will be described under the different physical treatments that may be used, in later sections of this book.

SUMMARY

As may be seen, the authors have grouped the psychiatric illnesses into six major headings. Each of these headings carries with it certain implications, not only as to appearance of the illness but also as to etiology, dynamic structure, and treatment. When careful examination of a patient has provided sufficient evidence to make a diagnosis, the physician who is aware of likely etiologic facts is able to concentrate his searching in the areas where he may expect to find the pertinent dynamic material. He is better able, thereby, to work rapidly and effectively with the illness which he has recognized. As will be seen in later chapters, however, information which can be obtained at this diagnostic level provides this help only in a broad and general fashion. It is the additional leads, which come from subdivisions of diagnostic categories, the patient's emotions, his symptoms, and other signs, that enable one to pinpoint the explicit and individual characteristics which must be used in understanding and treating the individual patient.

3

PATHOLOGIC EMOTIONS, MOODS, AND SEXUAL UNREST

Having once established a diagnosis, or at least arrived at a tentative formulation, the next step in the evaluation of a patient for therapy is to determine the presence of pathologic emotions and moods or of sexual unrest. These factors are capable of profoundly affecting his immediate clinical condition. It is apparent that careful examination of a number of patients with identical diagnosis will often reveal striking differences in the quality and intensity of symptoms and in the ways in which the patient's ability to function may be impaired. Moreover, within a single patient marked fluctuations in the clinical picture frequently occur. These fluctuations possess great significance with regard to therapeutic planning, yet in no way change the basic ingredients of the illness which permit diagnostic classification.

For example, there is a great difference between the paranoid schizophrenic patient with violent rage outbursts whose perception of his environment is crippled by delusions, in which the very doctors who are trying to help him have become members of a conspiracy to harm him, and the paranoid schizophrenic patient with transient, mild ideas of reference, in whom the most prominent symptoms are apathy and lack of drive and spontaneity. At one time a schizophrenic patient may be in a state of extreme excitement characterized by intense sexual unrest, anger, anxiety, and persistent overactivity. At another time, the same patient may be bland, vague in his thinking, and withdrawn.

The three leading emotions which are known to affect seriously the clinical state of any patient within any diagnostic setting are anxiety, fear, and hostility. The two basic pathologic moods which can be seen in any patient are depression and elation. Equally significant and effective in coloring the clinical picture is sexual unrest.

Each of these factors, alone or in combination, will frequently influence not only the presenting symptomatology of the patient's condition, but also his ability to utilize personality assets, cope successfully with his environment, or participate effectively in psychotherapy. Each factor has certain identifying characteristics. Hence it can often be readily recognized and incorporated into the plans for therapy.

There are a number of ways in which each factor can manifest itself in patients. The end results of its presence may vary widely. At times, it may actually be beneficial to the progress of treatment. For example, the anxious or depressed patient is more often motivated to pursue a dynamic investigation of contributing psychologic conflicts while he is anxious or depressed than after these intense feelings have subsided. At other times, pathologic emotions or moods may produce serious obstacles to successful psychotherapy and rehabilitation. Anxiety may so intensify a thinking disorder that a patient may be helpless to use constructively the psychotherapeutic experience. Depression may facilitate the misunderstanding of interpretations, the patient taking each as further evidence of his inner worthlessness.

Rarely do these emotions occur in isolation, and in most patients a combination of these factors is found. The anxious patient may also reveal resentment. The angry patient may, at times, become afraid of the intensity and consequences, real or imagined, of his profound hostility. The elated patient may demonstrate admixtures of sadness and hopelessness associated with his otherwise remarkable buoyancy of spirits. The patient with marked sexual unrest may be frightened by his excitement; he may react with anger and rejection toward erotically stimulating objects; he may be elated or oppressed with guilt and futility.

There may or may not be an accurate correspondence between the subjective awareness of these emotions by the patient and their overt manifestations in his appearance and behavior. Some patients report well-defined anxiety to the physician, and this is readily corroborated by their facial expression, posture, motor activity, and general behavior. Other patients describe intense feelings of fear but lack any obvious external evidence of this emotion. Still others will appear markedly anxious and yet remain unaware of the inner feelings which their behavior reflects; if they are aware, they are able to describe their emotions only in the most vague terms. What is true of anxiety is equally true of fear, hostility, mood alterations, and sexual unrest. It is not uncommon for an angry patient sincerely to deny any recognition of his hostility, even though this pathologic emotion is obvious to anyone in contact with him. Certain patients entertain feelings and fantasies containing either strong hostility

or sexual desires, but they manifest none of these features in their behavior. A flirtatious patient may be honestly unaware of the gestures,
tone of voice, posture, and dress which betray the hidden, powerful drives.
The seriously suicidal, depressed patient, whose appearance suggests only
fatigue and who smiles when speaking with his doctor, may report in no
uncertain way the awful intensity of his inner suffering. The determina-
tion of the presence or absence of these pathologic factors depends,
therefore, on an integration of the subjective descriptions of the patient
with the observations of his appearance and behavior made by the physician.

Emotions, moods, and sexual unrest obviously may vary widely in intensity. In some patients it is possible to secure an accurate estimate of
the degree to which these factors are present, but in others it is often difficult to arrive at such an estimate. One of the reasons for this is that
patients differ extensively with regard to their ability to tolerate certain
emotions. One person may interpret the experience of anxiety as an "un-
masculine and cowardly" feeling. He may, therefore, be inclined to hide
it from everyone, including himself if possible, behaving stoically until
a state of near panic develops. Another patient, to whom the slightest
feeling of anxiety or depression implies impending loss of sanity, may
plead loudly and constantly for reassurance or medication, giving the
impression of being severely agitated indeed. The depth of the emotion
may, at times, be hidden by the presence of associated psychopathologic
features, such as delusions. A severely depressed patient may be relatively
unaware of the extent of his sadness and hopelessness, offering minimal
external evidence of this mood change as long as paranoid delusions are
prominent. A very fearful schizophrenic patient may be withdrawn and
unable to communicate clearly, manifesting marked interference with
logical thought processes. As long as these features are in the forefront,
the presence and degree of his fear may be difficult to detect.

These facts are very important in planning therapy. There are certain
patients, with mild or moderate anxiety, for example, in whom one would
refrain from using medication in an attempt to encourage tolerance of
undue emotions and simultaneously facilitate a working through of the
dynamic problems involved. This is a difficult position for a therapist to
maintain successfully unless he is able to recognize and deal adequately
with the tendency of certain patients to exaggerate the degree of their
distress. There are other patients, who require immediate somatic intervention, in whom such treatment may unfortunately be postponed because of failure to recognize the depth of the emotional state, concealed,
as it might be, by the patient's pride or the development of other symptoms.

In the following pages, the authors will attempt to describe each of these factors in such a way as to facilitate its recognition and to convey the manner in which it may interfere with personality function or with the progress of treatment.

Anxiety

Psychopathologic and psychoanalytic investigations have clearly established anxiety as a major factor contributing to the development of many psychiatric illnesses. Certainly anxiety is not the only significant pathologic emotion. Although in certain conditions, such as psychoneurotic reactions, it occupies a central position, in others, such as certain schizophrenic states and disorders of mood, it may be of more peripheral importance.

Anxiety may be described as a state of apprehension. It becomes pathologic when it is inappropriate to its object or unduly strong or prolonged in relation to the stimulus apparently giving rise to it. For a person to be concerned for his welfare and that of his family when reading newspaper reports of international tensions in this day and age would hardly be considered evidence of disease. However, if this same man became so worried about these matters that he was unable to concentrate on his work, ate poorly and lost weight, required sedation to sleep at night, and could not rid himself of intense fears of atomic war, a deeper, hidden source of anxiety would have to be considered as the explanation for his disturbance.

ORIGINS

One of the most important origins of pathologic anxiety is to be found in the conflict between the timeless and often turbulent unconscious and the ego or superego structures of the personality. As a simplified example of this, let us suppose that a woman has literally repressed all awareness of her sexual desires. She has done this, not because of ethical considerations, but because these feelings are incompatible with her concept of herself as an intellectually motivated human being. This self-concept is an important element in her superego structure. Whenever forces arise which threaten to stimulate her erotically, the basic conflict between unconscious and superego is activated and anxiety is produced. This pathologic emotion at one and the same time signals distress and serves to reinforce the repressive mechanisms which protect her from facing the fundamental contradiction in her personality.

This type of formulation, as a dynamic explanation for the generation of abnormal anxiety, is generally well known. What is not so widely realized is the fact that anxiety can also arise as a result of conflict between entirely conscious factors. It is not uncommon to see patients engaged in patterns of behavior which are opposed to their ethical expectations of themselves, who, instead of directly experiencing guilt, describe manifestations of anxiety which they do not connect with the inherent disparity between what they would like to be and what they are.

The precipitating factor leading to a state of anxiety often arises from the environment. Such an event or series of events must possess qualities to which the particular patient is sensitive. The stressful situations capable of stimulating the pathologic emotional reaction need not be universally traumatic, such as loss of work, endangered prestige, or threat of injury or death. In fact, they may often be characterized by features which in the ordinary sense might be considered beneficent. The circumstances giving rise to the pathologic anxiety reaction, therefore, may be characterized by real elements of pleasure or success, such as the birth of a child, the day of graduation, learning of promotion to an important post in business, or receiving a large sum of money.

Pathologic anxiety, therefore, arises largely from dynamic psychologic conflict and is unrealistic in quality, degree, or both. It is likely that there are several types of anxiety which are relatively indistinguishable with present methods of biological investigation. This opinion is held by many who have studied anxiety as experienced by certain schizophrenic patients and have compared it with that seen in other schizophrenic patients and in patients with affective or psychoneurotic disorders. This consideration can have little immediate role in planning therapy, but no doubt partly explains the resistance of certain patients demonstrating anxiety to therapeutic methods established for the relief of anxiety.

MANIFESTATIONS

There are many ways in which a patient may experience and manifest anxiety. Subjectively he may be aware of a general state of uncertainty or apprehension, with no clear explanation for his discomfort. Frequently his anxiety becomes attached to apparently real objects, and he may worry about his health, his financial status, or his personal relationships at home. He may present these concerns to himself and to others in a most convincing fashion, thereby concealing the pathologic nature of his disturbance. At times, the objects of his anxiety are more clearly unrealistic. He may describe being afraid of certain thoughts or feelings which recur within himself. He may be anxious in such apparently neutral situations as crowded stores, telephone booths, or high bridges. Sometimes, by avoiding these special circumstances, he may be completely free of anxiety. Often, however, anxiety is present in a relatively continuous manner, ignoring the need for well-defined external precipitating causes. It is not uncommon for anxiety to be periodic or recurrent, yet still lacking in external stimuli sufficient to account for the experience. A patient with anxiety attacks may awaken at night fearful, perspiring, with heart racing, with no recall of any nightmare or upsetting experience of the previous day. It is important to keep in mind the fact that, although neither the physician nor the patient can offer a satisfactory explanation for the pathologic experience, such an explanation usually exists, deeply hidden in the patient's unconscious. For example, an anxiety attack at night may reflect a highly successful maneuver to separate the emotion from its legitimate object. On the other hand, the timing of this painful experience may possess symbolic meaning. Sleep and death are often intimately connected on a preconscious or unconscious level. The apparently inexplicable disturbance of sleep by anxiety may therefore reflect in certain patients an attempt to cope with hidden death wishes directed toward persons who are close to and loved by the patient. This example is only representative of the manner in which the actual precipitating factors for an anxiety reaction may be concealed in a complex manner from both the patient and his physician.

In addition to the subjective reports of the patient, there are certain overt manifestations of anxiety which may readily be recognized by the clinician. The anxious patient often presents a worried expression. His speech may be pressured, as he talks of himself and his concerns in a harassed, rapid, repetitious manner. At other times anxiety may be associated with blocking or other difficulties in verbal communication. The patient's ability to concentrate may be impaired. His difficulty in carrying out complicated mental activities as well as his inattentiveness during discussions with the doctor can indicate this. Motor restlessness may often be prominent, ranging from slight trembling to a serious inability to sit still for more than a few minutes. Conversely, in certain patients, motility may be decreased when anxiety is present; however, this phenomenon may often be due to associated tension, as the patient struggles to control his emotions.

When one becomes familiar with the eating and sleeping habits of individual patients, these too may serve as barometers for the presence of this emotion. Certain patients overeat, while others lose their appetites when anxious. Sleep is often affected by anxiety, this change being characterized by frequent awakening during the night and, occasionally, terrifying dreams.

Physiologic changes may also accompany anxiety. Sometimes these constitute the primary complaints of the patient, even in the absence of a clear awareness of apprehension. The most frequently observed concomitants of anxiety include gastrointestinal distress, in the form of nausea, vomiting, pain, or diarrhea; palpitations or shortness of breath, which the patient usually refers to his heart or lungs; perspiration, generalized or localized, often affecting the hands and feet. The pulse rate may frequently be elevated, rising to levels of 90 to 120 beats per minute and even higher; this change may be characterized by periodic shifts from normal to accelerated rates and is then described as *spiking*. Certain patients may demonstrate a substantial rise in blood pressure when anxious.

CONSEQUENCES

What are the consequences of anxiety on function and on participation in treatment? As already indicated, anxiety may impair concentration. If, for example, a patient's livelihood depends upon a high degree of mental activity, such as chemical engineering or creative writing, even moderate degrees of anxiety can seriously cripple his ability to work. The exercise of sound judgment, as in the making of significant business decisions, may be limited. A patient may be paralyzed by ambivalence in matters in which he is ordinarily quite proficient. In the psychotherapeutic interview, a serious impairment of concentration may render the production of dynamically significant material difficult and delay the acquisition of meaningful insight.

When a patient experiences anxiety in apparently neutral but actually dynamically sensitive situations, the result may or may not be a serious impairment of function. If a man lives near his place of work, anxiety experienced only in trains and airplanes is relatively inconsequential. If, on the other hand, his job requires him to travel to various parts of the country, such a manifestation of anxiety would have disastrous consequences. From time to time anxiety may become focused primarily on the doctor or the place at which psychotherapy is carried out. If the emotion becomes sufficiently powerful in such circumstances, it may constitute a most effective and destructive resistance to further progress in treatment.

In many psychoneurotic conditions, anxiety is the central psychopathologic disturbance. In other conditions, such as schizophrenic disorders and mood disturbances, it may be a fundamental factor of greater or lesser importance, but it usually serves to aggravate the basic psychopathologic state. For example, in a schizophrenic patient, the thinking disorder may become quite marked when the patient experiences anxiety, leading to an aggravation of looseness in logical associations and a decrease in coherence. The depressed patient may become much more aware of the intensity of his sadness under the pressure of anxiety and may tend to focus more attention on his morbid preoccupations. The hypomanic patient, with mildly elevated spirits, may be driven to a severe manic excitement by strong anxiety.

These ways in which anxiety may interfere with function, exaggerate other psychopathologic manifestations, or impede the progress of treatment are illustrative and by no means complete. Moreover, anxiety must not always be considered an undesirable feature of a patient's illness. Just as pain constitutes a signal, informing patient and doctor that an appendix is infected and giving the impetus to operate and remove the basic cause of the physical disturbance, so too anxiety is a signal of psychologic inflammation. The painful emotion cries out that something is amiss. The suffering serves as a motivation to participate in psychotherapy and to produce conscious and unconscious alterations which are essential for the restoration and preservation of well-being. Therefore, the premature or complete removal of anxiety by somatic methods may be, at times, exceedingly unwise.

Fear

Although it is sometimes difficult to distinguish between intense anxiety and pathologic fear, it is important to realize that there are fundamental theoretical and practical points of distinction between these two emotions. Whereas anxiety usually originates as a result of conflict between conscious and preconscious or unconscious factors within the personality, signaling the presence of potential danger but also enhancing the forces of repression which protect the patient from being confronted with that danger, fear is the immediate, intense reaction to a terrifying stimulus which is present here and now and seems inescapable. Anxiety may affect certain dimensions of function, but fear is an all-encompassing emotion which disrupts the total balance of the personality.

ORIGINS

The "dreadful" stimulus precipitating a reaction of fear may arise from the environment or from within the patient. Fear becomes pathologic when it is inappropriate to its object or is unduly intense or persistent and can, therefore, be understood only in terms of the dynamically determined sensitive factors within the person experiencing the reaction. For example, as long as the forces of repression remain active, a patient with an unconscious homosexual conflict may withstand an overt attempt at seduction successfully, developing only symptoms of anxiety. If the protective mechanisms break down, however, and he is faced with the sudden, immediate emergence of his own threatening impulses, he may be overwhelmed with intense, pathologic fear.

MANIFESTATIONS

If the fear reaction has not yet reached an intensity which would disrupt the integrity of personality functioning, the patient may be able to describe his emotional state to the doctor. Frequently, however, it is necessary to depend upon his appearance and behavior and associated psychopathologic features in order to detect the presence of fear. The emotion is often clearly reflected on the face of the patient. Motility is usually influenced, the patient being either hyperactive, restless, and at times assaultive or underactive, withdrawn, motionless, and even mute. His ability to attend to routine affairs is markedly diminished and often completely destroyed. Thinking may be seriously impaired, even in the absence of an underlying schizophrenic disorder. In a state of maximal fear, called *panic,* a serious break in contact with reality occurs, facilitating the formation of delusions, illusions, and hallucinations. The content of these psychopathologic features usually indicates the nature of the conflict generating the fearful reaction.

CONSEQUENCES

It is apparent from the foregoing description that any patient in a state of pathologic fear will be unable to carry out his daily responsibilities. One of the most serious consequences of unabated fear is suicide. In his attempt to escape the terrible danger which confronts him, the patient may impulsively seek the most convenient exit, even if it happens to be a window on the sixteenth floor of an apartment house.

In like fashion, the patient is seldom able to respond to psychotherapeutic measures. He is relatively untouched by reassurance and often afraid and suspicious of those trying to aid him. He frequently misinterprets the physician's questions and answers. The physician should secure knowledge of the sources of the patient's fear from the content of his verbal and behavioral productions and then, whenever possible, eliminate those stimuli in the environment which tend to foster his reaction.

In contrast to anxiety, therefore, fear is hardly a positive source of motivation to participation and progress in treatment. Fear is nearly always destructive, and somatic intervention is usually indicated.

Hostility

Hostility is a broad term used to describe several different emotional responses, all of which possess certain common characteristics. In contrast to anxiety and fear, which constitute a flight from offending stimuli, hostility implies an attack upon the person or thing which threatens the patient. Hostility may be considered constructive in the sense that it protects the patient. It may be considered destructive in the sense that its aim is to annihilate the factors provoking him. Hostility becomes pathologic when it arises in the absence of adequate irritation, is unduly intense or prolonged, or loses its constructive quality and becomes primarily destructive toward its object, the patient experiencing it, or both. To become angry when one has been cheated of a substantial amount of money by an unscrupulous business associate could hardly be considered pathologic. If, however, this hostile response becomes so strong and persistent that the victim of the swindle is unable to clear his mind of murderous fantasies directed toward the perpetrator, cannot sleep, loses his appetite, ruminates over the experience, and is overwhelmed by his emotions to such an extent that he is able neither to accept his unfortunate experience nor to take constructive measures to correct the situation, his plight must clearly be considered unhealthy and a more complex dynamic explanation for his reaction must be sought. It is not unusual for a person to experience hostility when rejected in love or barred from desirable social situations. However, this person is to be contrasted with the painfully sensitive human being who perceives rejection where none exists and reacts with hostility which is grossly undeserved. In extreme states of disturbance, hostility may reach such an intensity that a patient becomes a real danger to himself or to others.

ORIGINS

The two major forms of hostility are anger and resentment. Anger is a strong, direct emotional reaction to a threatening stimulus arising from the environment or from within the patient himself. It is usually, though not always, circumscribed in time. This can be contrasted with resentment. Resentment is essentially a prolonged reaction, usually of less strength, characterized by sullen bitterness, and not requiring an immediate provocation. The type of situation giving rise to resentment is more often chronic in duration and frequently relates to past as well as present experiences of the patient. For example, when denied something he wants and needs, the frustrated angry patient may flare up vigorously but briefly, directing his anger toward the person refusing to accommodate him. On the other hand, the resentful patient repeatedly expresses his bitter feelings about a number of current or old deprivations: "never enough love; never enough money; never enough luck."

Anger or resentment may be directed outwardly, toward the environment, or inwardly, toward the patient. The direction of the emotion may carry with it certain specific dynamic and physiologic correlates influencing the selection and outcome of psychologic and somatic therapy. To illustrate this simply, it can be stated that pathologic anger directed outwardly may result in murder, whereas pathologic anger directed inwardly may lead to suicide. The resentful patient may shake his fist at God, his family, his doctors. On the other hand he may gnaw away at himself, denying his abilities, castigating himself for past mistakes, and repeatedly attacking his self-esteem.

A lack of conscious, constructive hostility may be considered as pathologic as an excess of this emotion. One of the central dynamic features in the development of certain psychopathologic reactions is an inability to experience and handle legitimately stimulated hostile feelings. If the patient described previously as reacting to the manipulations of his business partner with prolonged, unduly intense rage did not react to this experience with any conscious hostility at all, the result might well be the development of psychoneurotic anxiety or depression. He might, for example, experience anxiety attacks, insomnia, phobic fears of crowded places, or difficulty in concentration. The therapeutic task might then be to liberate the hidden hostility and free him of those dynamic forces which prevented him from reacting appropriately in the first place. Just as there is probably a psychodynamic and biological difference between hostility directed outwardly and hostility directed inwardly, so too there is a meaningful difference of great importance in planning treatment between hostility which is directly and consciously experienced and hostility which is automatically repressed and beyond the awareness of the patient.

MANIFESTATIONS

The presence of overt hostile emotions can be detected from the subjective expressions of the patient and objective notations of his appearance and behavior. The angry patient often leaves little doubt about his emotional state: "I'm damned mad." The resentful patient may continually voice his sullen protest against the world and the circumstances of his life.

Frequently, however, the patient may not be an accurate reporter of his inner psychologic experiences. The physician may have to depend upon the indications of hostile countenance, motor activity, and behavior when formulating a diagnosis. Hostility is clearly written on the faces of many patients. The tone of voice of a hostile patient changes, sometimes becoming very loud, at other times becoming barely a whisper. Activity may be increased or decreased. The patient may restlessly pace the floor and, if sufficiently disturbed, strike out at persons and break fragile objects within reach. On the other hand, certain hostile patients are retarded, remain aloof from others, hardly speak, and refuse to eat. Severe hostility, handled through such marked withdrawal from the environment, has been called an aversion reaction. Certain schizophrenic patients, particularly those in catatonic reactions, may express hostility through negativistic responses, doing the direct opposite of whatever is requested of them.

CONSEQUENCES

Hostile emotions may profoundly influence a patient's ability to function, his basic psychopathologic state, and his participation in treatment. The seriousness of the consequences of anger in a frustrated manic patient who tears his telephone from the wall and burns valuable personal documents is obvious. The more subtle effects of hostility often have equally enduring and disastrous results. The chronically resentful salesman may not only fail to conclude vital contract negotiations, but he may so alienate his prospective buyers and his fellow employees that he will be fired, only to find that his reputation has preceded him when he seeks a job elsewhere. The wife who constantly nags and flares up if her husband arrives home a few minutes late for dinner may soon find herself in a divorce court. The bitter young woman who complains that no man has ever proposed to her may communicate her hostility to potential suitors and thereby destroy any opportunities for a sound love relationship.

In a more direct way, hostility may so absorb the attention of the patient that he may become unable to concentrate constructively on other topics. His ability to utilize his imagination and intelligence may be seriously impaired as long as the intense reaction persists. If other psychopathologic features are present, such as a schizophrenic thinking disorder or a profound mood depression, these may be intensified by hostile emotions. As with fear, maximal hostility may lead to the formation of delusions, usually of a paranoid nature, in which the patient explains his intense emotional state to himself as the result of antagonistic forces in the environment attempting to harm him.

Pathologic hostility can also destroy progress in psychotherapy. Unlike the anxious patient, the hostile patient frequently lacks any awareness that he is sick and in need of help. Suggestions to enter psychotherapy are often rejected. The hostility may become intimately interwoven with the universal phenomenon of resistance, presenting a far more difficult obstacle to overcome than such manifestations of resistance as forgetting dreams or being late for appointments. The establishment of rapport with the physician can often be prevented; once established, it can be demolished by pathologic hostility.

Unlike anxiety, hostility seldom motivates a patient to participate actively in treatment. However, inasmuch as there are constructive aspects to certain hostile emotions and the therapeutic goal is frequently to help the patient accept, tolerate, and handle his hostile emotions, the decision to use somatic intervention requires careful consideration.

Elation

Elation is an elevation of spirits. It is an unusual sense of well-being, which is considered pathologic when it lacks a sound reason to explain it or is inappropriately intense or prolonged. For a person to feel remarkably jubilant after overcoming a difficult problem, such as successfully completing a series of college examinations, is not unusual. However, when such a response is seen in the presence of an ordinarily tragic experience, such as immediately following the death of a close, beloved parent, its pathologic nature is at once apparent. If the change of mood is mild, as in hypomanic states, the patient may be unusually cheerful and outgoing, jovial, and friendly. He may be overtalkative and somewhat self-centered. He may frequently be able to utilize his mind and imagination in a profitable fashion. When the mood change is intense, however, and the patient enters a state of manic excitement, the extent of his disturbance disrupts the total integrity of his personality.

ORIGINS

The fundamental dynamic mechanism contributing to the development of elation is denial—denial of the painful aspects of the patient's contemporary life situation, of the loss of the object of love, of the limitations of time and space, of deeply buried early frustrations and deprivations. It is a reaffirmation of infantile omnipotence and omniscience in which the predisposed patient has never really stopped believing. The dynamic biological factors contributing to elation are essentially unknown, although the remarkable efficacy of chlorpromazine and electroconvulsive therapy in terminating manic states strongly suggests that in elation, as in depression, such physiologic factors are present.

MANIFESTATIONS

Elation can be detected from the verbal productions of the patient as well as from objective changes in his behavior. The friendly, outgoing, and cheerful qualities of the mild hypomanic state have already been mentioned. Such a patient will usually describe a sense of optimism and well-being. He may even, occasionally, recognize certain unreal qualities about his mood. Emotional responsiveness is prominent. The patient may laugh easily, cry readily, or become intensely angry when frustrated in his desires or contradicted in his opinions. His self-esteem and estimate of his abilities are elevated. Indeed, at times, his ability to function may be enhanced. Sexual unrest is often present, with the patient describing sexual dreams and fantasies in abundance. Sexual references may be frequent in his conversation, and flirtatiousness may be prominent. He usually tends to be overactive in speech and motor activity.

When this mood change reaches maximal intensity, a state of manic excitement exists. In such a condition, the warm, friendly, and pleasant aspects of the elation are less apparent, and the self-centered, demanding, tense, easily frustrated, and enraged qualities are in the forefront. When angered, the patient may readily strike out at the offending person. When sexually aroused, instead of being mildly flirtatious, the patient may become frankly obscene and even masturbate openly. Still he describes his spirits as good, if he is willing to discuss them at all, and insight into the pathologic nature of his experience is lacking. Rather than being heightened, his intellectual capacities are seriously impaired, and his apparently imaginative productions become repetitious and stereotyped. His attention span is gravely reduced, and he shifts rapidly from one subject to another, often at the suggestion of the sound of a word or syllable. At times he is frankly incoherent. His grand ideas become grandiose and often delusional. His scheme for improving his business becomes a plan for transplanting all the major manufacturing industries from New England to the middle of the Sahara Desert. Anyone who disagrees with his ideas becomes a member of an international plot to destroy his ambitions. He sleeps poorly, eats little, and is extremely overactive. Occasionally tearfulness and sadness may be intermingled with his elation.

CONSEQUENCES

The consequences of elation are varied and depend upon its degree and the life circumstances of the patient. In a hypomanic state, as indicated, the patient may actually function at a higher level than usual. However, he may also exert poor judgment as a result of his unduly optimistic outlook. Therefore, if he is responsible for large amounts of money or important political negotiations, the results could be disastrous. This is particularly true when his mood change is difficult to detect, since the patient can be most convincing in the eyes of his associates. The destructive effects of a severe manic excitement are self-evident.

When the mood change constitutes the central psychopathologic feature of the patient's condition, an affective disorder is present. Similar mood changes of varying intensity can occur in psychoneurotic patients and in the setting of schizophrenic reactions. In the latter group the elation may, for a time, be the most obvious presenting symptom of the disorder.

The patient in psychotherapy who experiences an occasional mild mood elevation, as is not infrequently the case after a release of conflicting tensions, may actually be encouraged to continue treatment by this sense of well-being which he has derived in the course of his psychotherapy. On the other hand, the denial associated with buoyant spirits may impede further progress. This is usually only temporary unless the elation is too fixed or intense. The decision to employ somatic intervention in such mild situations depends, therefore, on many variables. In the more serious manic excitements, however, some form of somatic intervention is practically always indicated, not only because the condition may result in exhaustion, death, or injury to others, but also because of the futility of attempting to persuade so disturbed a human being of the desirability of treatment and his obvious inability to utilize purely psychologic approaches to his condition.

Depression

Depression is an alteration of mood characterized by a loss of self-confidence and realistic outlook for the future and the presence of feelings of sadness, hopelessness, or futility. It is the direct antithesis of elation. Such a mood would be considered normal if there were reasonable grounds for its existence. To grieve after the death of a child, to be saddened and discouraged after a significant defeat in the pursuit of one's career, to feel guilt when one acts in opposition to one's own ethical standards—these are normal universal human experiences. To have such feelings in the absence of any obvious tragedy, however, would be clearly pathologic. So, too, would be depression which continues for so long a time or reaches such a degree that it profoundly affects the total personality, rendering daily function difficult or impossible. Such a severe depression is often associated with such features as marked anorexia and weight loss, disordered sleep, and suicidal attempts.

ORIGINS

The origins of depression of mood are complex. Psychologic factors, such as unconscious identification with and ambivalence toward a recently deceased person, undoubtedly contribute strongly to the reaction. It is quite common, for example, to note the onset of a pathologic depression shortly after the death of a parent or spouse. Moreover, there also appears to be an intimate connection between depression and unconscious hostility directed toward the patient himself, at times linked with masochistic needs. Nonetheless, the results of electroconvulsive therapy in certain depressed patients indicate the presence of significant physiologic factors as well.

Although the dynamic differences have yet to be worked out, there are undoubtedly various types of depression of mood, each of which may possess specific psychologic and biochemical characteristics. Although the presenting symptoms may be identical, there does appear to be a meaningful difference between the depressed patient with hypochondriac complaints and the depressed patient with marked resentment, suspiciousness, or paranoid delusions. There is a definite difference between the depressed schizophrenic patient who experiences hopelessness after many years of therapeutic failure and whose life has become disrupted beyond repair by his illness and the psychoneurotic patient whose depressive mood rapidly subsides as unconscious hostility and sexual fantasies emerge through layers of defenses and resistances in the course of psychoanalytic psychotherapy. These variations are real and possess great significance in the establishment of a program of therapy for an individual patient. These observations may also account, in part, for the often contradictory experimental results obtained from studies of anti-depressive medications.

Nonetheless, there are certain characteristics of depression of mood which are seen regardless of the setting in which the pathologic mood occurs. It is the purpose of this section to describe these and to discuss the complications which they may produce in the adjustment of the patient and his participation in therapy.

MANIFESTATIONS

If a patient is able to perceive his mood correctly, he may offer a description of depression in clear terms. He may speak of feeling low, depressed, discouraged, unhappy, sad, or miserable. At times he may not be able to identify his current mood, but the depressive affect may be revealed in his preoccupation with morbid topics, such as failure or death, lack of self-confidence, or guilt over transgressions which may be slight or which may have occurred years before his present illness. Suicidal ideas may be present and will often be revealed to the physician.

These subjective considerations are frequently substantiated by changes in the appearance and behavior of the patient. His face seems tired and sad. Tearfulness may be prominent. His gait may be slow and his posture characterized by an attitude of one burdened with sorrow. Motor activity may be retarded, but if pathologic emotions of anxiety, fear, or hostility are also present, the patient may be overactive, restlessly pacing, and unable to sit still. There may be a decrease in appetite with an associated loss of weight. Sleep may be disturbed, with the patient often awakening early in the morning and experiencing the most intense hopelessness at that time of day. Constipation may occur.

CONSEQUENCES

Depression of mood carries with it a series of complications ranging from poor judgment, influenced by the patient's lack of confidence and pessimistic outlook for the future, to serious suicidal attempts. The manner in which the depressed patient manifests his condition often discourages the very love and attention which in one way he requires and in another he feels worthless to receive. This often leads to rejection by his family and further reinforcement of his depressed mood. Concentration is often impaired, so that the patient cannot carry out complex work activity. Not only are his mental processes slowed and the content and flow of thoughts sparse, but he tends to concentrate much of his energy and attention on the morbid, bleak topics associated with his mood. There is a withdrawal from human contact and from stimuli beneficial to him which might serve to distract him from his preoccupations.

Depression of mood, like anxiety, may facilitate the patient's participation in psychotherapy. It is, however, just as likely to create certain difficulties for the therapeutic process. Changes do not usually occur readily, and the depressed patient may go through session after session with no demonstrable relief and only the physician's reassurance that the dynamic investigations are worthwhile. When the discussion comes close to particularly sensitive material, the depressive mood may be intensified and the hazards of impaired function or suicide increased. The patient tends to distort past and present in terms of his mood. He denies or minimizes real achievements and meaningful human relationships. He exaggerates guilt and misjudgments. The therapeutic situation itself may become the victim of the patient's hopeless attitudes. He may terminate treatment prematurely, or he may interpret the therapist's remarks and silences as confirmation of his own worthlessness and the futility of his life. At times, the patient may assume that his low opinion of himself is also the opinion of the therapist. The patient may show strong resistance to leaving the topics which preoccupy him to move along avenues of constructive analysis. Spontaneity is limited, and use of the technique of free association is often undesirable and impossible. Many of these considerations can be successfully met and mastered by the psychotherapist. Often, however, if the depression is intense, if suicidal trends are prominent, or if associated emotional features of anxiety or hostility are marked, somatic intervention of a limited or extensive degree may become necessary.

Sexual Unrest

It is generally accepted that absence of sexual drives or deviations from the normal pattern of heterosexuality, such as overt homosexuality, fetishism, or sadomasochistic aspects of the sexual act, constitute important symptoms and contributing dynamic factors in many psychiatric conditions. It is not as widely recognized, however, that the existence of strong and persistent sexual drives which often dominate the thinking and behavior of a patient may also be considered pathologic. This phenomenon is called sexual unrest.

ORIGINS

Inhibition of sexual desires may be limited or extensive. This condition is often strongly influenced by complex psychologic factors within the patient as well as by the environmental setting. Some men, for example, are impotent only with women whom they respect and yet can carry out the sexual act successfully with prostitutes. Others have so eliminated their sexual needs that they are unable to obtain an erection in any situation, and their fantasies and dreams are absolutely devoid of erotic content. In like manner, the patterns of sexual unrest vary widely. One patient may experience increased drives whenever anxiety is precipitated, even in the apparent absence of an erotic stimulus. Another may become intensely excited only when exposed to dynamically significant environmental factors; for example, such a change can be noted in certain hospitalized patients when a patient with an overt homosexual difficulty is admitted to their unit. Some patients may enter a state of extreme sexual excitement which continues long after the initial stimulation has disappeared and during the course of which erotic manifestations constitute the leading feature of their intensely disturbed condition.

As indicated, environmental factors also contribute to the development of sexual unrest, but only when acting upon a person who is psychologically sensitive to them. The dynamic origins of such sensitivity are not entirely clear. There appears to be a relationship between the abrupt removal of repressive defenses and the emergence of sexual unrest. Moreover, there appears to be a close link between sexual unrest and the experiencing of anxiety, fear, or hostility; this is particularly true of sexual panics and sexual excitements. The striking response of these conditions to chlorpromazine or electroconvulsive therapy argues in favor of a physiologic origin as well.

MANIFESTATIONS

It is important to distinguish between behavior which is directly influenced by sexual unrest and behavior which seems to be erotic but is, in fact, determined by motivations unrelated to sexual drives. For example, one patient may expose himself and take every opportunity to touch the female nurses during a sexual excitement. On the other hand, the exhibitionism and aggressive flirtatiousness of another patient may have no direct relationship to sexual unrest and may be primarily motivated by a need to provoke anger and rejection in those taking care of him. Similarly, sexual fantasies of an obsessive type may be described by certain patients. These may not be a reflection of excitement but rather stem from other dynamic conflicts, such as the fulfillment of a need for punishment in a person to whom such fantasies are unacceptable.

The presence of sexual unrest may or may not be recognized and reported by the patient. He may describe vivid fantasies or dreams rich in erotic content. Conscious sexual desires associated with pleasurable genital sensations may be revealed. At times, the patient may only be aware of the physical components of excitement, such as erection, tightness in the pubic area, or increased vaginal secretion, without any corresponding recognition of the fantasies themselves. There may be no clear connection between an environmental stimulus and the somatic sensation. At times, the description of the physical changes may be vague and only suggestive of strong sexual tension.

Since sexual unrest, like pathologic emotions and moods, may exist without the patient's awareness or willingness to admit its presence, the subjective descriptions of the patient should be complemented by observations of his appearance and behavior. The excited patient will often dress in a seductive or revealing fashion. Conversation may be filled with sexual references. Flirtatiousness and erotic overtures toward persons of the same or opposite sex may be prominent. If the disturbance is sufficiently extreme, frank exposure and open masturbation may occur.

Sexual unrest rarely occurs in isolation. It is usually accompanied by other psychopathologic phenomena, such as anxiety, fear, hostility, or an alteration in mood. If it is accompanied by intense fear, delusions or hallucinations may develop and the patient's condition is then called a sexual panic. Sexual unrest of maximal intensity is called sexual excitement, and is usually accompanied by profound hostility, marked agitation, and, at times, the formation of delusions or hallucinations. Sexual panics or sexual excitements appear to be more common among patients diagnosed as schizophrenic, but they may occur in any diagnostic setting.

CONSEQUENCES

From the foregoing, it is apparent that the consequences of severe sexual unrest can be devastating. Milder states of sexual unrest may also have undesirable results. Preoccupation with sexual needs and fantasies may be associated with impaired concentration and an inability to utilize intelligence and imagination along constructive avenues. In a morally sensitive person, such a change may be accompanied by marked guilt, which, in turn, may only serve to intensify the state of sexual unrest. A lonely schizophrenic patient may seek human contact through injudicious sexual activity in such a state, later suffering guilt and self-recrimination and occasionally an unwanted pregnancy.

Extreme sexual unrest often militates against the initiation of constructive psychotherapeutic rapport, since the patient usually lacks insight into the pathologic nature of his state. During a panic or excitement psychologic therapy is usually limited to the removal of erotically disturbing stimuli from the patient's environment and the acquisition of as much dynamic knowledge as possible from his behavior. Milder degrees of sexual unrest can also present difficulties in therapy. A patient's preoccupation with sexual themes may encourage him unwisely and destructively to seek sexual formulations for all his conscious and unconscious motivations. Thereby he may prevent analysis along lines which are exceedingly important but not sexual in nature. He may invest essentially neutral topics with sexual overtones. He may incorrectly perceive sexual meanings in the attitudes and interpretations of the therapist. The rapport and transference aspects of the doctor-patient relationship may be seriously disturbed by a patient's tendency to contaminate the therapeutic situation with inappropriate sexual meaning. Whereas in certain patients the revelation of sexual dynamics is an essential part of treatment, in others it may constitute a serious resistance to progress in therapy. At times it is necessary to allow sexual unrest to continue, in order to investigate its dynamic origins and assist the patient in handling his erotic drives; at other times, however, sexual unrest is essentially injurious to the patient's progress, and somatic treatment is required.

SUMMARY

The second step in the evaluation of an individual patient for treatment is to determine the presence of prevailing emotions, moods, and sexual drives which can significantly affect his clinical condition, regardless of the diagnostic setting. Anxiety, fear or hostility, elation or depression, and sexual unrest, occurring singly and in combination, may profoundly influence the basic psychopathologic state of the patient, his ability to utilize his personality assets and to cope with his environment, and his participation in psychotherapy. Each of these dynamic factors possesses subjective and objective characteristics allowing its identification in the majority of patients. Each must be considered in the establishment of a correct psychologic and somatic approach to treatment.

4

ASSOCIATED PSYCHOPATHOLOGIC FACTORS

The diagnosis has been established. The role of pathologic emotions, abnormal moods, and sexual unrest has been determined. It is now necessary to evaluate the status of each patient with regard to certain psychopathologic symptoms which can occur in practically all diagnostic settings and which have an important bearing on the selection of treatment methods. Not infrequently they seem the result of pathologic emotions rather than a reflection of the basic disease process. For example, when a patient is beset with anxiety, he may experience this emotion directly as a state of apprehension. His anxiety may or may not have physiologic concomitants. It may be either generalized or attached to a specific object. On the other hand, he may also react to the anxiety through the formation of dissociative symptoms, phobias, obsessions, or compulsions. In a state of intense fear or rage, particularly when his capacity for reality testing is seriously impaired, owing either to an underlying schizophrenic disorder or to the extent of the emotional upheaval, a patient may develop delusions, hallucinations, and paranoid features. Certain patients who turn to alcohol as a method of relieving distressing emotional symptoms may become habituated to it. Thereby chronic alcoholism may be superimposed on the original psychopathologic state, continuing long after the initial illness has subsided.

In addition to the specific manifestations of anxiety in the form of dissociative symptoms, phobias, obsessions, and compulsions, these relevant psychopathologic factors include delusions, hallucinations, paranoid features, insomnia, tension, apathy, depersonalization, significant variations in motor activity, eating difficulties, suicidal trends, and habituation or addiction to alcohol or drugs.

Each of these psychopathologic factors has certain identifying characteristics; each may interfere with the patient's ability to function in life or may impede efforts at psychotherapy. As with pathologic emotions, their recognition depends upon combining the subjective descriptions of the patient with an objective evaluation of his appearance and behavior. Some of these factors, such as depersonalization, can only be revealed to the examiner by the patient. Others, such as underactivity and overactivity, are estimated entirely on a behavioral basis. Evaluation of the misuse of alcohol may require a careful history obtained from family members to complement that secured from the patient.

These psychopathologic factors may occur singly, but more often several are present at the same time in an individual patient. For example, the acutely disturbed patient with paranoid delusions is frequently anorexic, markedly tense, unable to sleep, and over- or underactive. In the following pages, these factors will be described and their consequences discussed in order to facilitate their inclusion in the evaluation of any patient for therapy.

Specific Manifestations of Anxiety

Pathologic anxiety has been described as an emotional state characterized by the presence of focal or generalized apprehension. In certain patients this feeling of dread is directly perceived and manifested. In others, it is handled through the development of symptoms which modify the anxiety experience. The major symptoms which may result from anxiety include dissociative phenomena, such as conversion reactions, amnesias, and phobias; obsessions; and compulsions. There are important dynamic and probably physiologic differences between patients who reveal one mechanism of handling anxiety, such as eliminating all awareness of the emotion and developing physical symptoms which lack any organic basis, and those who utilize another method, such as experiencing a compulsive, irresistible need to comb their hair whenever it is slightly out of place. The selection of the particular symptoms seems to depend upon dynamic factors affecting the patient during his childhood. A patient with obsessions or compulsions has usually experienced serious psychologic trauma between ages 2 and 4, at which time he was learning that certain patterns of behavior were acceptable and others unacceptable to his parents. Because toilet training is an important event at this phase of growth, the period has been called the anal period. The patient likely to handle anxiety through the formation of phobias usually has experienced psychologic disturbances during the genital phase of childhood, occurring between ages 4 and 6 and characterized by the

involvement in and eventual resolution of the Oedipus complex. Physiologic factors contributing to the selection of anxiety symptoms are largely
unknown.

All symptoms of anxiety possess important qualities which must be considered in planning therapy. First, each serves to repress the basic
anxiety and conflicts from which it stems well beyond the patient's awareness. Second, the content of the anxiety symptom will usually reflect the
nature of the underlying difficulties, but in a way which escapes the
recognition of the patient. For example, if he is attempting to cope with
unconscious hostile emotions, he may well develop a phobic fear of
guns or obsessive ideas of a violent nature. A patient with pathologic guilt
about unconscious sexual desires may handle his anxiety by the formation
of phobias, the objects of which may be persons, places, or things which
could arouse him sexually.

In addition to enhancing repression and secretly reflecting the nature
of the hidden conflicts, these symptoms may also effectively express or
communicate the very feelings which the patient is attempting to
eliminate. By repeatedly telling his wife of his obsessive fears of failing
in business, a patient may succeed in disturbing her greatly. He may
thereby express the unconscious hostility toward her which constitutes
the central conflict he is attempting to deny. The secondary gain to be
derived from the symptoms is readily seen in the example of the patient
who, temporarily at least, obtains attention and sympathy from his relatives by informing them repeatedly of his concern over his physical
health.

In setting up any program of therapy, psychologic or physiologic,
aimed at the removal of these anxiety symptoms, it is essential to keep
their complex nature in mind. In spite of the suffering which he experiences, the patient often prefers his symptom to the necessity of facing
the conflicts which account for it. Premature relief of anxiety symptoms
may meet with strong resistance or may force the patient to fall back on
other lines of defense, such as severe depression, which are more disastrous, yet essential to the preservation of his psychologic balance.

DISSOCIATIVE SYMPTOMS

When dissociative mechanisms are brought into play, the patient wards
off the painful experience of anxiety by eliminating it from consciousness,
i.e., repressing it beyond awareness. Characteristically such a patient will
be unaware of the conflict threatening him and of the anxiety resulting
from this conflict. He will substitute either a physical or psychologic
symptom in place of the pathologic emotion. This is the type of reaction
often referred to as hysterical. A patient who dissociates anxiety may
develop paralysis of an arm or leg, inability to speak, blindness, deafness,

paraesthesias, or anesthesias, none of which have any structural basis. There may be, as in amnesia, a circumscribed or extensive loss of memory for sensitive events or complete forgetting of an entire segment of a person's past life. Occasionally, the dissociation is so complete that no anxiety is evident, and the patient exhibits a bland, indifferent attitude toward his physical or psychologic deficit, called *la belle indifférence.* Occasionally the dissociation is only partial, and the patient is indeed anxious, his concern being focused largely on the hysterical symptom.

The same mechanism of dissociation is involved in the development of a phobia. In such a state, the patient not only shuts out the true source of his disturbance but also projects his apprehension onto an otherwise neutral object in the environment. By avoiding the thing which he fears, he is able to maintain a state of relative well-being. Common examples of phobias include fears of closed or open spaces, high places, animals, knives, and other weapons of violence. With the current cultural emphasis on the importance of "getting along well with others," a frequent, but often unrecognized, object of a phobia may be another human being, particularly someone in close daily contact with the patient. Accordingly, distress experienced in the presence of a mother, father, sister, brother, husband, or wife need not always indicate a basic defect in the relationship but, in fact, may be the reflection of anxiety handled by the formation of an insidious phobia.

OBSESSIVE-COMPULSIVE SYMPTOMS

An obsession is defined as a disturbing idea recurring again and again in the mind of the patient and which he is unable to dismiss without extreme effort, since to do so would expose him to the more threatening source of his painful anxiety. The content of obsessive thinking varies widely and often, in a hidden way, reflects the actual nature of the underlying conflicts. These ideas may be sexual, with the patient disturbed by intruding fantasies of perversions or homosexual and autoerotic activities. They may be essentially hostile, containing images of mutilated or dying persons who are actually close to and loved by the patient. They may fill his mind with doubts, feelings of worthlessness, guilt, and self-recrimination, of which he is unable to free himself.

Closely akin to obsessions are compulsive activities. These are patterns of behavior which the patient is forced, by anxiety, to perform over and over again, in order to avoid experiencing the more awful fear attached to his basic conflicts. The more dramatic types of compulsions are well known and easily recognized, such as hand washing 20 or 30 times daily. When the compulsive pattern deviates from the flamboyant and particularly when it becomes colored by cultural factors, it may be more difficult to detect. Masturbation, for example, is often overlooked as a compulsive activity. Instead of being the direct release of sexual tension, there are times when it is anxiety-driven, performed as often as half a dozen times in a single night and serving to protect the patient against the disturbing realization of his impotence with women.

CONSEQUENCES OF ANXIETY SYMPTOMS

The manner and extent to which a patient's life adjustment will be impaired by these symptoms of anxiety will depend upon the type of symptom, its intensity, and the demands which are placed on the patient by his responsibilities. Mild forgetting, a form of dissociation, may in no way interfere with his ability to work. Extensive amnesia, however, may make it impossible for him to function at all. The plight of a history instructor with a paralyzed left hand is quite different from that of a high-voltage lineman with the same conversion symptom. Many patients with mild phobias do not even experience sufficient interference with their lives to come to the attention of a physician. However, if the anxiety experienced is sufficiently intense, the number of phobic objects large, or the nature of those objects specifically disabling to the patient, the consequences can be severe. If a woman, responsible for the care of her home, is unable to shop in stores because of phobic anxiety in crowded places, her life may become chaotic. For some, air travel is a luxury; for others, it is necessary for earning a living, a ready target for a crippling phobia. Obsessive ideas may be so intense as to make constructive concentration impossible. Compulsive activities may be so extensive as to leave the patient little time for anything else. They may also be benign, such as the need to empty ash trays whenever they become dirty, and might well go unnoticed. If mild, and not characterized by a content that is strikingly absurd, obsessive ideas may not even be recognized as abnormal by the patient and hence may influence his judgment and behavior. Obsessive doubts concerning his ability to carry responsibilities could lead a sensitive man to turn down an important opportunity for advancement in his career. An obsessive concern over her attractiveness could lead a woman to avoid important social activities.

These anxiety symptoms may also constitute obstacles to psychotherapy. A fear of traveling could prevent a patient from being able to visit the psychiatrist's office. The tendency to continue in compulsive modes of behavior can successfully maintain resistance to therapeutic progress and enhance the forces of repression. Thereby dynamically significant conflicts are prevented from emerging in the treatment setting. It is often difficult to separate an obsessive patient from his fixed and recurrent ideas in order to pursue other important but unrelated topics for analysis. In most instances, however, anxiety symptoms succumb to psychotherapeutic ingenuity and skill, without the need for somatic intervention.

Delusions

A delusion is defined as a conviction contrary to fact and at variance with the cultural setting, but tenaciously held by a patient regardless of attempts to persuade him of its falsity by the presentation of reasonable evidence. There are several common types of delusions, distinguishable by their content. These include delusions of grandiosity, persecution, guilt, and bodily disturbance. A patient with delusions of a grandiose nature may be utterly convinced, for example, that he has been sent by God to save mankind from the dire consequences of evil. The paranoid patient may believe that his food has been poisoned by the doctors, who, in his eyes, are the agents of malicious relatives ambitious to inherit his estate. Concrete evidence of former achievements and generosities will fall on deaf ears when presented to a patient with delusions of guilt and worthlessness. A man in his fifties in the course of a depressive illness may be overwhelmed with morbid guilt concerning marital infidelities which never actually occurred. The mother of four children may remain adamant in regarding herself a failure as a parent, despite the frequent reassurances of her own family. Bodily delusions may be subtle and almost convincing. A patient with such a symptom may attribute his constipation to bowel cancer even though repeated examinations have failed to demonstrate any disease. On the other hand, somatic delusions may be quite complex and bizarre, containing such ideas as "concrete slowly hardening in the lungs" or "arms and legs changing from muscle and bone to rubber."

Many factors, psychologic and physiologic, known and unknown, contribute to the formation of delusions. A defect in reality testing is usually necessary. This factor may be part of the basic disease state itself, as in certain schizophrenic reactions. It may occur in association with profound pathologic emotions, such as anxiety, fear, or hostility. In patients whose perception of things as they are is seriously impaired, even mild anxiety may facilitate the development of delusions. Panic, in an otherwise well-organized human being, may often be associated with delusions of persecution. An extremely depressed patient is sometimes subject to false convictions of guilt, which serve to explain and confirm his terrible suffering. The excited manic patient often reveals grandiose convictions of being in possession of strange and mysterious powers for doing good. He may believe, for example, that he has discovered a new drug capable of prolonging human life for 500 years.

The psychodynamic factors contributing to the patient's conflict, and thereby to the generation of his psychopathologic reaction, are frequently reflected in the content of his delusions. For example, if a patient is threatened by the emergence of overwhelming homosexual urges, he may, in his state of intense fear or excitement, project these complexes onto the environment, forming delusions of persecution in which he is convinced that several business competitors have tried to discredit him by circulating rumors that he is homosexual. A schizophrenic patient, struggling with deep guilt-ridden hostile emotions, may believe that his stomach and intestinal tract have been brutally removed.

CONSEQUENCES OF DELUSIONS

It is apparent that the presence of delusions will usually seriously interfere with a patient's ability to function. Occasionally, a patient may be able to turn his attention away from his delusions most of the time and thus can work and live with his family as long as he is not disturbed by provoking situations. The degree and manner of impairment depend on the nature of the delusional thinking, as well as on its intensity. As already indicated, a patient with a paranoid delusion may refuse to eat if he fears his food has been poisoned. Delusions of guilt and worthlessness may encourage a patient to arrive at decisions adversely affecting his financial affairs or to end his life by suicide. The patient with grandiose ideas may become enraged and strike out against anyone contradicting his imaginative concepts of himself.

The presence of delusions may impede therapy. Patients with somatic delusions may be willing to frequent the office of the radiologist, but they are seldom convinced that psychologic factors contribute to their condition. Inasmuch as delusions serve to protect a patient against the awareness of his underlying conflict, there may be marked resistance to relinquishing the false convictions in the course of therapy. Grandiose delusions, in particular, contain obvious elements of wish fulfillment and, although pathologic, may provide a patient with important satisfactions. It may be difficult to distract a patient from his delusional preoccupations long enough to pursue constructive analysis. Sometimes the content of the delusion shifts, incorporating the therapist and the treatment situation, thereby endangering and defeating the physician's attempts to restore the patient to his previous health. Somatic intervention, when available, is almost always indicated.

Hallucinations

A hallucination is a sensory perception of an object outside the patient occurring in the absence of any real environmental stimulus to induce or even suggest such a response. This is to be contrasted with an illusion, which is an incorrect perception of an external object which requires some stimulus to provoke it. A patient with a hallucination may see another person in an empty room. A patient with an illusion perceives the outline of the bedpost as if it were another person in the room with him.

Hallucinations may affect the visual, auditory, olfactory, gustatory, or tactile modalities of sensation. The particular type of hallucination which occurs often indicates the underlying disease process giving rise to it. For example, olfactory hallucinations frequently are associated with damage to the temporal lobes of the cerebral cortex. Toxic conditions caused by such agents as bromides or alcohol may often be characterized by the development of tactile hallucinations. Auditory and visual hallucinations are most frequently seen in psychopathologic reactions of psychogenic origin, in which no known organic factors can be demonstrated with present methods.

Hallucinations are the products of known and unknown psychologic and physiologic factors. A defect in reality testing is required. This may occur either as part of the basic disease process, as in schizophrenic reactions, or as a result of intense pathologic emotions or toxic factors. The content of the hallucinatory experience may be pleasant or unpleasant, simple or elaborate, and nearly always reflects the nature of the dynamic conflicts giving rise to the psychopathologic state. An elated patient may hear voices commending him on his bravery and skill. A depressed patient may hear God reminding him of his guilt. A patient threatened by his hostile emotions may visualize men and women being cruelly tortured. Sexual unrest may lead to images of persons engaging in various types of erotic practices.

CONSEQUENCES OF HALLUCINATIONS

In rare instances, patients with hallucinations may be able to tolerate their pathologic experiences and function in life in a limited fashion. Usually, however, such a patient is severely disturbed and unable to attend to his personal needs. Inasmuch as certain patients occasionally hear voices forcefully instructing them to kill themselves or injure others, this state can be hazardous. The loss of contact with the environment demonstrated by many patients whose attention is absorbed by their hallucinations can be extensive. Communication with them may be very difficult and hence psychotherapeutic efforts thwarted. Some patients will readily communicate the nature of their experiences to the physician. Some will hide their hallucinations, afraid of acknowledging to themselves or others the extent of their illness. Others may want to preserve the pathologic satisfaction derived from their hallucinations. The voices some patients hear may instruct them to keep their presence secret.

Somatic intervention is nearly always indicated. The timing of such treatment, however, is exceedingly important. The hallucinations often contain material which is essential for an understanding of the nature of the dynamic factors contributing to the patient's illness. Once the acute reaction subsides, either spontaneously or as a result of therapy, the patient may no longer recall his unusual sensory experiences and, therefore, will be unable to inform the doctor of their vital content.

Paranoid Symptoms

In the discussions of delusions and hallucinations, examples of these symptoms were mentioned in which patients falsely perceived persons in their environment as threatening to their well-being. Further examples, such as the patient who may be convinced that his wife has been unfaithful to him and is plotting to take his life and the patient who may hear voices accusing him of dishonesty and threatening him with punishment, can be cited. In these examples, the psychopathologic manifestations have been colored by the presence of paranoid features. The term *paranoid* is used to describe the phenomenon in which a patient perceives an unfounded threat from the environment. The fundamental psychologic mechanism employed in the formation of a paranoid symptom is projection. The conflict which is the source of the patient's disturbance is removed from his innermost self and transported into the world around him. For example, a patient attempting to cope with unconscious homosexual strivings or hidden hostility may protect himself from the recognition of these factors by perceiving effeminate traits or angry countenances in the appearance of various men around him, although no such characteristics actually exist among his associates. Paranoid features are often closely related to pathologic emotions of anxiety, fear, and hostility; patients experiencing them may readily project these feelings onto others.

The quality and intensity of paranoid features vary widely. In some patients, they may be evidenced only by an indiscriminate distrust and suspiciousness of others. In a subtle fashion, patients with paranoid features may explain subjective feelings of anxiety, resentment, or depression to themselves by blaming contemporary environmental difficulties which are real, but insufficient to account for their emotional states. For example, a woman whose hostility stems from deeply buried unconscious sources may erroneously attribute her suffering entirely to her husband's slightly irresponsible behavior. In a hospital setting, a patient with paranoid trends may misinterpret the actions of the medical staff, exaggerating their human frailties, and attributing boredom and unhappiness to the therapeutic program, feeling at times that it has been deliberately designed to make him more miserable.

In a more striking way, patients may demonstrate paranoid symptomatology in the formation of ideas of reference. In such a state, a patient refers essentially neutral stimuli to himself in a derogatory fashion. He may pick up a novel lying on a table, note that it is open to a passage describing the misfortunes befalling a man who has betrayed his friends, and instantly feel that this book was deliberately placed there by someone for him to find. He may walk into a crowded room, observe that several of his friends are involved in a heated conversation, and for a moment feel that they are talking about him in a malicious fashion. There is but a shade of difference between this fleeting psychopathologic experience and the construction of paranoid delusions.

Delusions, it will be recalled, are fixed beliefs which are untrue but beyond appeal to reason. Paranoid delusions may be highly organized and persistent or loosely organized and shifting. One patient may believe in a highly elaborate scheme in which his wife has been carrying on an affair with his lawyer, the two of them conspiring to have him committed to a psychiatric hospital so that they can obtain legal control of his financial matters. Another patient may feel one day that his wife has betrayed him, deny this the next day, and on the day after that be convinced that business rivals have surreptitiously gained entrance to his home in order to kill him. Paranoid features may also be apparent in hallucinations, with the patient perceiving threatening images or hearing abusive voices.

Paranoid symptoms may be the result of pathologic fear and hostility. Conversely, a patient with paranoid symptoms may react to his misinterpretations with expressions of fear and hostility. For example, a patient with persecutory delusions or hallucinations may become terrified, and withdraw into himself, or enraged, and attempt to assault his family or the medical staff. Such emotional reactions tend to complicate and reinforce the basic dynamic factors which originally prompted the paranoid state. When paranoid symptoms are the result of pathologic emotions, the therapeutic reduction of these emotions will usually be associated with the disappearance of the paranoid features. On the other hand, the reduction of anxiety, fear, or hostility secondary to misinterpretations of the environment will ordinarily leave the persecutory concepts intact.

Consequences of Paranoid Features

Paranoid features often complicate a patient's life and obstruct psychotherapeutic treatment. In addition to the obvious dangers of suicide during a state of panic or bodily injury to others, there are more subtle but also serious complications. The paranoid patient, because of his exquisite sensitivity and readiness to distort the motivations of others, is usually a very difficult person with whom to live or associate. His behavior often leads to divorce or unemployment. His ability to project and attribute subjective distress to external causes prevents him from realizing that he is sick and in need of help. Once involved in therapy, he may have great difficulty trusting the physician and confiding in him. He tends to become intensely dependent on his therapist and yet often remains prepared to turn against him at the slightest provocation. Stirring up sensitive dynamic factors may enhance the paranoid features, preventing their analysis. Occasionally a delusional system involving the doctor may be constructed. The physician, instead of being there to help him, becomes sexually seductive or cruel and merciless in the eyes of the paranoid patient. Somatic means to reduce the intense emotions so often associated with paranoid features are often required in order to proceed with psychotherapy and to reconstruct the patient's life.

Insomnia

Mild or severe psychopathologic disturbances frequently affect the sleep patterns of patients. Interference with normal sleep is called insomnia and is generally recognized by the clinician as evidence of emotional distress. It is not as widely realized, however, that there are various types of insomnia, each possessing certain characteristics which are dependent upon the nature of the pathologic emotions and specific dynamic factors contributing to the development of this symptom.

Insomnia may be characterized by difficulty in falling asleep, interruptions during sleep, early morning awakening, or a combination of these features. Tension often prevents the adequate relaxation required to enter a state of sleep. Pathologic anxiety is usually responsible for restlessness and frequent awakening during the night. Depressed patients often wake early in the morning, before daylight, feeling most distressed at the time but unable to fall asleep again. These considerations have important practical implications. If tension keeps a patient awake, measures designed to induce relaxation, such as warm baths or short-acting sedatives, may be all that is needed to ensure a good night's sleep. On the other hand, control of anxiety-disturbed sleep or the early morning awakening of a depressed patient may necessitate long-term or repeated sedation. In certain patients with intense sexual unrest, psychotherapeutic and pharmacologic reduction of this feature may be required before a normal sleep pattern can be reestablished.

Insomnia may also be determined by specific psychodynamic factors which are largely unconscious and hence cannot always be managed as directly as pathologic emotions, tension, or depression of mood. For example, insomnia is often observed in patients whose unconscious sexual conflicts are largely unresolved. These patients are to be differentiated from those experiencing sexual unrest, which is a conscious experience. The patient with unconscious sexual conflicts may automatically resist sleep with remarkable vigor in spite of sedation because of his deep, hidden fear of being sexually molested while unconscious or because of passive homosexual wishes which to him are symbolized by the sleep experience. As a second example of this phenomenon, the common association of sleep with death may produce marked insomnia in a patient with unconscious death wishes directed at himself or at others. There are certain patients who invest great significance in their dream life. They may utilize insomnia to avoid awareness of disturbing feelings which might make themselves known through dreams. Some patients, who are convinced of the importance of sleep for their physical and psychologic well-being, may find insomnia a most effective method of punishing themselves for unconscious guilt-ridden desires. These examples are but representative of the manner in which unconscious psychodynamic factors may contribute to sleep difficulties. The correction of such conditions depends on satisfactory analysis of these factors.

CONSEQUENCES OF INSOMNIA

A human being can tolerate extensive sleep deprivation without endangering his psychologic or physical health. On the other hand, sleep does seem to facilitate the alleviation of many psychopathologic states. In fact, sleep therapy, which will be described later, is effectively used in certain very disturbed patients. The fatigue, tension, and irritability which often follow a distressing night of tossing and turning without relaxation may be sufficient to impair a patient's ability to work efficiently and add to his general state of emotional distress. The depressed patient, early in the morning, alone with his hopelessness, may be more prone to commit suicide than at other times of the day.

As with anxiety and tension, insomnia often spurs on a patient to seek relief through psychotherapy, but it can also, at times, interfere with treatment. Failure to achieve early relief from this symptom may encourage certain patients to terminate therapy and seek remedies elsewhere. Resistance may be expressed through insomnia, preventing the patient from being able to report dreams for analysis. Continuation of the symptom of insomnia may be a method for expressing concealed transference hostility toward the therapist. Hypochondriac patients, for example, may harp on their insomnia, obstructing progress in the analysis of significant dynamic factors, much as they might utilize physical complaints in therapy. These problems, however, are usually best handled by psychotherapeutic methods, using somatic intervention judiciously when really necessary.

Tension

Tension may be described as a state of increased alertness, heightened sensitivity, and hypertonicity of voluntary musculature. Conflicting forces giving rise to tension may exist within the patient or emanate largely from the environment. For example, this reaction may often be seen in anxious or hostile patients who are attempting to control these emotions and to hide them from others. Tension is not uncommon in patients who are struggling to free themselves of obsessive ideas or interrupt compulsive patterns of behavior. It is often present in patients who experience intense and persistent sexual unrest. It may be experienced by the conscientious person who is burdened with more responsibility than he can handle adequately. Tension may be seen in the rigid, perfectionistic person who is expected to make important decisions rapidly, at unexpected times, and with little preparation. It may constitute the major feature of a patient's condition, or it may be quite incidental in the setting of a severe psychopathologic reaction.

The ability of the tense patient to utilize his intelligence and imagination may be temporarily increased, unless the condition is so marked that concentration is impaired. Irritability and impatience are common associates of tension. Muscular involvement may be localized or general. Posture and gait may appear rigid and unspontaneous. Motility may be increased or decreased. In some patients the neck and scalp muscles are affected, with vascular involvement and the development of headaches. In others, pain and tightness in the arms and legs may be observed. It has been suggested that the groups of muscles involved indicate the underlying dynamic factors responsible for the tension, but such a concept is not sufficiently defined to assume therapeutic significance.

Tension often results in fatigue, in spite of which relaxation is difficult to obtain. Physical distress, irritability, fatigue, and insomnia are the most commonly seen complications of tension. When concentration is affected and the tense patient is no longer able to utilize his abilities efficiently, his life adjustment may be moderately impaired. When a patient recognizes the psychologic basis of his tension, psychotherapy is ordinarily facilitated, since relief is eagerly desired. The fact that the dynamic and physiologic nature of tension differs from that of anxiety is often important in the selection of somatic treatment methods.

Apathy

The leading manifestation of certain psychopathologic states, in particular chronic schizophrenic reactions, is apathy. Apathy is characterized by a decrease or absence of apparent emotional responsiveness, associated with a lack of spontaneity and drive. The apathetic patient may describe a marked loss of interest in any form of mental or physical activity. He may spend hours and days in a state of disinterested idleness. In milder degrees and for short periods of time, apathy may appear in any diagnostic setting. It is important to distinguish between apathy and the withdrawal and loss of interest so often seen in depressed patients. Depression of mood is, in fact, an intense feeling-state, and the associated loss of drive observed is the result of the patient's absorption in his hopelessness and suffering. True apathy is a fundamental lack of affective investment in any object, including the patient himself. He is neither anxious nor hostile, neither sexually aroused nor depressed. His mind may be "blank," and he is often unresponsive to efforts to engage him in conversation. When not so extreme, some patients may be quite apprehensive and discouraged by the experience of apathy, recognizing it as an abnormal state of being.

The basis of apathy is unclear. Extensive dissociation of conflicts and associated emotions contributes to its development in certain cases. In others, it may be a complication of many years of inactivity forced upon the patient by the presence of a chronic illness and environmental neglect. The human being seems to require stimulation in order to be stimulating. In psychoneurotic states, boredom, which is painful apathy, may be the result of unconscious dynamic factors, such as guilt and punishment or masochism. Physiologic factors, which undoubtedly contribute to the development of many apathetic states, are largely unknown.

The complications of apathy depend upon the degree and psychopathologic setting of this phenomenon. A mild lack of spontaneous interest and drive may often be compensated by a deliberate, conscious effort on the part of the patient. He may force himself to attend a conference, play golf, accept social invitations, even though he is tensely working against a lack of desire to do these things. Extreme apathy may reduce a human being to a state of near vegetation in which he requires continual encouragement to carry out the simplest daily hospital routines. Obviously, apathy undermines the motivation of certain patients to begin or continue in therapy. There may be no inclination to communicate with the physician about their personal lives. There may be no drives or emotions with which to work in the therapeutic sessions. It is often necessary for the psychotherapist to play a very active role for a very long time before he begins to see a glimmer of responsiveness from an apathetic patient.

Depersonalization

In many psychopathologic states patients experience a distinct and frequently distressing alteration in their perceptions of themselves or of the world around them. The former symptom is called depersonalization, the latter derealization. The ways in which these changes may be described by patients are so numerous that only a few examples can be presented in illustration. The depersonalized patient may feel that his mind or body has undergone a strange metamorphosis, as if it is no longer his own. He may complain of being unable to feel emotions. He may describe peculiar sensory experiences, emanating from various parts of his body, which are often difficult to differentiate from somatic delusions. He may feel as if a heavy weight is pressing on his brain and producing numbness through his entire body; yet he remains quite aware of the fact that no such change has actually taken place. In states of derealization, perceptual alterations occur with regard to the outer world. The patient feels that his room, his house, his office is no longer the same, but he cannot clearly identify the nature of the change. At other times, his sense of color may be affected, and the whole world assumes a gray appearance, reflecting his inner mood.

The basis of depersonalization and derealization is only partly understood. That a patient who is depressed or severely anxious should state that he is no longer his old self or that the world no longer seems the same to him seems like a natural consequence of his altered condition. Dissociative factors appear to contribute strongly to some states of depersonalization, especially when this symptom appears to replace evidence of pathologic emotions or depression of mood and serves to hide provoking conflicts. For example, a patient in a state of severe depression may appear quite bland, revealing the alteration of mood in the morbid content of his thinking but denying any feelings of sadness or hopelessness. In schizophrenic patients, in whom reality testing is impaired and autism is prominent, depersonalization phenomena may be quite bizarre and difficult to distinguish from somatic delusions. In analytic psychotherapy, depersonalization experiences often accompany the emergence of previously repressed infantile dynamic material.

The degree of impairment induced by this symptom depends on its intensity, accompanying psychopathologic features, and the degree to which it distresses the patient. Some patients experience depersonalization in an obsessive manner, their attention constantly being focused upon the disturbing sensations. Others may tolerate these experiences without undue influence on their behavior. Depersonalization may conceal the depth of the underlying emotional disturbance and mislead the physician with regard to various dangers, such as suicide in a depressive reaction. In some patients, this symptom is intimately connected with the repression of important feelings and dynamically sensitive material which can not emerge for analysis as long as depersonalization persists.

Variations in Motor Activity

Pathologic emotions and moods, sexual unrest, and other psychopathologic phenomena may or may not be accompanied by alterations in motor activity. It is often incorrectly assumed that a given emotional state produces a particular type of change in activity. The depressed patient is often expected to be hypoactive, while the angry patient is expected to be overactive. This may be the case. Frequently, however, opposite reactions can be seen; that is, the depressed patient may be agitated and the angry patient withdrawn and underactive.

Changes in activity may be mild or severe. One patient may feel restless but may be able to control all evidence of it with ease. Another may tap his fingers repetitiously on the edge of his chair, while still another may feel the need to stand up and walk around the room several times in the course of an hour's interview. A severely agitated patient may pace the corridors constantly, unable to sit still or to concentrate on anything for more than a few minutes. At times, the change in activity may be revealed only in certain dimensions of behavior, such as in increased or decreased rate of speech.

A particular pathologic emotion may result in either overactivity or underactivity in different patients and in one patient at different times. The direction of change seems to depend upon the personality structure of the patient, the intensity of the driving emotion, the setting of the psychopathologic experience, and the nature of associated symptoms. Let us use hostility to illustrate these considerations. One patient, when moderately angry, may readily lose his temper, shake his fist, talk loudly and rapidly, and pace about until this emotion subsides. If his anger reaches a maximal intensity, however, he may become afraid and suspicious of those around him, construct paranoid delusions, withdraw into his room, and refuse to eat, speak, or move. The origin of his reaction in each instance is pathologic hostility, but activity is affected in completely diverse directions.

Pathologic states in which activity is affected in either direction often impair the ability of patients to function adequately. Therapeutic planning is influenced by the nature and degree of change in activity. For example, the extremely overactive patient who becomes assaultive may have to be prevented from injuring himself or others. The extremely withdrawn, underactive patient may have to be fed, clothed, and stimulated to reestablish contact with the environment. In formulating a plan of treatment, however, the factors contributing to the change in activity must be carefully considered as well.

Eating Difficulties

Alterations in eating habits are often associated with pathologic emotions and psychopathologic states and, when present, may have to be considered in the evaluation of a patient for treatment. Some patients overeat; some undereat; some become extremely selective with regard to what they will eat. Loss of appetite or conscious refusal to eat is called anorexia. This symptom may, at times, lead to a state of malnutrition which imperils the life of the patient, as in certain cases of anorexia nervosa.

Pathologic emotions may be directly associated with eating abnormalities. The particular patterns which develop depend on the personality of the disturbed patient. Anxiety, for example, may lead to a loss of appetite or a craving for specific foods. Anorexia is common among depressed patients and may reflect physiologic changes as well as suicidal desires. Schizophrenic patients, suffering pangs of loneliness, may eat bulky foods to relieve their inner emptiness and hollowness. Abnormalities in eating are also frequently associated with sexual unrest.

It is important to distinguish between changes in eating habits which are directly associated with pathologic emotions and related psychopathologic features and those resulting from unconscious dynamic factors. In the latter instance, for example, a young woman's unconscious guilt and pregnancy wishes following a sexual experience may facilitate overeating and an increase in weight resembling that which occurs in the pregnant state. Overeating can also be utilized, in an unconscious manner, to make a woman obese and consequently unattractive to men.

Eating difficulties may be mild or severe. Anorexia can lead to death. Obesity can result in marked self-consciousness, social rejection, and habitual use of dietary medications. Either can constitute a difficult resistance in psychotherapy which a patient may be unable or unwilling to modify.

Suicide

The ultimate complication of a psychiatric illness, placing the patient once and for all beyond any therapeutic measures, is suicide. There are many methods, simple and complex, for accomplishing this purpose. The selection of the manner of death may be influenced by the nature of the psychopathologic reaction, the personality of the patient, and the cultural milieu in which the suicide occurs. In a panic, a patient may leap from a high window or in front of an oncoming truck. A depressed patient, concerned about the effect of his act on his family, may drive his automobile over an embankment to make his death appear accidental. For a number of years, carbon monoxide poisoning or barbiturates may be the most common methods employed; then, for a while, pistols or plastic bags may replace these in frequency.

The motivations for suicide are many. Some patients end their lives because of the overwhelming hopelessness which they experience as part of a depressive illness. Others, in a rage, use this weapon to revenge themselves lastingly on friends and relatives. In certain cases, the patient desires to rejoin deceased loved ones and at the same time punish himself for resentment which he has felt toward them. The disorganized or poorly organized patient may die as a result of self-mutilating sado-masochistic impulses. The alcoholic patient may kill himself in a state of intoxication or upon realizing the extent to which his behavior has destroyed his life.

Many patients experience suicidal thoughts and impulses but do not make any overt attempts on their lives. Such feelings may be described in various ways: as obsessive ideas of self-destruction, as phobic fears of injuring oneself, as fantasied relief from inner suffering and turmoil. Some patients will hide these impulses, whereas others are willing to talk about them. At times, suicidal threats are utilized by patients to secure attention and manipulate others to fulfill their needs and desires. An adult woman may employ suicidal threats to obtain the worried solicitousness of her parents and distract them from giving love and attentiveness to her siblings. The rejected suitor may speak of killing himself unless his girl friend agrees to marry him.

It is sometimes difficult to determine if and when the patient who is deeply depressed or speaks of suicidal impulses will make an attempt on his life. If the psychopathologic state is intense and the force of the impulses strong and if the setting of the patient's life is disturbed and he is rejected by his family, he is more likely to carry out his threat. If a patient has actually tried to commit suicide, he may well make a second attempt, particularly if his emotional state or life circumstances have not changed in a fundamental way. A family history of suicide, particularly if a parent or sibling has died when the patient was a young child, seems to increase the danger.

The presence of suicidal trends clearly will influence the establishment of a therapeutic program. The physician must decide whether protective measures, such as hospitalization, are indicated. The patient may or may not be amenable to following his advice and frequently cannot be forced to do so. The selection of a particular method of somatic intervention may depend on the certainty and rapidity of its effects.

Alcoholism and Drug Addiction

The indiscriminate use of alcohol is a frequent concomitant of many psychopathologic conditions. At times, it may constitute the major feature of the patient's condition. The heavy use of alcohol may lead to the development of the syndrome known as chronic alcoholism. Chronic alcoholism is characterized by the use of alcohol to an extent which interferes with the patient's personal, social, or work adjustment in a manner which he either does not recognize or is unable and unwilling to modify.

In order to determine whether the use of alcohol is pathologic in nature or degree, it is necessary to determine the amount of drinking which the patient does, the frequency or periodicity of his intoxications, and the effects which it has on his emotional state. Certain patients use alcohol, as they might use a tranquilizing medication, to relieve themselves of disturbing pathologic emotions, such as anxiety, tension, or resentment. In others, it reduces awareness and dilutes the impact of the superego, thereby permitting them, for example, to manifest profound emotions of rage or to carry out otherwise inhibited sexual activities. Angry outbursts and assaultive or destructive behavior may occur under the influence of alcohol in persons who, when sober, reveal little evidence of hostility. A patient who is ordinarily faithful to his wife may engage in promiscuous activities when intoxicated. Paradoxically, at the same time that it increases or liberates sexual unrest, alcohol seems to diminish the patient's ability to complete the sexual act.

A true craving for alcohol is probably rare. Although patterns of excessive drinking may be fixed and resistant to modification, they are not ordinarily considered compulsive. The patient may offer many rationalizations for his behavior, such as the sedative benefits of alcohol, social pressures to drink, or the enhancement of self-confidence. However, these reasons are often self-deceptive, and the true motivations remain deeply hidden. For instance, there seems to be a seriously self-destructive, punitive aim in excessive drinking in certain patients which can be seen in the effects it has on the patient and his family.

The physical complications of prolonged, heavy drinking are well known. These include damage to the liver and the central nervous system. Organically determined changes in intellectual function and memory may result. Dissociative factors may combine with brain damage to account for black-outs, experiences in which a patient behaves in an apparently conscious and purposeful manner, but later, when the effects of alcohol have disappeared, he demonstrates a total amnesia for the events.

The complications of alcoholism transcend physical dimensions. It may seriously obscure the true psychopathologic disturbance of the patient, thereby delaying corrective therapeutic measures. Pathologic emotions, schizophrenic thinking disorders, and intense mood alterations may be concealed by the drinking pattern, emerging clearly only after it has been interrupted. Occasionally the underlying psychopathologic state is aggravated by alcohol, and the patient manifests such features as depression and suicidal intent or paranoid delusions only when intoxicated.

The continued use of alcohol often impairs progress in psychotherapy. The patient may use it to blot out significant affective experiences and dynamic content. Meaningful developments in the transference relationships may be discharged outside the interview situation; for instance, the patient may drink heavily as an expression of pathologic resentment toward the therapist. At times, even small amounts of alcohol may lead to difficulty in thinking and impaired judgment. Therefore, the role of alcohol should be clarified with any patient with a psychiatric illness and not merely when chronic alcoholism is the presenting syndrome.

The use of opium, morphine, heroin, or cocaine may lead to states of addiction. Addiction is considered to be present when a patient demonstrates increased tolerance, and hence requires progressively larger doses of a given drug to produce the same effects, and when he cannot be deprived of the drug without experiencing profound withdrawal symptoms. Drug addiction may begin in the setting of medical treatment, during which some of these compounds are administered for the relief of pain. Other patients become involved with their use in the setting of antisocial behavior. Conscious and unconscious motivations combine with physiologic factors to promote the development of addiction. As long as the patient uses the particular drug to which he is addicted, he may be successful in avoiding confrontation with his basic conflicts, discharging his pathologic emotions in his behavior, denying the need for medical assistance, and further complicating the social and environmental aspects of his life. The presence of addiction strongly influences the outcome and plan of therapy in any patient, regardless of the diagnostic setting or contributing pathologic emotions.

Addiction is to be distinguished from habituation, which may develop as a result of prolonged injudicious use of such drugs as barbiturates, bromides, and perhaps some of the new tranquilizing medications in psychologically sensitive patients. Habituation is characterized by severe difficulty in terminating the use of these drugs, but the development of tolerance and the withdrawal phenomena seen with addicting compounds are lacking. Habituation is also an important determinant in the selection of treatment methods.

SUMMARY

There are a number of psychopathologic features which may be seen in any diagnostic setting. These symptoms often result from or are associated with the presence of pathologic emotions, moods, and sexual unrest. They can be identified by certain characteristics. In various ways they may impair personality function and obstruct psychotherapy. Therefore, these symptoms must also be considered in the selection of treatment methods.

5

THE DYNAMIC SETTING OF ILLNESS

The dynamic setting in which the psychopathologic reaction occurs will influence strongly the decision to use a somatic method of treatment and the selection of the particular therapeutic agent. This consideration exists independently of the diagnosis, pathologic emotions, and associated symptoms of the illness. It includes (1) the nature of those factors precipitating the reaction, (2) the personality structure of the patient, (3) the period of his life in which the illness takes place, (4) the presence of unrelated but important physical disorders, (5) his contemporary environment, (6) previous therapy which he has received for the same or other psychopathologic disturbances, and (7) his over-all attitudes toward psychiatric treatment.

Precipitating Factors

Traumatic experiences giving rise to psychiatric disorders vary widely in quality, intensity, and duration. Some may be well defined and easily recognized; others may be obscure except after extensive psychologic investigation. Some may exist concurrently with the illness; others may have subsided long before the illness began. For example, in certain predisposed patients, landing on the Normandy beaches during the World War II invasion of Europe generated acute psychopathologic disturbances. The obvious precipitating factor was the threat of injury or death. No one would question the reality and severity of the stimulus. The duration of the traumatic situation was limited to the time required to secure a foothold on the continent and drive out the last of the enemy. This type of precipitating factor contrasts markedly with one such as the death of a parent. Although each is well defined and realistically distressing, the latter lacks the sharp intensity of the battle situation and, perhaps more importantly, represents a permanent change in the patient's life. In many patients the precipitating factors are much more obscure. It may take weeks or months to discern the relationship between a middle-aged man's depressive illness, characterized by pathologic guilt about sexual indiscretions of his youth, and the onset of puberty in his adolescent son. Such conditions are often mistakenly dismissed as entirely endogenous in origin, that is, lacking contributing psychogenic causes, because of premature termination of the search for dynamic factors. Likewise, it may be difficult to recognize immediately the connection between a traumatic experience, such as an automobile accident or enforced unemployment, and a psychopathologic reaction which developed later, after the physical injuries have healed or the patient has obtained a new job.

Personality Structure

The second element contributing to the dynamic setting of the illness is the personality of the patient. Let us assume that two patients demonstrate phobic anxieties originating largely from similar dynamic conflicts. In spite of the resemblance between the diagnostic and psychopathologic components, there may be marked differences between the patients with regard to intelligence and imagination. One may be unusually talented and capable of a high degree of mental activity, with a history of having completed a leading university first in his class. He may demonstrate warmth and a singular ability to make and keep friends. He may communicate his feelings readily. He may incorporate and synthesize new ideas with ease. The other may be aloof and lacking in the development of any particular skill. He may reveal difficulties in completing the second year of high school and be unable to recognize inner emotions. He may be limited by a poverty-stricken vocabulary and may be practically devoid of synthetic powers. Such variations as these undoubtedly will influence the therapeutic methods employed by the physician in his management of patients, even though the diagnosis and leading emotional considerations are very similar.

Period of Life

The selection of treatment methods will also be affected by the time of life at which the psychopathologic illness occurs. The ordinary psychotherapeutic techniques applied in adults are modified by the use of the playroom and the emphasis on behavior in children. The adolescent experiences wide emotional swings. He lacks experience. His judgment is immature, and he requires direction. Psychotherapeutic techniques must be adapted to his needs and will differ substantially from those employed in the treatment of an aging patient. In the later years of life, interests may narrow. The patient's personality may be rigid and resistant to change. He may be keenly aware of the immediacy of disabling disease or death. His thinking and memory may be impaired by arteriosclerotic brain damage. The institution of prolonged psychotherapy in a young man of 24 who has the development and application of his talents and abilities still stretching ahead of him may be a most sensible goal. To establish such a plan for a retired executive in his late sixties who has already been subject to two heart attacks would indeed be unrealistic. Certain phases of life seem to be particularly critical in the development of psychiatric disorders; these include puberty, the postpartum state, and menopause. In addition to psychodynamic considerations, such as the onset of overt sexual drives and the struggle for independence during early adolescence, the activation of a mother's unconscious rejection of her new infant after its birth, or the reluctance to part with the erotic charms of youth by the narcissistic woman to whom menopause symbolizes their loss, there may be significant endocrinologic factors which contribute to the nature and extent of reactions occurring at these times. Thyroid, steroid, pituitary, and other hormonal imbalances may unduly complicate the psychopathologic picture.

Physical Status

The physical health of a patient may also influence the selection of treatment methods. An emotionally disturbed man in his fifties who also suffers with inoperable carcinoma of the lung or who has experienced an extensive cerebrovascular accident from which he is in the process of recovering will hardly be managed in the same fashion as the middle-aged patient whose illness has interrupted an active, productive life and whose physical status is excellent for his age. Certain organic disabilities constitute contraindications to the use of available somatic methods of treatment. For example, chlorpromazine cannot be given to a patient with infectious hepatitis; electroconvulsive therapy cannot be used in a patient with a known aneurysm of the circle of Willis.

Environmental Factors

The environmental situation of any patient at the time of his illness is vitally important. The management of a patient whose condition prompts violent rejection by his family differs from that of a similar patient whose family offers him support, reassurance, and love. Attempts to resolve marital conflicts will be facilitated when both partners are eager and willing to make necessary adjustments. On the other hand, they will be severely handicapped when the couple is already on the verge of divorce or when one of them is totally uncooperative and adamantly rejects the suggestion of seeking psychiatric assistance. It is one thing to treat a successful individual suffering with serious doubts about his abilities and lacking self-confidence, whose responsible position waits for him after his discharge from the hospital. It is entirely different to work in therapy with a patient whose employment history is erratic and disorganized and who has seriously alienated his co-workers and faces unemployment. Financial considerations warrant attention. For some patients hospitalization means the end of the regular income which is necessary to provide for their family. Some patients are fortunate enough to have savings, medical insurance policies, or family assistance to help them in their critical times. Some patients are unfortunate in having such large amounts of money at their disposal that they can readily live out their conflicts, discharge pathologic emotions, and avoid coming to grips with themselves. They can change jobs, homes, or wives at will rather than make the adjustments necessary for good health. All too often, the inevitable psychopathologic reaction occurs, but only after many years of complications which then severely limit the prognosis for readjustment. These instances are but illustrative of the manner in which the patient's family, working circumstances, financial condition, and other environmental considerations may influence the course of his illness and the selection of treatment methods.

Previous Therapy

The evaluation of the dynamic setting also includes careful analysis of previous treatment which the patient has received for his current or earlier episodes of illness. A 40-year-old patient, in a state of marked panic with associated paranoid delusions developing acutely in the setting of a specific environmental trauma, may reveal a history of successful treatment in his twenties for an anxiety psychoneurosis. It is not unusual for a depressed patient to describe substantial but fleeting relief obtained early in his illness through the administration of a series of electroconvulsive treatments unaccompanied by psychotherapy. One patient may enter an acute schizophrenic reaction in the course of intensive psychotherapy for what appeared to be a psychoneurotic reaction with obsessive-compulsive and phobic features. Another may have received no psychotherapy whatsoever while maintained with dubious success on a number of tranquilizing drugs, stimulants, or antidepressive medications. The nature and extent of these measures will strongly influence what the doctor will do at present for the patient.

Attitude to Treatment

Finally, the attitude of the patient and his family toward treatment must be considered. Some patients readily accept psychotherapy but reject any suggestion of drug treatment or electric shock. Others insist that there is a physical basis for their disorder and request or demand somatic therapy. In hospitalized patients a failure to secure the cooperation of the close relatives may be very damaging. They may, for example, object to the use of insulin or electroconvulsive therapy and refuse to grant permission for these procedures. They may encourage the patient to sign out of the hospital, their pride preventing them from accepting the emotional nature of the illness and their unconscious selves fearing that their relationship with the patient may be altered by treatment.

All these factors combine to constitute the dynamic setting of the illness. They must be considered in the evaluation of any patient for treatment, since they will significantly influence the selection and efficacy of somatic as well as psychotherapeutic regimens.

Part Two

THE CLINICAL EFFECTIVENESS
OF SOMATIC THERAPIES

6

CHLORPROMAZINE AND RELATED
PHENOTHIAZINE DERIVATIVES

Chlorpromazine (Thorazine, Largactil) was first used in clinical psychiatry in 1951 in France. Within a short period of time, it was established as a vital adjunct in the management of patients with severe psychiatric disturbances. Early reports rapidly confirmed the fact that the drug differed materially from other sedative compounds then available. Acute, intense reactions, such as manic and catatonic excitements, could be promptly and reliably terminated with chlorpromazine. In custodial hospital settings, the number of assaults by disturbed patients decreased, interpersonal contact and socialization among patients increased, and many patients could be discharged to their homes. The number of electroconvulsive treatments administered fell dramatically. In all but a few hospital centers insulin treatment was prematurely abandoned altogether.

Since that time thousands of patients have received chlorpromazine and related phenothiazine derivatives. Many have been hospitalized patients. Others have been treated in psychiatric outpatient departments or by psychiatrists in private practice. Still others have received these drugs from their general physicians. In the past 5 years several other pharmacologic agents, each containing the basic phenothiazine nucleus, have been developed and marketed.

Although the importance of these drugs is beyond question, the present state of their use is unfortunately confusing to the physician who is confronted with an individual patient and a particular clinical syndrome. In general, the indications for the use of these drugs have remained poorly defined. Terms such as "disturbed," "overactive," and "uncooperative" still

89

appear in the literature, offering little or no information about the exact nature of the emotional conditions which respond well to the phenothiazine compounds. A more precise knowledge of specific emotional and psychopathologic effects of these drugs is clearly required if they are to be employed efficiently. Some basis for separating those patients who are likely to respond well from those who are likely to respond poorly to phenothiazine therapy is essential.

Inasmuch as chlorpromazine is the oldest member of this group and hence has been more widely used and studied than any other single phenothiazine, it seems desirable to discuss in some detail the methods and complications of its administration and its influence on specific emotions and associated psychopathologic features. At a later point, the authors will compare its usefulness with that of some of the newer phenothiazine compounds. However, until such time as evidence to the contrary develops, it appears reasonable to assume that the *principles* underlying the effective use of chlorpromazine may be applied to phenothiazines in general.

MECHANISM OF ACTION

The mechanism of action of chlorpromazine and other phenothiazine derivatives in producing clinical improvement in psychiatric patients is largely unknown. These drugs do possess certain established physiologic and biochemical properties. There is evidence that they affect the reticular substance of the central nervous system, particularly in the hypothalamic area. Undoubtedly there are also cortical effects, but consciousness is usually not affected, as it is with the barbiturates. Electroencephalographic changes are often observed, and the phenothiazine derivatives are known to reduce the seizure threshold of the central nervous system. The actions of other drugs which influence the nervous system, such as barbiturates, anesthetics, and morphine, are potentiated by phenothiazines.

Experiments with chlorpromazine demonstrate that this compound possesses a moderate adrenolytic action and is a weak inhibitor of serum cholinesterase. In animals it will block the action of small doses of injected epinephrine, but this effect cannot be seen when large doses of epinephrine are administered or when norepinephrine is used.

Other important metabolic effects of these compounds have also been reported. In the cerebral tissue of animals, intracellular enzymatic activity is reduced. There is a diminution in oxygen uptake and in the activity of phosphorylase, cytochrome oxidase, and adenosinetriphosphatase. Adenosinetriphosphate accumulates in the midbrain tissue. Aerobic and anaerobic glycolysis, oxygen and phosphate uptake, and pyruvate oxidation are inhibited.

A decrease in blood pressure and an increase in pulse rate are frequent concomitants of chlorpromazine administration in human beings. These changes may not be as marked with certain other phenothiazine derivatives, an important consideration in the treatment of psychiatric patients with cardiovascular disease. Hypothermia may often be seen. Menstrual suppression and at times the initiation of lactation suggest an influence on the endocrine system, possibly at the pituitary level. It is not clear whether the weight gain which so often accompanies the administration of chlorpromazine is related to an increase in appetite and dietary intake, an enhancement of anabolic processes, or a reduction in catabolic factors which may be associated with strong and persistent emotional states.

In summary, chlorpromazine and related phenothiazines not only affect the central nervous system but also possess a wide range of physiologic activities throughout the body. These cannot as yet be correlated with the clinical effects of these drugs.

METHOD OF ADMINISTRATION

When the control of an acute, intense reaction is urgently required, the intramuscular route of administration may be utilized. On the first day of treatment 100 mg chlorpromazine is given in four divided doses. This amount can be increased by 100 mg daily until the desired clinical effect is obtained. Rarely will the maximal dosage by this method exceed 500 mg daily. The patient may then be placed on oral medication, in doses twice the intramuscular dose to allow for absorption differences. The maintenance dose is then secured by gradually decreasing the amount given until a level which permits sustained control of the emotional state with a minimum of undesirable side effects is achieved. The maintenance dosage of chlorpromazine usually falls between 200 and 600 mg per day. In rare instances, where the intramuscular route is insufficient to obtain immediate control, intravenous doses of a related phenothiazine derivative such as promazine may be utilized. The starting dose of intravenous promazine is usually 50 mg, and a total of 300 mg may be given within the first 10 minutes.

Under less urgent conditions, chlorpromazine may usually be started in oral dosage of 100 to 200 mg per day. This amount is increased by 100 or 200 mg daily until the desired effect is achieved. Rarely will the maximum level by this method exceed 600 mg daily, and the usual maintenance dosage is about 300 mg per day in four divided doses. When chlorpromazine is terminated, the dose is usually reduced gradually, at a rate of 100 to 200 mg daily. The drug may be stopped abruptly, but only if necessary, as in the case of agranulocytosis or jaundice.

For long-term administration, Spansule forms of chlorpromazine and related derivatives are available, reducing the number of individual doses required each day. In a hospital setting, the liquid form of medication is preferable, to avoid hoarding and to ensure that the patient consumes the medication.

The duration of treatment with chlorpromazine varies markedly, depending upon the nature of the condition and the goals of therapy. An acute reaction may require only 14 to 21 days of chlorpromazine therapy. On the other hand, if intensive psychotherapy is to be carried out, several months of drug treatment may be necessary. Chlorpromazine may also be used for months and even years when supportive management of a chronic psychopathologic condition is required.

Sleep Treatment

In the management of severely agitated, excited, manic, or schizophrenic patients who fail to respond satisfactorily to the routine administration of chlorpromazine or electroconvulsive therapy, the ability of chlorpromazine to potentiate the activity of barbiturates may be successfully employed in the maintenance of sleep therapy. This is a specialized form of treatment in which a patient is kept in an almost continual state of sleep for approximately 15 to 20 days. During this time his pathologic emotions may subside, and his personality may become reintegrated. He is awakened for short intervals, two or three times each day, so that the total hours of sleep approximate 20 out of every 24. When awake, he receives nourishment and medication. Careful observations of his cardiovascular status, including determinations of the pulse, blood pressure, and respiration, are carried out. Regular temperature readings are done to avert the development of undue infectious processes. Renal and intestinal function must be preserved. Constant vigilance against oversedation must be maintained. It is customary to depend upon a long-acting barbiturate, such as barbital, to maintain the state of unconsciousness, although amobarbital may also be added if additional sedation for a short phase of the treatment is indicated. Certain clinicians advise the use of a mixture of various barbiturates, but the superiority of this method has not been established. In a 24-hour period, the patient will ordinarily receive about 1.2 Gm barbiturates, combined with 200 to 400 mg chlorpromazine, in two or three divided doses, orally or intramuscularly. In carrying out this procedure, it is important not to reverse the roles of chlorpromazine and the barbiturates, since the former is incapable of inducing the somnolent state by itself. Because of its potentiating effects, it allows the utilization of lower amounts of barbiturates than would be otherwise required.

SIDE EFFECTS AND COMPLICATIONS

Drowsiness, lethargy, weakness, and motor retardation are frequent concomitants of phenothiazine treatment. These are usually most marked during the first few days of treatment, and they often disappear if the dosage is sufficiently lowered. Hypochondriac and hysterical patients may readily utilize these changes, incorporating them into their psychopathologic structures.

Parkinsonlike side effects, characterized by rigidity of muscle tone affecting facial expression, stature, and gait, shuffling walk, tremors and loss of fine movements of fingers and hands, blurring of vision, and complaints of difficulty in speech, may often be seen in patients receiving high doses of these drugs. These changes also appear to be related to the amount of the drug being used and will usually decrease with lowered dosage. However, it is important to note that the incidence of severe motor involvement is much greater in patients whose conditions are characterized by the presence of dissociative mechanisms, as in catatonic states and hysterical reactions, and among those patients with organic cerebral changes, as in arteriosclerosis. If the dosage of the drug cannot be lowered without endangering the control of the psychopathologic state, anti-Parkinson drugs, such as trihexyphenidyl hydrochloride or benztropine methanesulfonate, may be employed to counteract the neuromuscular changes.

The two most dangerous complications resulting from the use of chlorpromazine are agranulocytosis, which is rare but can be rapidly fatal, and hepatic damage. No patient should receive chlorpromazine unless physical examination and laboratory investigation reveal intact hepatic function. During the course of treatment, temperature should be taken regularly. Any unexplained fever should be considered as early evidence of agranulocytosis or liver damage until laboratory investigation clarifies the situation. The drug should be terminated at once if any undue complication appears, since these reactions are *unrelated to dosage* and can occur as readily with 100 mg as with 1,000 mg. Drug-induced jaundice is usually reversible and, in most instances, disappears after termination of chlorpromazine.

Allergic phenomena, such as exfoliative dermatitis, are occasionally seen. These often clear quickly when the treatment is stopped. It is frequently possible to reinstitute the same drug within several weeks after such an episode without producing a recurrence of allergic symptoms.

The hypotensive action induced by chlorpromazine indicates the need for caution when using this drug in patients with extensive cardiovascular disease.

In patients suffering with epilepsy or extensive brain damage convulsions may be precipitated by the administration of phenothiazine derivatives. This does not preclude their use in this group of patients, however, when the emotional state indicates such a course of treatment. Anticonvulsant drugs, such as phenobarbital or diphenylhydantoin sodium, should be administered simultaneously to these patients. Moreover, chlorpromazine should be terminated as early as possible once the goals of treatment have been achieved.

The combined use of chlorpromazine and electroconvulsive treatments at first promised to reduce the number of shock treatments required to alleviate certain psychopathologic states. It is now considered desirable to allow a minimum period of 72 hours to elapse between the termination of drug treatment and the institution of ECT in order to reduce the risk of cardiovascular complications. Moreover, when shock treatments are given within 1 week after the end of chlorpromazine treatment, post-ECT confusion and memory loss occasionally seem to be more severe.

There is no conclusive evidence that addiction to any of the phenothiazine derivatives can occur as a result of prolonged administration. Experience suggests, however, that habituation may develop, as with barbiturates, presenting an equally complex management problem.

CLINICAL EFFECTIVENESS OF TREATMENT

In order to utilize chlorpromazine and similar drugs efficiently, it is necessary to understand the diagnostic and psychopathologic conditions in which the drugs are likely to produce a satisfactory response, and to be able to differentiate these settings from those in which the response to the drugs is likely to be limited or poor.

Diagnostic Considerations

General diagnostic considerations will be of some value in prognosticating the desirability of chlorpromazine treatment. Good clinical effects may be expected in patients diagnosed as having paranoid reactions, manic or catatonic excitements, and paranoid schizophrenic reactions. Patients diagnosed as having depressive mood disorders, psychoneurotic reactions, or simple, undifferentiated types of schizophrenic states may react satisfactorily to the drug to a more limited degree. Toxic confusional and delirious conditions often respond well to chlorpromazine; it is a useful adjunct, for example, in the management of acute alcoholic intoxication and delirium tremens. Patients diagnosed as having catatonic stuporous reactions or hebephrenic reactions will usually fail to show any substantial degree of improvement on chlorpromazine.

It is important to realize that within any diagnostic group considerable variations in response can be observed. Paradoxical reactions in which a manic excitement will actually be intensified during the administration of chlorpromazine are occasionally seen. Some patients diagnosed as hebephrenic reactions will receive substantial benefit from a course of chlorpromazine therapy. The authors' own experience confirms that repeatedly reported in the literature. For example, moderate or marked improvement may occur in about 85 per cent of paranoid reactions, 80 per cent of manic excitements, 70 per cent of paranoid schizophrenic reactions, and 65 per cent of catatonic excitements. It is essential to possess indicators which will facilitate identification of those patients falling within these diagnostic groups who will respond adequately to chlorpromazine from the 15 to 35 per cent of patients in these groups who will fail to be substantially influenced by a course of treatment.

The authors have noted, for example, that about 40 per cent of patients with depressive mood disorders show substantial clinical improvement on chlorpromazine, although the drug clearly does not affect the central depressive mood. It is important that the nature of such an influence be understood and that this minority be separated from the 60 per cent of patients with depressive mood disorders who would not improve significantly on chlorpromazine.

Emotional and Psychopathologic Considerations

In addition to the diagnostic considerations, the influence of chlorpromazine can be analyzed in terms of emotions and psychopathologic features that occur individually and in combination. Knowledge of the effects of chlorpromazine and related phenothiazines on such features will permit more precise utilization of these drugs. Chlorpromazine appears to be most effective in reducing strong emotions of fear, hostility, and sexual unrest. It often alleviates psychopathologic symptoms, such as paranoid features, delusions, hallucinations, insomnia, variations in motor activity, and eating difficulties resulting from these emotions. The drug does not usually relieve anxiety, specific manifestations of anxiety, apathy, depression, and depersonalization, and it may occasionally intensify these symptoms.

FEAR

The striking ability of chlorpromazine to alleviate intense fear, such as seen in panic reactions, is illustrated in the following case.

Case 1. In the setting of family conflict, a 42-year-old single woman became increasingly threatened by the emergence of previously unconscious sexual strivings. Her concentration was markedly impaired. It was difficult for her to continue her secretarial work. She became depressed, with strong feelings of inadequacy and hopelessness about the future. She felt that her co-workers were watching her continuously and disapproved of her. These changes became more intense over a 1-month period. Forty-eight hours before her hospitalization she became acutely withdrawn, markedly fearful, and suspicious. Auditory and visual hallucinations were present. Hostile, condemning voices abused her, and she visualized frightening sexual scenes. She was placed on barbiturate sedation for 6 days, combined with prolonged relaxing baths, without any substantial influence on her condition. Chlorpromazine treatment was instituted and rapidly increased to a level of 400 mg daily intramuscularly. On the fourth day of chlorpromazine treatment fear subsided remarkably, with complete disappearance of hallucinations and paranoid delusions. At the end of 1 week of treatment, her psychopathologic symptoms had improved markedly. Residual feelings of anxiety and guilt were still apparent. It was then possible to pursue an active investigation of the dynamic factors which had precipitated the panic reaction. The drug was continued for 17 days at a maintenance level of 400 mg daily. Her improvement continued following termination of treatment, and it was possible for her to be discharged shortly thereafter.

The fear which this patient experienced appeared to be a fundamental feature of her condition. This strong emotion led to the development of delusions and hallucinations which subsided when the fear was relieved by the administration of chlorpromazine. In other patients, such as those whose contact with reality is markedly defective, chlorpromazine may reduce strong emotions, but delusions and hallucinations may persist.

HOSTILITY

Chlorpromazine is often successful in reducing strong hostile emotions which are directly experienced and manifested. However, the drug does not seem to influence hostile emotions which are repressed, secondary to anxiety, or expressed in a symptomatic fashion, as through hypochondriac ruminations or psychopathic behavior. The following patient illustrates a case in which hostility was a central emotional feature and chlorpromazine markedly alleviated the clinical condition.

Case 2. A 38-year-old businessman, engaged in a vicious competitive struggle within his corporation, developed a 1-week episode of severe tension, suspiciousness, and profound rage. Paranoid ideas of reference were prominent: "Why did you hide the newspapers that have those terrible stories about me in them?" During the first week of hospitalization, barbiturates were used in an attempt to control his condition, but without success. Chlorpromazine was then given intramuscularly and rapidly increased to 500 mg daily. On the fourth day of treatment, his rage was markedly reduced. Shortly thereafter his entire clinical picture was cleared. The drug was terminated after 2 weeks, and the improvement persisted, allowing him to be discharged from the hospital shortly thereafter.

In this patient the intense pathologic hostility preceded and contributed to the formation of paranoid concepts. Accordingly, when chlorpromazine therapy led to a reduction in his rage, the paranoid ideas of reference also subsided.

The next patient illustrates a case in which chlorpromazine also reduced strong hostility, thereby producing a significant but somewhat more limited clinical improvement.

Case 3. A 56-year-old married woman reacted to separation from her husband and children with a "feeling of emptiness" and "no desire to ever get well." Depression of mood was prominent, with marked insomnia and anorexia, a 20-lb weight loss, anxiety, and restlessness. She reluctantly accepted hospitalization. Shortly thereafter her depression increased. When psychotherapeutic efforts began, she became angry and resentful, denying the need for treatment and refusing to offer essential information. She entered an aversion reaction and refused to speak or cooperate with the daily routine. She would neither eat nor drink. Chlorpromazine was begun in daily oral doses of 400 mg and continued for 3 months. Within 10 days after the initiation of treatment, hostility diminished markedly. She ate well and cooperated with environmental and psychotherapeutic efforts. In spite of these extensive changes, however, apathy and depression of mood persisted.

In this patient, chlorpromazine reduced pathologic hostility which had led to an aversion reaction. The patient's suffering was alleviated and she was able to participate in the total treatment program. Her depression of mood, however, was not significantly influenced. It was necessary to administer a series of electroconvulsive treatments several months later in order to produce a more complete clinical improvement.

This patient illustrates the fallacy of thinking of "hypermotility" as a primary indication for the administration of chlorpromazine. Although many patients with extreme fear or rage may be overactive, it is equally possible for them to be retarded and withdrawn.

As already described, chlorpromazine is effective in reducing hostile emotions only when these emotions are overt. If hostility is unconscious and its presence must be inferred from the nature of the presenting symptoms, the drug is not likely to influence the psychopathologic condition. The next patient clearly illustrates this point.

Case 4. A 24-year-old single woman, diagnosed as a psychoneurotic anxiety state, developed over a 1-month period marked anxiety with phobic preoccupations in a setting of conflict with her mother. She was afraid of going insane, hurting herself, screaming, or becoming physically ill. Following her hospitalization, her hidden resentment was expressed through uncooperative behavior. She was late for activities. She would not dress in accordance with routine expectations. She smoked in prohibited areas. When directly questioned about her emotions, she profoundly denied any hostility and did not display any direct manifestations of anger or resentment. Chlorpromazine was instituted in an attempt to control her behavior. For 2 weeks 500 mg of the drug was given daily by mouth. On this regimen her uncooperative behavior was actually intensified. Anxiety increased, and strong feelings of depersonalization appeared. Lethargy and fatigue were prominent. After termination of the drug, she returned to her initial state. Psychotherapy was continued without somatic intervention for 6 months, resulting in a gradual emergence of hostile feelings and the eventual resolution of her phobic anxieties.

The failure of this patient to improve on chlorpromazine illustrates the inability of the drug to alleviate repressed hostility or manifest anxiety. These observations may partly explain why chlorpromazine is more useful in the treatment of schizophrenic and affective disorders than psychoneurotic reactions. In the latter, repression of hostile emotions is often extensive, and anxiety is usually the leading manifestation of the disorder.

SEXUAL UNREST

One of the most important properties of chlorpromazine is its ability to reduce sexual unrest. The next patient illustrates this effect.

Case 5. A 25-year-old housewife, diagnosed as a psychoneurotic reaction, presented a 2-year history of anxiety occurring in the setting of her husband's infidelity. She was often preoccupied with sexual fantasies and masturbated frequently. During psychotherapeutic investigations, her sexual unrest increased. She became openly flirtatious with her male therapist, insisting that he could not help her unless he attempted to satisfy her sexual demands. Her concentration was markedly impaired. A severe sleep disturbance developed. Chlorpromazine was instituted in daily oral doses of 200 mg. Sexual stirrings rapidly subsided. Concentration improved, and a normal sleep pattern was established. The drug was continued for 8 weeks; following its termination, her psychopathologic state did not recur. Anxiety was essentially unaffected throughout.

In this patient, chlorpromazine promptly reduced intense sexual unrest and probably prevented the development of a severe panic or excitement. In spite of the beneficial effects of drug therapy, her anxiety persisted, subsiding only after many more months of psychotherapy.

The following case illustrates this effect of chlorpromazine on sexual unrest in a different dynamic and diagnostic setting.

Case 6. A 51-year-old electrician was hospitalized for a depressive reaction of 1 year's duration, which began shortly after his son's marriage. His condition was characterized by extreme agitation and anxiety, with strong feelings of hopelessness. He described pleasurable erotic sensations around his pelvic area. He repeatedly pressed his thighs together in a masturbatory manner. Three months prior to hospitalization he had received seven electroconvulsive treatments (ECTs). These had produced a temporary alleviation in his condition. Within 1 month, this improvement had disappeared. Insomnia was marked and he required heavy sedation. At the time of his admission, barbiturates were instituted, but these were ineffective in controlling his agitation. He was therefore begun on chlorpromazine, which was raised to a level of 800 mg daily by mouth. Within 2 weeks his agitation disappeared. The sexual sensations in the pelvic area and the masturbatory activity ceased. Feelings of hopelessness and depression remained. The drug was continued for 6 weeks. Following its termination, anxious agitation again became marked but without sexual features. Chlorpromazine was reinstituted at a level of 800 mg daily. This time the drug completely failed to influence his clinical state. It was necessary to terminate chlorpromazine and administer a series of 10 ECTs, in the course of which his depression and agitation cleared.

This patient offered an unusual experimental situation. He served as his own control for the evaluation of chlorpromazine given in two different dynamic settings. At no time did the drug influence the depression of mood itself. Chlorpromazine markedly reduced his agitation when sexual unrest was prominent. Reinstitution of chlorpromazine failed to influence his agitation when sexual unrest was no longer a factor and his overactivity was primarily the result of intense anxiety.

Table 1   Therapeutic Effectiveness of Chlorpromazine: Emotional and Psychopathologic Considerations

Psychopathologic feature	Expected response	Enhanced combined with	Reduced combined with
Hostility	Good	Fear Sexual unrest Paranoid	Anxiety Depression
Sexual unrest	Good	Fear Paranoid Hostility	Depression
Anxiety	Poor	Fear Sexual unrest Hostility	Paranoid Depression
Depression	Poor	Paranoid Hostility Sexual unrest Fear	Anxiety
Paranoid	Good	Fear Sexual unrest Hostility	Anxiety

It is evident from the foregoing examples that chlorpromazine may often produce marked clinical improvement in certain patients. In others, the drug may alter the emotional state significantly without affecting the basic psychopathologic condition. For example, in the first case, an acute paranoid panic state subsided rapidly under the influence of chlorpromazine. In those patients presented with diagnoses of depressive mood disorders, chlorpromazine did not affect the basic mood alteration, but it did significantly reduce rage leading to aversion reactions, fear associated with paranoid delusions, and sexual unrest associated with

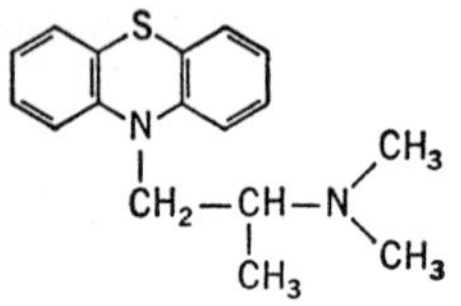

Promethazine

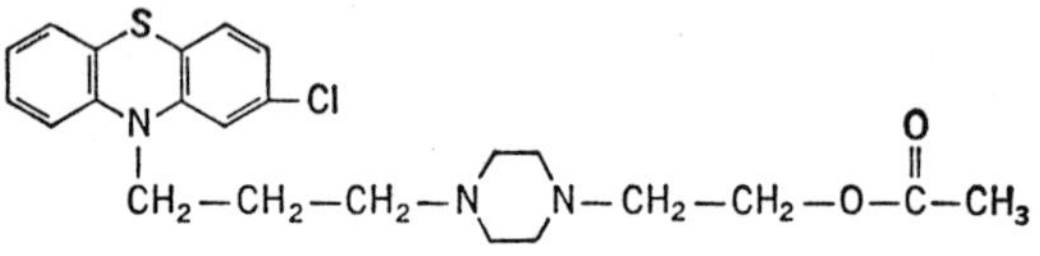

Thiopropazate

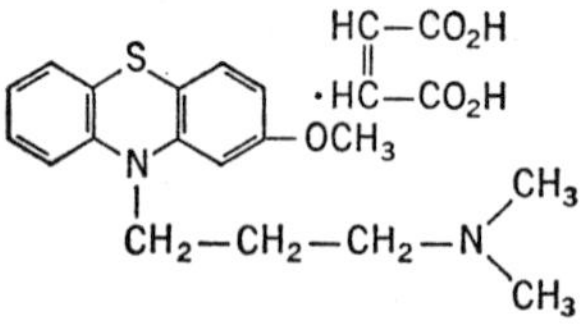

Methoxypromazine

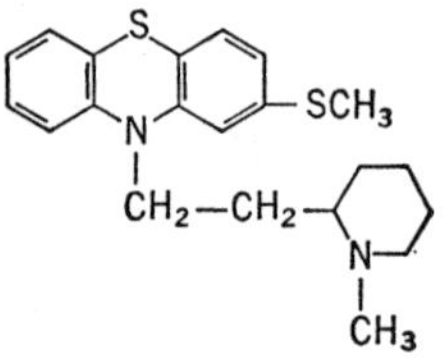

Thioridazine

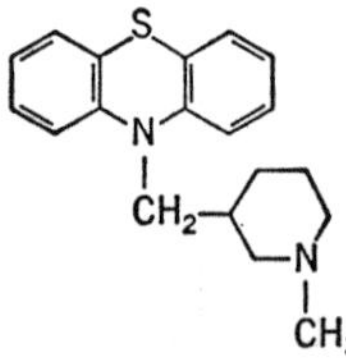

Mepazine

marked agitation. In these ways the drug relieved the patients' suffering and allowed them to participate in psychotherapy.

In order to use chlorpromazine effectively, it is therefore essential to know not only the diagnosis of the patient, but also the dynamic psychopathologic structure of his condition at the moment of deciding upon the course of treatment. As summarized in Table 1, chlorpromazine is most effective in those conditions in which strong emotions of fear and hostility are overtly manifested. It has a unique effect in reducing sexual unrest. Paranoid delusions and hallucinations, when they are associated with strong emotions, are strikingly reduced. In patients in whom hostility or sexual unrest has been repressed, with the consequent development of pathologic anxiety, the drug is relatively ineffective. In fact, in such cases, chlorpromazine may actually intensify distressing symptoms.

RELATED PHENOTHIAZINE COMPOUNDS

There are 10 phenothiazine derivatives besides chlorpromazine which have received wide attention as psychopharmacologic agents. These are perphenazine, thiopropazate, promazine, promethazine, prochlorperazine, mepazine, thioridazine, triflupromazine, trifluoperazine, and methoxypromazine. The chemical structure of each of these drugs is presented for comparison with chlorpromazine.

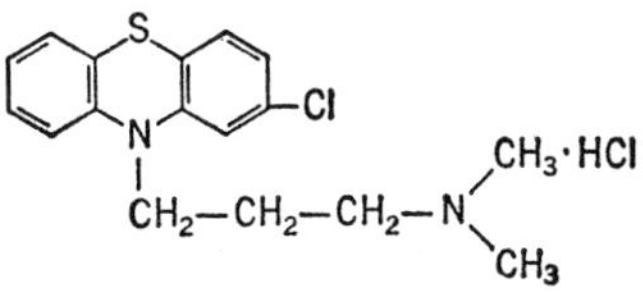

Chlorpromazine

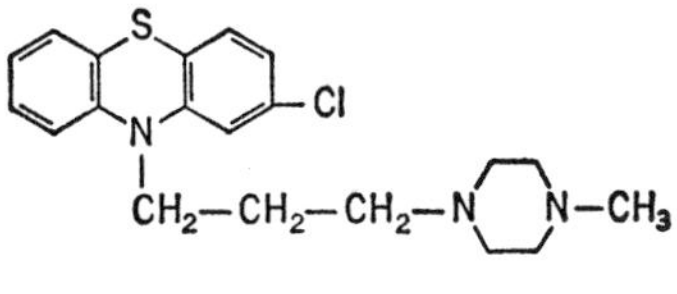

Prochlorperazine

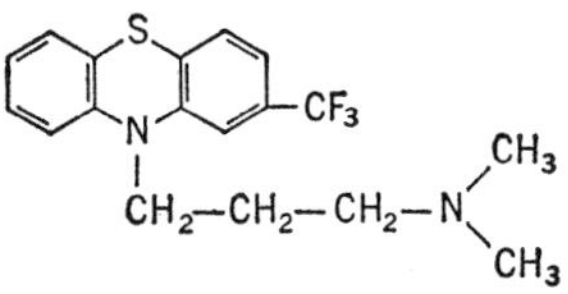

Triflupromazine

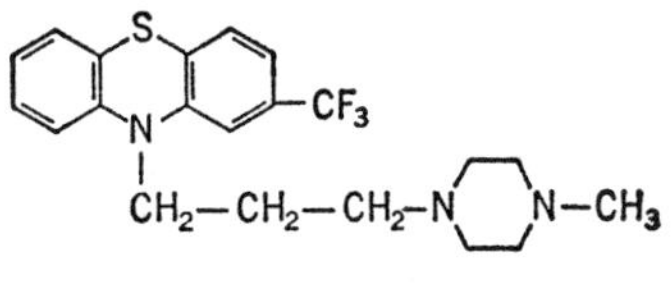

Trifluoperazine

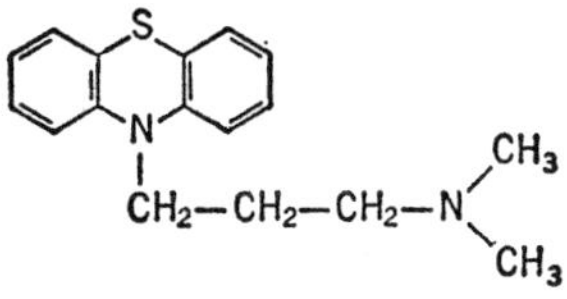

Promazine

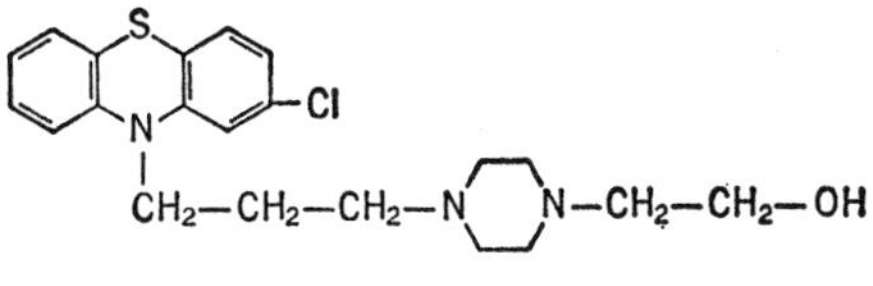

Perphenazine

It is apparent that there are two significant modifications of the original phenothiazine structure differentiating these derivatives from chlorpromazine. The first affects the central nucleus. Chlorpromazine, prochlorperazine, perphenazine, and thiopropazate are all chlorinated compounds. Chlorine has been removed from promazine, promethazine, and mepazine. Fluorine replaces chlorine in triflupromazine and trifluoperazine. In thioridazine, the chlorine has been replaced by a thiomethyl radical, in methoxypromazine by a methoxyl group.

The second important modification affects the side chains. These segments are quite similar in chlorpromazine, promazine, triflupromazine, methoxypromazine, and promethazine. However, a piperazine ring has been introduced into the side chains of prochlorperazine, perphenazine, thiopropazate, and trifluoperazine, and a piperidyl ring in thioridazine and mepazine.

It has been reported that the phenothiazine compounds in which fluorine has replaced chlorine or which possess a piperazine or piperidyl side chain are less inhibitory to the central nervous system than chlorpromazine and those phenothiazines without fluorine or with a simple side chain. If this observation is correct, then the former group of phenothiazines would seem more desirable for patients undergoing intensive psychotherapy and less so for severely disturbed patients in whom a swift and reliable agent is required. However, a drug such as trifluoperazine, which combines a fluorine group with a piperazine side chain, has been successfully used in large doses to reduce pathologic fear and hostility and associated paranoid delusions in acute schizophrenic reactions, although it is more commonly reserved for the treatment of milder psychopathologic states.

The complications produced during the administration of these phenothiazine drugs resemble those associated with chlorpromazine therapy. These include cardiovascular changes, in particular hypotension, tachycardia, and palpitations; gastrointestinal distress, such as nausea, vomiting, or constipation; dry mouth and nasal congestion; endocrinologic changes, such as the initiation of lactation or cessation of menstruation; liver damage; blood dyscrasias, such as agranulocytosis; allergic reactions, in particular dermatitis; photosensitivity; increased appetite and weight; and central nervous system effects, characterized by weakness, drowsiness, motor and coordination impairment, agitation, dizziness, slurred speech and blurred vision, the precipitation of convulsions, and the potentiation of depressants such as barbiturates or morphine. The introduction of a piperazine or piperidyl ring into the side chains of phenothiazines often seems to reduce the frequency of jaundice and blood dyscrasias, but it often increases the tendency to develop parkinsonlike motor and coordination dysfunction. Liver damage and blood dyscrasias have not, thus far, been reported in association with the use of thiopropazate, trifluoperazine, and thioridazine and seem to occur rarely with perphenazine or prochlorperazine. Inasmuch as serious side effects appear to be less frequent in this group, these agents may be preferable for nonhospitalized patients.

In Table 2, the approximate dosage ranges for these phenothiazines are outlined. It is apparent that a marked difference in the dosage required to produce clinical effects exists between those phenothiazines which have simple side chains and those with piperazine rings. Chlorpromazine and promazine, for instance, must be used in daily oral dosage ranging from several hundred to a thousand milligrams or more in order to alleviate pathologic emotions. Other compounds, such as prochlorperazine, perphenazine, and thiopropazate, are given in daily oral dosage in the neighborhood of 30 mg.

Table 2 *Approximate Dosage Ranges for Various Phenothiazines: Dosage per 24 Hours (Oral, in Milligrams)*

Compound	Low	Moderate	High
Chlorpromazine	100–200	200–600	600–1,000
Promazine	100–200	200–600	600–1,000
Triflupromazine	50–100	100–200	200–300
Promethazine	100–200	200–600	600–1,000
Thioridazine	100–200	200–400	400–800
Mepazine	50–100	100–300	300–600
Methoxypromazine	50–200	200–600	600–1,200
Prochlorperazine	10–30	30–60	60–200
Thiopropazate	5–10	10–20	20–40
Trifluoperazine	2–4	4–10	10–30
Perphenazine	8–16	16–24	24–64

These dosage schedules must remain approximate. The actual amount of medication used in a particular patient will depend to a great extent on the intensity of his psychopathologic condition and the urgency of obtaining control over his disturbance. When immediate alleviation of the patient's state is indicated, the parenteral route of administration is usually preferred. The parenteral dosage range is occasionally lower than the oral. For example, in the case of chlorpromazine, one-half the oral dosage is used when the drug is given intramuscularly. It is usually desirable to change to the oral route of administration as soon as the clinical state has been adequately controlled, but this modification should not be introduced prematurely in the treatment of severe disturbances.

Although certain investigators feel that a qualitative difference can be discerned between one phenothiazine and another with regard to their influence on psychopathologic symptoms, the evidence for this is, as yet, unconvincing. Indeed, there are certain patients who demonstrate improvement when one phenothiazine has been terminated and another instituted. In these reports, however, such basic considerations as comparative dosage levels or the degree of absorption following ingestion do not seem to have been thoroughly explored. Moreover, the exact nature of the observable improvement, in terms of pathologic emotions and associated symptoms, has rarely been described sufficiently. Until further studies have been completed, it is prudent to assume that the actual influence of these phenothiazines on emotions and psychopathologic features resembles that of chlorpromazine, namely, that they are more effective in the presence of overt fear, hostility, and sexual unrest and of limited usefulness in states of pathologic anxiety or depression.

SUMMARY

In addition to chlorpromazine, there are a number of phenothiazine compounds which have been established as useful psychopharmacologic agents. Some of these seem to have a lower incidence of serious side effects, in particular hepatic damage and agranulocytosis, than chlorpromazine.

For the management of intensely disturbed patients within a hospital setting, chlorpromazine remains the most reliable and effective agent in this group. Other phenothiazines which have less inhibitory effect on alertness and energy may be preferred for the treatment of patients who are involved in intensive psychotherapy.

Although there are reports of certain patients responding more adequately to one phenothiazine than to another, there is no convincing evidence that a qualitative difference exists among these compounds with regard to their influence on pathologic emotions and associated psychopathologic features. In sufficient dosage each seems capable of reducing pathologic hostility and fear, sexual unrest, elation, and associated delusions, hallucinations, and paranoid features. None are clearly effective in combating pathologic anxiety or depression of mood.

For the physician, confronted with the need to choose from so many phenothiazine derivatives, the soundest course of action is to familiarize himself well with the application of several of these drugs rather than to attempt to master the entire field, at least until the superiority of one or more of these compounds becomes indisputably established.

7

RESERPINE

Derivatives of the powdered root of *Rauwolfia serpentina* (Benth), such as reserpine, were initially introduced as effective agents in the management of hypertension. These compounds had been used for many years in the treatment of a number of clinical conditions in India. The calming effect which they seemed to produce in certain patients encouraged more extensive investigations of their psychopharmacologic potentials. Great excitement accompanied the early reports of their clinical effectiveness. The most dramatic results were obtained when the rauwolfia compounds were used in patients presenting severe management problems because of overactivity and assaultiveness. Some patients with long-standing anxiety and tension symptoms appeared to benefit substantially during the administration of the drugs. At first, there did not seem to be any qualitative difference between the action of rauwolfia derivatives and the phenothiazines, but as clinical experience grew, it became apparent that the latter group of drugs was much more dependable and possessed a much wider range of effectiveness. Moreover, with the introduction of meprobamate, which is useful in controlling anxiety and tension in many nonhospitalized patients, and with restored confidence in the barbiturates and insulin therapy, the need for a drug with the actions of the rauwolfia group markedly decreased. Gradually its use was restricted to the treatment of agitated patients in whom chlorpromazine was contraindicated because of the presence of liver damage or severe allergic reactions. With the subsequent development of phenothiazines less likely than chlorpromazine to induce hepatic dysfunction, the indications for resperine and related compounds in the treatment of psychiatric patients disappeared almost entirely.

Inasmuch as these drugs are still being used in the treatment of patients with hypertension and since they are still employed to alleviate tension and anxiety in many settings, even though better agents are available, it is desirable to review the pharmacologic and clinical aspects of these drugs. The beneficial and undesirable psychologic changes which they seem to induce will be illustrated.

The four rauwolfia derivatives which have received most extensive attention are reserpine, alseroxylon, rescinnamine, and deserpidine. Of these, reserpine has been most widely studied. Differences may exist between the pharmacologic and psychologic effects of these compounds, but none have been established which are of any practical significance. Therefore, the discussion will be centered largely around the use of reserpine, but it will be representative of this entire group of rauwolfia alkaloids.

Mechanism of Action

The formula for reserpine is illustrated, along with those of serotonin and the antagonists of serotonin, lysergic acid diethylamide and yohimbine, to demonstrate differences and similarities among these compounds. It has been postulated that the physiologic and emotional changes noted during the administration of reserpine may be related to the effects of this drug on serotonin metabolism in the central nervous system.

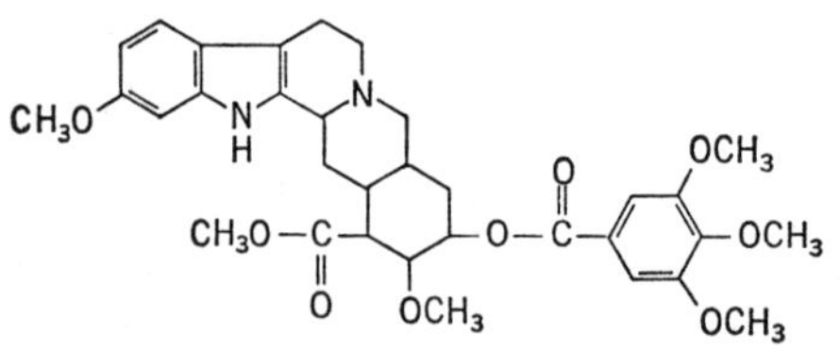

Reserpine

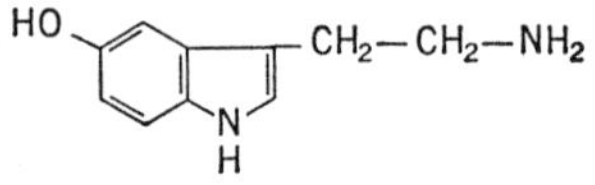

Serotonin

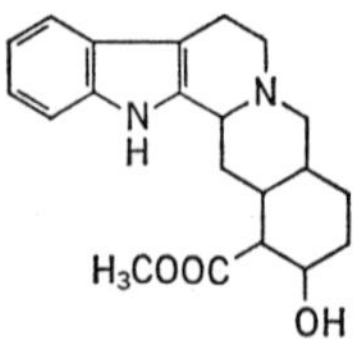

Yohimbine

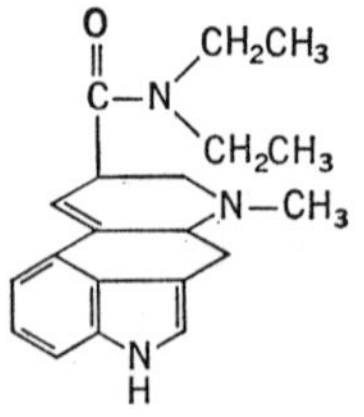

Lysergic acid diethylamide

Serotonin may or may not be significantly involved in the regulation of normal mental processes. The administration of lysergic acid diethylamide, which is a potent antagonist of serotonin, usually leads to the development of psychopathologic reactions in otherwise healthy human subjects. These states are characterized by the formation of hallucinations and depersonalization experiences and resemble certain schizo-phrenic conditions. Lysergic acid diethylamide may induce such changes by competing with serotonin for serotonin receptors or by blocking nerve transmission in the central parasympathetic system, antagonizing ser-otonin at crucial synaptic junctions. On the other hand, the intracerebral administration of serotonin itself in animals produces a lethargic, drowsy, motionless state. Reserpine may act by releasing 5-hydroxytryptamine, thereby producing an excess of this compound. Reserpine also seems to possess parasympathomimetic activity, as it allows a constant flow of free serotonin to stimulate appropriate centers.

By contrast, monoamine oxidase inhibitors, which will be discussed in Chap. 11, seem to produce central nervous system stimulation, possibly by inhibiting the enzyme which destroys serotonin, thereby allowing an accumulation of this compound. Many antagonists of serotonin, however, possess no ability to produce any kind of mental changes whatsoever.

The biological roles of serotonin and drugs affecting the metabolism of serotonin, therefore, remain unclear. Many studies are filled with con-tradictory observations. It may well be that the clinical changes induced are not related to changes in serotonin at all or that there are still many unknown factors which determine whether a shift in the amount of free serotonin will lead to sedation or excitability. Clinical experience, in which some patients are agitated, others calm, and still others alternately disturbed and at ease during the administration of reserpine, tends to confirm this impression.

The resemblance between yohimbine, an antagonist of serotonin, and reserpine is interesting. The former compound was used in primitive societies as an aphrodisiac, and certain patients receiving reserpine ap-pear to develop sexual unrest.

Method of Administration

One of the major problems complicating the use of reserpine is the difficulty in establishing an adequate dosage level for an individual patient. For some, 0.5 to 1.0 mg daily, given orally, is sufficient to produce emotional changes. Others may require as much as 15 to 30 mg daily, given orally or intramuscularly, and even then only slight alteration in the psychopathologic condition is common. Moreover, in addition to determining the initial effective dose, there is considerable difficulty in obtaining a maintenance dose which will continue the beneficial effects with a minimum of side effects. Frequently, it is necessary to administer large amounts of reserpine, thereby producing marked motor retardation, in order to control disturbed behavior. When the dosage is lowered in order to alleviate these distressing complications, control over the clinical state is often lost. Once having established an average maintenance dose of about 6 mg daily, it may be necessary to vary the amount of the drug used, increasing and decreasing it every few days, in order to keep pace with the emotional aberrations which the patient demonstrates.

In contrast to the phenothiazines, which are excreted from the body in about 72 hours, reserpine requires between 1 and 2 weeks and perhaps longer to be completely metabolized and eliminated. This clearly limits the control which the physician has over the treatment. It also leads to complications in the management of patients who are being shifted from drug therapy to electroconvulsive therapy. It is now generally held that ECT should not ordinarily be given to patients while they are receiving either phenothiazines or rauwolfia derivatives, because of the risk to cardiac function. When ECT is contemplated, these drugs should be terminated. It is possible to initiate ECT within 48 to 72 hours after the last dose of chlorpromazine, but it may be hazardous to begin shock treatment in less than 1 week and even 2 weeks after the end of a course of reserpine. In the latter instance, therefore, it may be necessary to delay adequate treatment for an undesirably long period of time.

Side Effects and Complications

The complications and side effects of reserpine therapy have been well documented. Reserpine slows the pulse and lowers the blood pressure; although this may be a medically desirable effect in hypertensive patients, it may be dangerous in others, for example, in the victim of a recent myocardial infarction. Motor restlessness, retardation, and extrapyramidal tract symptoms, such as tremor and impaired coordination, may occur, resembling side effects of phenothiazine administration. These may often be eliminated by reducing the dosage level, but all too often control of the patient's disturbance is lost at the same time. Anti-Parkinson drugs, such as benztropine methanesulfonate and trihexyphenidyl, have been successfully employed to counteract these complications. In small doses, such as 0.5 to 2.0 mg daily, reserpine may induce a subtle restlessness which so resembles the effects of anxiety that it escapes attention as a drug-induced phenomenon. However, this is often so uncomfortable that it nullifies any calming influence which the medication might have.

Other side effects include increased appetite and weight gain; excessive salivation and drooling; rarely, severe allergic dermatitis or peripheral edema; and increased gastric secretion, endangering the health of any patient with a history of peptic ulcer.

One of the most serious complications of the use of reserpine is the appearance of moderate or severe depression of mood. Many investigators feel that this pathologic mood results directly from the action of the drug on the central nervous system. It is equally possible, however, that many patients who have become depressed during reserpine therapy have reacted to the removal of one psychopathologic symptom with the formation of another. For example, it is not uncommon to see a 50-year-old man, complaining of multiple phobias, such as fears of heights, crowded places, and vehicles, experience marked anxiety in the presence of these objects and deny any depression of mood. The administration of reserpine may substantially reduce his anxiety, and he may be able to expand his range of activities. Within several weeks, however, he may begin to notice fatigue, a lowering of spirits, periods of tearfulness, and the onset of severe inexplicable hopelessness. While it is possible that his mood disorder is intimately associated with physiologic changes induced by reserpine, it is just as likely that his original anxiety symptoms served to protect him against becoming aware of his underlying depressive illness and the contributing conflicts within his personality. When this armor was prematurely removed by the use of reserpine, the depressive illness then manifested itself in full force. Depressive reactions associated with the administration of reserpine are sometimes quite intense and prolonged, necessitating the use of electroconvulsive therapy to alleviate the pathologic mood.

Clinical Effectiveness of Treatment

Careful analysis of the specific emotional and psychopathologic changes occurring in patients during the administration of reserpine strongly suggests that the degree to which this drug is effective in producing improvement in psychiatric patients depends largely upon the importance which anxiety and tension play in the development of the condition, regardless of the diagnostic setting. In certain patients anxiety constitutes a central pathologic factor; in others it is only incidental. The effects of reserpine appear to be fundamentally different from those of the phenothiazines, which are of limited usefulness in many situations where anxiety is a prominent consideration.

The following cases illustrate the manner in which reserpine, by means of its ameliorating effect on anxiety, may substantially alleviate the psychopathologic state of patients in various diagnostic settings.

ANXIETY IN MANIC REACTIONS

The first case is of a manic excitement, complicated by pathologic anxiety.

Case 1. A 42-year-old married woman with a diagnosis of manic excitement was admitted to the hospital with a 2-week history of marked tension, anxiety, and restlessness, developing in the setting of conflict with her adolescent daughter. Her mood fluctuated between mild elation and depression. Tearfulness and angry outbursts occurred from time to time. She had some difficulty falling asleep and awoke frequently during the night. She was slightly flirtatious and would expose herself in subtle ways. Her pulse ranged from 80 to 100 beats per minute. Concentration was seriously impaired. Overtalkativeness and pressure of speech were prominent. Her history revealed two previous episodes of elation during the preceding four years; the first had been terminated successfully with six ECTs; the second had lasted only 3 weeks and was adequately managed with barbiturate sedation.

Two weeks after hospitalization, reserpine therapy was instituted. The patient received 10 mg intramuscularly the first day, 20 mg the second day, 15 mg on the third and fourth days, and a maintenance dose of 6 mg beginning on the fifth day of treatment and continuing for 8 days. During this period, her pulse was reduced from its high level to a range of 60 to 75 beats per minute. Restlessness, mood lability, overactivity, pressure of speech, and insomnia disappeared. The intensity of her sexual unrest, hostility, and elation was definitely reduced, but these features could still be easily detected in her appearance and behavior.

The side effects of treatment included drowsiness and lethargy, trembling and restlessness, staggering gait, and poor coordination, all of which decreased significantly when the maintenance dose of 6 mg was established.

On the twelfth day of therapy, her excitement was again intensified by anxiety, stirred partly by dynamic investigations and partly by the effect of certain visitors, and it was necessary to increase the daily dose of reserpine to 15 mg orally. Several weeks later, her family acquiesced to her demands for discharge from the hospital.

The response of this patient to reserpine indicates its effectiveness in the control of manic excitements in which anxiety is prominent and intensifies the basic psychopathologic state. Although it was possible actively to carry out dynamic investigations while she was on reserpine and her social adjustment improved significantly, it is important to note that the essential features of her condition, namely, eroticism, hostility, and elation, were modified but still qualitatively unchanged. This effect is in contrast to that seen in many manic patients who receive phenothiazines, in whom not only a decrease in the intensity of these psychopathologic features but also the actual disappearance of elation, sexual unrest, and hostility can be observed.

ANXIETY IN SCHIZOPHRENIC REACTIONS

The next case illustrates the efficacy of reserpine in the treatment of a patient in an acute paranoid schizophrenic reaction, with marked anxiety.

Case 2. In the setting of conflict with her mother and sexual difficulties with her husband, a 31-year-old woman experienced the gradual development of tension and anxiety. Her apprehension was focused on her ability to run her home and cope with her job at the same time. She felt disturbingly confined within the small apartment in which they lived. Several weeks before her hospitalization her anxieties expanded to include fears of crowded places. She frequently noted palpitations and shortness of breath. Sleep was restless and interrupted, with occasional nightmares. During the week before admission, paranoid delusions developed. The patient was convinced that her neighbors were accusing her of being a liar and troublemaker and of having misplaced important secret documents. She believed that her phone had been tapped, that the Federal Bureau of Investigation had assigned men to follow her everywhere, and that her husband, who in her delusion was a member of an anti-American organization, was responsible for her dilemma. She appeared bewildered, and thinking was impaired, at times to the point of incoherence. A diagnosis of paranoid schizophrenia was apparent.

On the third day of hospitalization, reserpine therapy was instituted. The dosage was increased by 5 mg intramuscularly each day until a daily dose of 20 mg was reached. She was maintained on this high amount of the drug for 16 days, at which time it was reduced to 6 mg orally per day. A striking reduction in anxiety was observed. The patient's pulse decreased from 100 beats per minute to a range of 50 to 75 beats per minute. Sleep improved markedly. Her delusions subsided, and she was able to recognize their inappropriateness. She was more active and spontaneous and made a satisfactory social adjustment.

Two weeks after the termination of reserpine, anxiety, tension, and suspiciousness, with some degree of social withdrawal, decreased spontaneity, and increased resistance to psychotherapeutic measures, recurred. Thereupon reserpine was again administered in daily oral doses of 4 mg and continued for 30 days. Again anxiety was reduced, and the patient was well controlled. This improvement continued for 6 weeks after the end of the second course of reserpine therapy. Then, in the setting of an argument with her husband and during active investigations of dynamic factors, intense anxiety returned. During a 3-week period severe paranoid delusions again developed; this time their content revealed sexual unrest. She believed, for example, that she had been impregnated mysteriously by a physician whom she had seen only once, many years before. She was withdrawn, unwilling to eat or attend activities, retarded, and mute. Nine ECTs were administered, with a rapid clearing of her delusions and a reduction in anxiety and sexual unrest. Her schizophrenic thinking disorder, however, was still evident at the time of her discharge.

This case illustrates the ability of reserpine to modify anxiety and the associated formation of paranoid delusions in an acute schizophrenic reaction. The schizophrenic features, particularly the disorder in thought processes, remained essentially untouched. Reserpine facilitated her social adjustment and participation in psychotherapy. The only significant side effects of therapy were restlessness and marked tension in her legs, which was relieved by keeping them elevated. Termination of the drug was associated with the return of her original psychopathologic condition. The use of electroconvulsive therapy rather than phenothiazines to alleviate her last period of disturbance, characterized by delusions with sexual content, was determined by the decision to terminate intensive dynamic investigations and concentrate on supportive, rehabilitative therapy.

ANXIETY IN DEPRESSIVE REACTIONS

The following case demonstrates the effects of reserpine in an anxious, agitated, depressed patient.

Case 3. Following the death of her older brother, this married 54-year-old woman became depressed, socially withdrawn, and indecisive. Anxiety was prominent; the patient worried about her finances and her future. She experienced some difficulty falling asleep, early morning awakening, and frequent interruptions of sleep during the night. She continued in this state for nearly 1 year, still able to do her housework and hide her disturbance from her family. Following a burglary attempt on her apartment her condition became worse. With the increase in her apprehension, paranoid delusions developed. She believed that the crime had been perpetrated by resentful neighbors in her apartment house and was convinced that it would be repeated. She incorrectly felt that her children had taken all her money and had been jailed for their unjust behavior. She was severely depressed, with suicidal ideas, although the depth of her depression was hidden by her bland countenance. Agitation was intense; the patient was unable to sit still for more than a few moments at a time. Her pulse was elevated to a range of 90 to 120 beats per minute.

When 3 weeks of hospital care failed to alleviate her psychopathologic condition, reserpine therapy was begun. The initial dose was 10 mg intramuscularly. The dose was increased by 5 mg daily until a level of 30 mg was obtained. At the end of the first week of treatment, an oral maintenance dose ranging from 6 to 10 mg daily was established and continued for 6 weeks. By the fifth day of therapy a striking reduction in anxiety and associated delusions was observed. She slept well without additional sedation. Her pulse fell to a range of 60 to 80 beats per minute. Overactivity was reduced, and her social adjustment improved substantially. Her appetite returned. In spite of these evident changes, her hopelessness persisted, and, in fact, depression was more obvious in her facial expressions. From time to time she manifested previously repressed or concealed resentment toward various members of her family.

Within 3 weeks after the termination of reserpine, anxiety, agitation, and paranoid delusions returned forcefully. It was then decided to end the psychotherapeutic investigations, and eight ECTs were administered, leading to rapid clearing of anxiety, paranoid features, and depression of mood.

This case illustrates the manner in which reserpine may relieve anxiety and symptoms associated with anxiety, such as paranoid delusions, insomnia, agitation, and anorexia, but without influencing the central mood depression. The indication for such pharmacologic modification of a depressive reaction is the desirability of carrying out dynamic investigations before the depression improves or is terminated by electroconvulsive therapy. In practice, such a procedure should be limited to hospitalized patients if the risk of suicide is present. Experience indicates that phenothiazines are more reliable than reserpine for this purpose. Interestingly, in this patient, manifestations of hostility appeared after reserpine had been instituted and her anxiety and delusions had subsided. This observation suggests that one of the purposes of these symptoms was to protect this patient from an awareness and expression of these hostile feelings. Unlike the phenothiazines, reserpine does not seem to reduce pathologic hostility, and, in fact, many patients demonstrate anger or resentment for the first time while receiving reserpine.

ADVERSE EMOTIONAL CHANGES DURING RESERPINE THERAPY

The three cases described above illustrate beneficial effects of reserpine. The administration of reserpine can also produce adverse emotional changes. Sometimes these may be transient and correspond to the so-called "turbulent phase" of reserpine therapy which may precede clinical improvement. At other times they seem to persist as long as the patient continues to receive the drug. Two instances of adverse psychologic alterations occurring during reserpine therapy will be presented. The first case illustrates the development of marked pathologic hostility, agitation, and depression of mood; the second, the appearance of sexual unrest and overactivity during the administration of the drug.

Case 4. A 55-year-old man presented a 3-week history of anxiety, expressed as acute attacks of apprehension and palpitations occurring at various times of the day and night. His sleep was interrupted. His concentration was impaired, and he demonstrated marked overconcern about his physical health in spite of several extensive examinations. This reaction developed in the setting of business conflicts and had been preceded by the death of his sister 8 months earlier. Hospitalization was recommended to provide freedom from daily pressures during the initial phase of psychotherapy. In spite of 10 weeks of hospital care, no significant improvement in his clinical condition was observed. Therefore, in order to relieve his anxiety symptoms, reserpine therapy was instituted. He received 10 mg orally each day for 4 weeks. By the end of the first week, his anxiety attacks had diminished, and his sleep was temporarily much improved. As these features subsided, however, the patient began to demonstrate intense depression of mood, pathologic hostility, and recurrent episodes of agitation. He described himself as hopeless, cried during his interviews, and appeared sad and tired. Suicidal ideas appeared. He frequently flared up angrily at the nurses, medical staff, and other patients, usually without sufficient provocation. He often paced the corridors restlessly. Concentration continued to be poor. His appetite decreased, and he lost 10 lb.

Following termination of reserpine, the patient's hostility and depression of mood continued unabated, although his overactivity decreased. After 3 weeks without medication, he was begun on chlorpromazine in daily oral doses of 400 mg. Pathologic hostility subsided. His appetite improved. He was better able to concentrate on uncomplicated subjects, such as reading the daily paper or playing cards. His depression of mood persisted, but he was better able to tolerate this state and turn his attention toward the analysis of dynamic factors in his psychotherapeutic sessions. Chlorpromazine was continued for 12 weeks. Following its termination, eight ECTs were given, with striking improvement in his clinical condition.

It is not possible to say whether the appearance of depression of mood in this patient was the direct result of the reserpine which he was receiving or whether this psychopathologic change was determined by the abrupt removal of anxiety, which had served to alert him to the onset of the depressive illness and yet protected him for a while against the awareness of depression and the contributing personality conflicts. Once it appeared, the pathologic mood persisted long after the reserpine had been terminated and eventually cleared only after the use of electroconvulsive treatments. The indication for employing chlorpromazine to reduce the pathologic hostility and alleviate the subjective suffering accompanying the depressive mood was again the pursuit of dynamic factors before the psychopathologic condition improved.

The agitation of this patient which appeared during reserpine therapy and subsided after the drug had been stopped may have been related to the hostile emotions which emerged at this time. However, this phenomenon could also have been the direct result of the action of reserpine on the central nervous system.

Case 5. A 24-year-old woman, diagnosed as a chronic paranoid schizophrenic reaction, presented a 5-year history of marked concentration difficulty; recurrent episodes of rage outbursts and depression of mood, occurring most often in association with her menstrual periods; severe disorganization of her daily routine; social withdrawal; and the excessive use of nicotine and coffee to maintain alertness. Her scholastic achievements, which had been impressive until the third year of high school, suffered, and she was unable to complete successfully her first college year in spite of three attempts to do so. She worried greatly about her physical health, fearing heart disease in particular. When not agitated, she appeared bland, bored, pale, and listless.

For 8 months prior to hospitalization, overactivity was prominent, with wide mood swings from mild elation to intense depression. Angry outbursts directed toward her parents were frequent. Depression of mood gradually became more marked and persistent. Thinking was impaired, and at times she was frankly incoherent. At the time of her admission she was withdrawn, mute, negativistic, and moderately anxious. Her pulse ranged from 70 to 90 beats per minute, and her sleep was interrupted.

Reserpine was instituted. She received 10 mg intramuscularly the first day of treatment, 20 mg the second, and 25 mg the third. Thereafter, she was maintained on oral medication, amounting to 6 to 30 mg daily, varying in accordance with changes in her clinical condition and the side effects of the drug. These complications were very severe, consisting of motor retardation, excessive salivation and drooling, and impaired coordination. During treatment, anxiety and tension were significantly reduced, and she was no longer withdrawn, mute, and negativistic. However, sexual unrest and pathologic hostility appeared, strongly influencing her behavior. She was flirtatious, exposed herself, and spoke often of sexual topics. She became enraged at the slightest provocation. Her restlessness was colored by repetitive demands for attention and reassurance.

Reserpine was continued for 5 weeks. Within 7 days after its termination, sexual unrest, hostility, and overactivity subsided, and she was strikingly improved. She maintained this level of adjustment for the next 5 months, while psychotherapeutic measures were carried out. The schizophrenic thinking disorder, now characterized by vagueness, rambling, and looseness of associations, remained unmodified. During a subsequent acute psychopathologic reaction, in which paranoid misinterpretations and delusions, depersonalization, and intense depression of mood with suicidal impulses were prominent features, this patient received 17 ECTs, administered over an 8-week period. This regimen produced marked improvement, which lasted, however, only for 3 weeks. Thereafter, suspiciousness, angry outbursts, and intense resentment were prominent. These features were controlled for nearly 3 months by 500 mg chlorpromazine given daily orally. She then received six more ECTs, which sufficiently alleviated remnants of her depressive mood to permit her discharge from the hospital.

In this patient, large doses of reserpine reduced anxiety and tension and alleviated associated features of marked withdrawal and negativistic behavior. Therapy was complicated, however, by the development of marked restlessness and overactivity, sexual unrest, and hostility. Only the neurologic side effects of reserpine administration controlled the manifest symptoms of her agitation. It is possible that the abrupt removal of anxiety facilitated the release of these intense emotions. It is also possible that the drug impaired her ego function, making it difficult for her adequately to control her impulses and feelings. On the other hand, the turbulent state may have been the direct result of the action of reserpine on the central nervous system; in this regard, it is worth recalling the resemblance between reserpine and yohimbine, the latter possessing aphrodisiac properties. After reserpine was terminated, the excitement disappeared and the patient's clinical condition was improved to a degree markedly surpassing her pretreatment state. Psychotherapy, which had been carried out during this entire period, also may have contributed to these beneficial changes. Moreover, the disturbing experiences may have served a cathartic purpose, allowing the patient to feel better after the liberation of her intense emotions. Although reserpine was influential in reducing anxiety and tension in this patient and the turbulent phase was followed by improvement, the changes did not involve the most essential elements of the schizophrenic disorder, particularly the disorganization of thought processes.

SUMMARY

Reserpine is a representative derivative of *Rauwolfia serpentina* (Benth). In spite of initially glowing reports of its beneficial effects in psychiatric patients, it now appears to have a very limited therapeutic role. The compound seems to influence psychopathologic conditions by reducing anxiety and associated symptoms dependent upon the presence of anxiety. If this pathologic emotion constitutes an important element in a patient's illness, the results may be impressive; if not, there may be little or no change in the clinical picture. The administration of reserpine and the consequent reduction of anxiety symptoms may, in certain patients, lead to or be associated with the appearance of depression of mood, which can often be very severe. Other patients may become agitated, excited, angry, or sexually aroused during the administration of the drug.

Unlike the phenothiazines, reserpine does not appear to reduce pathologic hostility and sexual unrest. The phenothiazines, as used in the treatment of manic or schizophrenic excitements, appear to eliminate many of the important pathologic emotions and symptoms. Reserpine, on the other hand, either because of its general sedative properties or through the reduction of driving anxiety, seems to reduce the intensity of these states without significantly influencing the central dynamic features of the excitement.

Meprobamate and barbiturates appear to be as effective as reserpine in the management of anxiety and tension in many settings. Moreover, they lack the complications and administrative problems inherent in reserpine therapy. In certain schizophrenic conditions, insulin therapy still appears preferable to any of these agents for the relief of pathologic anxiety.

Therefore, the indications for reserpine in the treatment of psychiatric patients are few, if indeed they exist at all.

8

THE BARBITURATES

Prior to the advent of tranquilizers, barbiturates occupied the most prominent place in the list of drugs used in psychiatry. Phenothiazines and other pharmacologic agents now appear to have taken the place of the barbiturates in some areas of treatment. It seems well assured, however, that the barbiturates will remain an extensively used group of drugs, because of their variety, potency, and inexpensiveness. By selecting the proper barbiturate, and by administering it in adequate dosage, a physician can use these drugs effectively in every psychiatric condition, from the most severe excitement to the mildest anxiety state. They can do this, moreover, with a much lower chance of complications, and a much lower cost, than with virtually any other group of drugs available.

Pharmacologically, the barbiturates may be regarded as central nervous system depressants. The exact site of action is uncertain, but it appears likely that they exert a depressive effect on cortical and subcortical levels. The former effect is seen in the confusion, impaired perception, and retarded thinking of the patient under the influence of barbiturates, while the latter effect is seen in the ease with which barbiturates produce sleep. The barbiturates may be administered orally or parenterally; most barbiturates suitable for oral administration may be obtained in capsules and in the form of an elixir. Once ingested, barbiturates are widely distributed throughout the body fluids; they are eliminated from the body by means of excretion through the kidneys or by being metabolized, chiefly in the liver.

The simplest classification of the barbiturates depends on their speed of action and duration of effectiveness. In general, barbiturates which act rapidly are excreted and metabolized rapidly, and vice versa. The commonly used barbiturates may thereby be classified as in Table 3.

Table 3   Classification of Barbiturates

Name	Oral sedative dose (given 4 times a day), Gm	Oral hypnotic dose, Gm	Optimal use
Long-acting barbiturates:			
Barbital (Veronal)	0.15	0.3–0.5	Sedation
Phenobarbital (Luminal)	0.045	0.2–0.3	Sedation
Moderate-acting barbiturates:			
Amobarbital (Amytal)	0.05–0.1	0.1–0.5	Long hypnosis
Pentobarbital (Nembutal)	. . .	0.1–0.2	Long hypnosis
Short-acting barbiturates:			
Secobarbital (Seconal)	. . .	0.1–0.2	Short hypnosis
Ultrashort-acting barbiturates:			
Thiopental (Pentothal)	. . .	. . .	Anesthesia

Clearly, the following discussion is limited to a consideration of the psychotherapeutic use of the barbiturates. Their anticonvulsant action will be considered in Chap. 14. Regarding the indications and contraindications which will be discussed, it is essential to remember that these depend on the assumption that the patient is in a satisfactory physical condition. The presence of hepatic or renal disease is a strong contraindication, owing to the impairment of barbiturate excretion and metabolism which accompanies these conditions. There is also serious danger in administering barbiturates to debilitated patients, where the central nervous system depression may precipitate respiratory failure. Similarly, the synergistic action of barbiturates with alcohol and opiates can easily lead to profound depression and circulatory collapse, when they are administered simultaneously. These are some of the factors which must be kept in mind as a base line in following the proper psychotherapeutic use of the barbiturates.

SIDE EFFECTS AND COMPLICATIONS

The major complications of barbiturate usage are overdosage and habituation.

Overdosage

Overdosage may occur when long-acting barbiturates are administered for a prolonged period of time and the blood level of the medication builds up faster than the drug is detoxified and excreted by the body. It can also result from accidental overdosage by the patient or from excessive intake in the course of a suicide attempt. One of the most frequent ways in which accidental overdosage occurs is in the use of barbiturates for sleeping. The story follows a typical pattern: A patient takes a prescribed dose of barbiturate and goes to bed; he is made drowsy by the barbiturate, and his thinking is cloudy, but he fails to go to sleep. Because of cloudy thinking, he does not remember whether or not he took a barbiturate, and he rises and takes another capsule. He then returns to bed, and the cycle of insomnia, uncertainty, and repetitive dosage continues, until the patient has finally taken a toxic amount. In order to minimize the possibility of overdosage, therefore, it is recommended that barbiturates be prescribed and dispensed in small amounts and that, preferably, they be administered by another family member, so that the patient cannot redose himself in the course of a night.

The treatment of barbiturate overdosage depends on the time at which the physician is called to the case. If he arrives shortly after the patient has taken the medication, the best treatment is gastric lavage, the administration of stimulants such as coffee, and forced physical activity. If the physician arrives later, when the medication has been absorbed into the blood stream, parenteral picrotoxin should be used if the patient's respirations become excessively slow. If the vital signs are normal, the patient should be kept under constant observation. Provided that they remain normal, it is just as well to allow the prolonged sleep to follow a natural course, with parenteral fluids and antimicrobial therapy to maintain the fluid balance and to prevent infection. Continued constant observations are indicated, with regular measurements of pulse, blood pressure, and other vital signs, in order that parenteral stimulants can be administered if necessary.

Habituation

Barbiturate habituation is a common problem in the treatment of psychoneurotic persons and in the treatment of persons who have been treating themselves with barbiturate medication. After repeated and prolonged dosage of any barbiturate, tolerance to the drug develops; when this happens, it is not uncommon for a patient to increase his intake until he is taking two to three times the usual therapeutic dose of a drug, without any effect. When sufficiently high levels are reached, the patient will begin to manifest withdrawal symptoms if the dosage is reduced. Psychologically, too, he can grow to depend on taking this large dose of medication in order to maintain the usual pattern of his life.

The interruption of such a course of habituation is not difficult, but it has some specific dangers. If the patient is regularly taking more than 1 Gm of barbiturates in every 24-hour period, the sudden cessation of this very high dosage of barbiturates will often produce epileptiform grand mal seizures, as well as very marked anxiety, tension, nausea, tremors, palpitations, and gastrointestinal disturbances. It is recommended, therefore, if habituation has reached this severe degree, that the patient be hospitalized for the period of withdrawal. Under conditions of hospitalization, the drug can be gradually removed. An appropriate reduction schedule will lower the daily barbiturate intake by 0.2 to 0.3 Gm every 3 to 4 days. By progressive stages, therefore, the daily intake is reduced and the patient gradually removed from drugs. Even with this gradual reduction program, the patient will have marked anxiety and will present a moderately serious psychotherapeutic problem in management.

In treating the patient who is habituated to barbiturates at a dosage level below 0.8 Gm per day, one need not be so concerned about the severe physical effects of withdrawal. One must still recognize, however, that the barbiturate is being used as a psychologic crutch and that the sudden removal of this crutch will precipitate intense psychologic symptoms. One must explore carefully the dependency needs which are being satisfied by the medication and help the patient to find better ways of satisfying these needs as one proceeds to eliminate the drug.

CLINICAL EFFECTIVENESS OF TREATMENT

Sedation

Sedation involves the prolonged use of frequent low doses of barbiturates throughout a patient's waking hours. The medication is used in order to slow the patient down or to alleviate his emotional turmoil. At the same time, the properly adjusted sedative does not greatly impair the patient's intellectual ability, psychomotor activity, or wakefulness. The barbiturates can serve as very effective sedatives for many patients.

A state of sedation can be achieved with virtually any of the barbiturates. The rapid-acting and intermediate-acting barbiturates, however, are able to produce this state only very briefly, because of the nature of their action. They also very frequently overshoot the mark and produce excessive drowsiness and impairment of intellectual function. The barbiturates most effective in producing the state of sedation, therefore, are the long-acting barbiturates: barbital and phenobarbital. Barbital appears to have a more benign and less restricting quality than does phenobarbital, but the difference is slight. These drugs can produce a state of sedation which can be controlled by minute adjustments in dosage. For each of these drugs, the production and maintenance of a steady state of sedation depends on the adherence to a regular therapeutic program, thereby maintaining a relatively stable blood level of the barbiturates. With phenobarbital, sedation can be achieved by administering 0.030 to 0.090 Gm of oral phenobarbital three to four times a day; by the end of the second day, the sedative effect should have reached its peak, and modification of the dosage level can be begun. With barbital, the dosage is 0.100 to 0.150 Gm, orally, administered three to four times a day; again the peak level of sedation will have been achieved by the end of 2 days.

There are many conditions in which the production of sedation, as described, is useful. These conditions may be found in any diagnostic category, and there appears to be no diagnostic contraindication per se to the use of barbiturates. It must be remembered, however, that the sedation achieved by the barbiturates can be utilized only when the patient is experiencing suffering due to emotional turmoil but when there is *not* any serious impairment in the patient's ability to recognize and deal with reality. In the presence of organic damage to the brain, for example, the preexisting impairment of intellectual function is a contraindication to the use of barbiturates. By the same criterion, sedation is contraindicated in such conditions as marked manic excitements, catatonic excitements or stupors, panic states, paranoid excitements, and organic brain disease; in all these conditions, thinking has already been impaired by the nature of the illness or the turbulence of the emotions, and to add the impairment of the barbiturate effect would only add to the patient's excitement.

With regard to the emotional characteristics which indicate successful use of sedation, it is characteristically most useful in psychopathologic states which are marked predominantly by anxiety and tension. Both the subjective experience of anxiety and the associated psychologic and physical symptoms will usually be greatly reduced by adequate sedation. Feelings of depression are usually unchanged by the administration of barbiturate sedation; the anxiety and suffering which accompany the depression, however, will frequently be made less severe. Feelings of anger and resentment do *not* usually respond favorably to barbiturate sedation; an angry or resentful patient, indeed, usually experiences the sedation as a restraint and becomes more angry and resentful as he attempts to cast off the effects of this restraint.

In achieving the state of sedation, in the areas which have been described, the limitations of barbiturate effectiveness must be recognized.

Whenever the illness and the level of emotional disturbance become excessively pronounced, the barbiturates do not have sufficient potency to deal with the problem. Moreover, if the condition continues for a prolonged period of time, the medication will gradually lose its effect as the patient becomes habituated to the drug. It is wise, therefore, to recognize that sedation produced by barbiturates should be used only in conditions which can be expected to terminate within 2 to 3 weeks. Under such conditions, when drug potency is sufficient, the patient will be relieved of much suffering during the period of drug administration, and psychotherapy may be helped by this process.

Hypnosis

The hypnotic effect of barbiturates may be used in order to produce sleep. For this purpose, the rapid-acting or intermediate-acting barbiturates are recommended. It is frequently observed that physicians who are not accustomed to dealing with psychiatric patients underdose patients with severe anxiety and other psychologic symptoms. The insomnia associated with tension is characterized by difficulty in going to sleep. Commonly it is necessary to use at least 300 mg pentobarbital, orally, or 200 to 400 mg Sodium Amytal, orally, to obtain sleep in this situation. Depression, on the other hand, is associated with a sleep pattern of easy falling asleep and wakefulness after 3 or 4 A.M.; a patient with both tension and depression may show both types of insomnia simultaneously. In the presence of depression, therefore, it is wise to use a combination of an intermediate-acting barbiturate and a long-acting barbiturate. Such a combination can include Sodium Amytal, at an oral dosage level of 300 mg, and barbital, at an oral dosage level of 200 mg; both these medications can be given in liquid form, at bedtime, and will usually produce a solid 6- to 8-hour period of sleep.

Certain aspects of the use of hypnotics should always be kept in mind. The need for sleep occurs in every kind of psychiatric illness and condition. It is most unusual, however, for the insomnia to be intermittent in nature. Only rarely does one find a patient who has sleeping difficulty on an unpredictable basis. Usually, patients have a continuing and regular pattern of insomnia, and it is with this that the patient must deal. Therefore, the problem for the physician is to destroy the pattern of insomnia and to substitute for it a healthy sleep pattern. If the physician remembers that this is his obligation—to produce a healthy pattern of sleep—the use of the barbiturates can be easily managed by following several simple rules, as follows.

USE AN ADEQUATE DOSAGE

If the dose of barbiturate administered is not sufficient to produce sleep, or to maintain the sleep for a sufficiently long period, the physician will find that his patient is having an interrupted and useless sleep pattern. It is better to withhold medication than to undermine the patient's confidence by inadequate treatment.

MAINTAIN THE PATTERN

It is sometimes difficult, especially when the patient is a physician or nurse, to convince the patient that it is necessary for a therapeutic program, once established, to be maintained. It is disastrous for therapy, especially when one is dealing with patients with a psychoneurotic reaction, to have the therapeutic program determined by the whims of the patient or *pro re nata*, "as things turn out." When the physician has assured himself that the prescribed dosage is adequate to provide the sleep the patient needs, the patient should receive this amount of medication each night at bedtime. Whether the day has been calm and quiet or riddled with anxiety, the therapy will go on and adequate sleep will be ensured; to establish a good sleep pattern, regularity is imperative.

Once an adequate dosage has been determined and the patient has begun to follow a regular sleep pattern, it is necessary for the pattern to be maintained for an adequate period of time. This duration will depend, of course, upon the nature of the patient's illness and the psychotherapeutic process. Medication may be used to provide an adequate sleep pattern during a period of excessive anxiety in psychotherapy, or to relieve the insomnia of a suicidal depressed patient, or to provide adequate rest for any excited manic patient. In each of these situations, the length of time over which the sleep pattern must be maintained will vary. In any case, once an adequate nightly sleep pattern is obtained, this pattern should be maintained for a minimum period of 2 weeks. Only after 2 weeks of satisfactory sleep have elapsed and the therapist has reason to expect that the patient will be able to sleep without the support of medication should an attempt be made to reduce or remove the medication.

TERMINATE THE MEDICATION GRADUALLY

When the time has arrived to terminate the artificial production of sleep, care must be taken that the established pattern is not destroyed at the last moment. The reasons for termination may be varied; the patient may have come out of a problem period during psychotherapy, or the excitement or depression may have been relieved. On the other hand, the patient may still be anxious but now ready to face the problem of insomnia without the support of the barbiturates. In any event, when termination is desired, the dosage of the medication should gradually be cut down, in regular stages. Whatever the total dosage of medication, no more than one-third or 200 mg, whichever is smaller, should be eliminated on a given night. Once the total dosage has been cut by such an amount, it should be maintained at the reduced level for a minimum period of 4 days. After the 4 days have elapsed a second cut in dosage may be made and after another 4 days, a third cut. As the medication is gradually reduced in this fashion, it will be found that the patient will maintain his drug-induced sleep pattern if the pattern has been established with sufficient firmness by virtue of the preceding steps.

If these simple procedures are followed in the use of barbiturates to induce sleep, many of the usual problems of habituation, anxiety, mutual frustration, and disappointment will be avoided.

When the problem is not a chronic one but involves an acute accident, a preoperative or postoperative condition, or other brief anxiety-producing stimulus, these principles may still avoid a great deal of difficulty. One of the most frequent causes of delirious reactions in postoperative or toxemic patients, for example, is insufficient dosage of barbiturates in order to produce sleep. When a patient is in pain postoperatively, he is experiencing marked anxiety. The usual dosage level of pentobarbital (100 mg) would not be nearly sufficient to produce sleep in this state. Instead, the administration of such a dosage (or even two or three times this dosage) is more likely only to impair the person's intellectual functioning and make him less able to deal with his pain and confusion and at the same time unable to go to sleep. In such a situation, the makings of a delirious reaction are present. Such dangers could be avoided by administering an amount of barbiturate which will definitely put the patient to sleep.

Prolonged Sleep Treatment

This treatment, which usually includes the phenothiazine compounds, has been described in Chap. 6. Classically, however, prolonged sleep treatment was carried on through the combined use of rapid-acting, intermediate-acting, and long-acting barbiturates; this treatment had an accepted role in the therapy of excitements for many years prior to the advent of tranquilizing drugs. The course, indications, complications, and effectiveness of this treatment with barbiturates are similar to those described under sleep treatment with phenothiazine derivatives.

Sodium Amytal Interviews

Since the dramatically effective utilization of interviews carried out under the influence of Pentothal Sodium and Sodium Amytal during World War II, the Sodium Amytal interview has occupied a recognized place in psychiatric diagnosis and treatment. In this procedure, the patient is given parenteral, usually intravenous, barbiturate to the point where he is not quite asleep but in a state of marked sedation, with slurred speech and greatly diminished control over his intellectual content. Such interviews are of use for purposes of diagnosis, exploratory psychotherapy, and directive treatment.

The techniques of the Sodium Amytal interview are relatively simple. The patient reclines on a sofa or bed in a quiet, darkened room. The physician is accompanied by a nurse or other attendant, especially when a woman patient is to be treated. Following explanation to the patient, Sodium Amytal is injected slowly into an antecubital vein, at a rate not to exceed 10 mg every 2 minutes. As medication is injected, the physician engages the patient in discussion. The injection is terminated at the time when the patient begins to demonstrate slurred speech and wandering thoughts, but great care must be taken that the injection does not proceed to the point where the patient's intellect becomes excessively confused. At the termination of the injection, the needle is left in place so that more Sodium Amytal can be injected if the patient should require it in the course of the interview or if the physician desires to put the patient into a state of sleep at the conclusion of the interview. Although Pentothal Sodium was used in earlier experiences in this kind of interview, the years have proved that Sodium Amytal best provides the desired effect. The dosage of Sodium Amytal required for such an interview will vary but will approximate 150 to 200 mg intravenously.

There are three purposes for which Sodium Amytal interviews may be utilized, and indications and contraindications vary according to these purposes.

ABREACTION

The first purpose of Sodium Amytal interviews is to ventilate and explore a single traumatic experience. This use originated in the acute war neuroses and psychoses, which had been precipitated by an outstanding traumatic event, such as an airplane crash. In such a situation, it is the purpose of the Sodium Amytal interview that the patient reexperience the traumatic event in a vivid fashion, in order that he may better learn to accept it and to live with its effects. The physician, in such an instance, recreates the dramatic situation, gradually pushing the patient into more and more detailed descriptions of the experience and finally into the state where he relives the experience. Repeated reliving is frequently necessary, in the course of repeated interviews. Usually it is necessary for the physician to discuss the material which has been reexperienced when the patient has awakened. This type of ventilating interview, used to explore a single traumatic event, can be utilized in any diagnostic category. Since its purpose is circumscribed and since the physician assumes a directing role, not allowing excessive rumination or wandering of associations, it can be used safely in schizophrenic, psychoneurotic, and depressed persons. Its use in civilian life, however, is relatively limited; catastrophes such as occur frequently to soldiers during war are not common in civilian life, and the occurrence of the psychoses and neuroses secondary to such traumatic instances is infrequent in peacetime living. The frequency with which this kind of interview is used in regular peacetime practice, therefore, is low.

SUGGESTION

A second purpose is to achieve a sedated state in which the physician may make quasi-hypnotic suggestions to the patient in order to control hysterical symptomatology. In the drowsy, somewhat obfuscated state to which the patient is brought in the course of a Sodium Amytal interview, it is very easy for the physician to assume a dominant and directive role. In such a situation, he may easily make suggestions which will produce the same effect as suggestions made during regular hypnotic interviews. He may alter the patient's perceptions in the course of the session, and he may clear up amnesias or other conversion phenomena. Similarly, he may implant posthypnotic suggestions, which will take effect after the posttreatment sleep has been terminated. In like manner, the physician may use one or two Sodium Amytal interviews in order to hasten the process of training the patient to respond rapidly to hypnotic suggestions, thereby helping a course of hypnotherapeutic interviews to be initiated.

The indications for this use of Sodium Amytal interviews are limited. It is most effective, obviously, in dealing with conversion symptoms, especially such troublesome ones as paralysis of extremities, nausea, vomiting, amnesia, blindness, or aphonia. When it is used in such situations, however, it has the usual disadvantage of suggestion and adds a few dangers specifically its own. The usual disadvantage of suggestion in controlling conversion symptoms is that the symptoms occupy a definite place in the psychologic economy of the individual; they serve a definite purpose in defending the patient against anxieties, fear, or conflicts with which he is unable to deal. When these defenses are rapidly stripped away by suggestion, the patient is left in an extraordinarily vulnerable condition and may easily enter a state of panic, where flight or suicide is likely. Controlling conversion symptoms with hypnosis, therefore, is an occasionally dangerous process; it must not be undertaken lightly or without knowledge of the patient's dynamic situation. This is as true with a Sodium Amytal interview as with hypnosis or other forms of suggestion.

When Sodium Amytal is used to help suggestion, however, several additional factors must be considered. On the credit side, Sodium Amytal will increase the effectiveness of suggestions. On the debit side, it will multiply the danger of the situation. Under the influence of Sodium Amytal, the patient has even less ability to control his behavior and to defend himself than he does when he is in the regular hypnotherapeutic session. It is therefore possible for the therapist to be much more ruthless and destructive in this situation than ordinarily. Secondly, the very nature of the Sodium Amytal interview, with an atmosphere which includes a darkened room, a mysterious injection, and a dominating therapist, may easily precipitate sexual panic or sexual excitement followed by many sexual accusations against the therapist.

The Sodium Amytal interview may be used for purposes of suggestion, therefore, but must be used with great caution. Such use should be limited to those patients who have conversion symptomatology in the setting of a well-organized personality, usually in a psychoneurotic reaction. When the patient has conversion symptomatology in the setting of a schizophrenic reaction and his ability to deal with reality has already been diminished, the dangers of the Sodium Amytal interview are multiplied enormously and it should be regarded as contraindicated.

EXPLORATION

The third use of the Sodium Amytal interview is for the purpose of exploration. When the patient has received 150 to 200 mg Sodium Amytal, his ability to think in an organized fashion is diminished and the freedom of his associations is increased. His defenses are less strong, and his suppressive and repressive resistances are weakened. As a consequence, it is possible for a patient under the influence of Sodium Amytal to be led into a discussion of meaningful dynamic material with much less difficulty than when he is awake. This holds true for repressed material and for consciously withheld material. Owing to the loosening of associations, the patient's productions surrounding known events of his life tend to be much richer, and the therapist may easily discover associations and historical material that are not produced in the course of the ordinary therapeutic interviews. Material that the patient has consciously suppressed because of shame or fear will also be brought out during Sodium Amytal interviews; this is particularly true of material in the sensitive area of sexuality, where the anxiety of the patient, or the reluctance of the therapist, frequently blocks progress.

The Sodium Amytal interview, therefore, may aim at exploring one of two areas: material which is unknown to the patient, or material which the patient is consciously withholding. It may be used for such exploration at those times in psychotherapy when the conscious or unconscious resistance is creating an insurmountable obstacle. In such a situation, it is easily possible to use a series of three to six Sodium Amytal interviews, given at a frequency of approximately twice a week. The therapist directs the discussion during the interview toward the material which he surmises is being hidden or toward the resistance itself. In doing so, he learns about the material discussed and obtains a rich fund of data, which can then be used to stimulate the patient in regular psychotherapeutic sessions.

In conducting Sodium Amytal interviews of an exploratory sort, several conditions must be maintained. The purpose of such interviews must be thoroughly explained to the patient. Careful notes and observations must be taken during interviews, so that the newly produced material can be utilized later. The importance of complete recording during the interview cannot be overemphasized. It is sometimes possible to obtain a degree of lasting benefit from the discussion of material during the Sodium Amytal interview itself; almost universally, however, this is not enough. It is almost always necessary for the dynamic material which is brought up to be rediscussed when the patient is free of the influence of medication.

Several factors must determine when to administer Sodium Amytal for the purpose of exploration. Obviously, interviews for this purpose are most effective in patients who have well-organized and even excessively organized defenses. They are most effective, therefore, when dealing with psychoneurotic situations, particularly those associated with rigid, obsessive defenses or with phobic defenses. In the hands of a skillful therapist who recognizes the danger, it is sometimes possible to utilize the Sodium Amytal interview with a schizophrenic individual, provided that the patient's over-all contact with reality is fairly adequate. In such a situation, the therapist must be extremely careful to avoid fostering looseness of associations or unrealistic interpretations of reality; he must limit the interviews to meaningful material which can be handled in subsequent regular interviews; he must be capable of handling the difficulties which new dynamic material may produce. In general, Sodium Amytal interviews for the purpose of exploration may unearth a very large quantity of psychopathology and result in a dangerous situation. They are never to be undertaken by anyone who is not prepared to deal with any amount of psychopathology which may be displayed during or after the exploration.

SUMMARY

The uses to which barbiturates may be put in psychiatric treatment are legion. By the proper selection of drugs, dosage, and mode of administration, the physician can use barbiturates to produce states which range from the mildest sedation to continual sleep. For every variation in effect, moreover, it is possible to find a specific psychotherapeutic use for the barbiturates. When this versatility is recognized in conjunction with the inexpensiveness and easy availability of barbiturates, the status which these drugs occupy in the psychiatric armamentarium may easily be understood.

The major uses for the barbiturates are as follows:

Sedation, in which the long-acting barbiturates may be used to relieve daytime anxiety and tension in patients who are not excessively disturbed, have not lost contact with reality, and do not suffer from organic brain disease

Hypnosis, in which the intermediate-acting and rapid-acting barbiturates may be used singly or in combination to produce sleep in patients who are suffering from insomnia

Prolonged sleep treatment

Sodium Amytal interviews, which may be used for purposes of abreaction, suggestion, or exploration

The very versatility and effectiveness of the barbiturates, paradoxically, adds some danger to their utilization. They can be used for so many purposes that not infrequently they are misused and abused. Familiarity breeds contempt, and these powerful drugs are often used lavishly and inappropriately. The results of such treatment may be seen in drug habituation, in exaggeration of organic brain disease, and in drug-induced panics and excitements. It behooves every physician who uses barbiturates, therefore, to become extremely familiar with these most common medications in order that he may use them to the extent of their capacity without danger.

9

MEPROBAMATE

Meprobamate (Equanil, Miltown, Meprospan) was first synthesized in 1950, as a result of investigations designed to develop a long-acting muscle relaxant. Not only did this compound induce prolonged relaxation of voluntary musculature, but it also appeared to have significant effects on thalamic structures in the brain and some anticonvulsant properties. The chemical structure differs from that of the phenothiazines and rauwolfia derivatives. In contrast to these groups of drugs, meprobamate does not appear to influence significantly the metabolism of acetylcholine, epinephrine, or histamine in animal experiments. The exact mode of action of this drug remains unclear.

$$NH_2-\overset{\overset{\text{O}}{\|}}{C}-O-CH_2-\overset{\overset{\text{CH}_2-CH_2-CH_3}{|}}{\underset{\underset{\text{CH}_3}{|}}{C}}-CH_2-O-\overset{\overset{\text{O}}{\|}}{C}-NH_2$$

Some investigators feel that the reported ability of meprobamate to reduce anxiety and tension in psychiatric patients is entirely dependent on the reassuring influence of prescribing any drug, even a placebo, to suggestible patients. Many studies, however, indicate that meprobamate is an effective agent in the alleviation of certain disturbing emotions. In contrast to the phenothiazines, this drug has little place in the treatment of severe psychopathologic reactions. Using meprobamate, even in massive doses, to control an acute catatonic excitement resembles a vain effort to put out a four-alarm fire with a bucket of water. Not only does this drug lack the potency of the phenothiazines, but its activity appears to be qualitatively different as well. In some patients, however, meprobamate appears to accomplish what the phenothiazines cannot.

Method of Administration

Meprobamate is administered orally. Ordinarily 400 mg is given every 4 to 6 hours during the day, the total daily dosage averaging between 800 and 1,600 mg. Certain patients may be instructed to use the medication only at those times or in those settings when he anticipates becoming anxious and tense. Occasionally, individual doses of 200 mg are sufficient to produce the desired clinical changes; frequently, however, this is too low a dosage level and may lead to premature abandonment of the treatment before it has been given a fair trial. It is sometimes necessary to use 800 mg or more in a single dose, totaling as much as 3,200 mg in 24 hours, to provide relief from severe anxiety.

Side Effects and Complications

Meprobamate has been so extensively used in general practice and psychiatric treatment that the complications associated with its use have been well documented. Serious toxic effects seem to be quite minimal, although rare instances of aplastic anemia, renal destruction resulting in uremia, leukocytopenia, fever, thrombocytopenic purpura, angioneurotic edema, and bronchial spasm have been reported. Several reported attempts at suicide in which patients have ingested large doses of the drug ranging from 10,000 to 40,000 mg have led to coma and vasomotor and respiratory collapse; fortunately, death was prevented by proper medical management in each instance.

No effect on pulse or blood pressure has been reported, although a reduction in the heart rate may be seen if the pretreatment level is elevated owing to anxiety. Drowsiness is the most common concomitant of meprobamate therapy, usually appearing when the patient is first started on the drug and vanishing when his tolerance increases or the dosage is reduced. Fainting is rare. Occasionally symptoms of gastrointestinal distress, such as nausea and vomiting, occur. Allergic dermatitis has been reported in less than 0.025 per cent of patients receiving this medication.

Although meprobamate possesses anticonvulsant properties, it is not directly effective in the management of epileptic disorders, except through its ability to reduce distressing emotions. Nonetheless, abrupt termination of large doses of the drug may lead to grand mal convulsions in a number of patients who lack any evidence of organic brain disease. Addiction to meprobamate has not been described, but habituation must be considered a potential hazard in patients who are prone to become dependent on such drugs as barbiturates or alcohol.

Clinical Effectiveness of Treatment

Meprobamate appears to reduce pathologic anxiety and tension, particularly when these two features occur in combination. The drug clearly lacks the broad spectrum of action of the phenothiazines and does not significantly influence hostile emotions, intense fear, sexual unrest and excitement, and related psychopathologic features such as paranoid sensitivity, delusions, and hallucinations. It does, however, often reduce the kind of anxiety and tension seen in psychoneurotic conditions, which the phenothiazines do not seem to alleviate. It is important to recall that anxiety may intensify other pathologic features. The anxious patient may reveal sexual unrest; the tense patient is often irritable and resentful. In such conditions, the pharmacologic reduction of anxiety and tension may also be associated with a decrease in the intensity of sexual unrest or hostility, but these factors are not directly affected, as they may be with phenothiazine treatment.

The striking results seen in some patients during the administration of reserpine seem to be related to the ability of the drug to reduce anxiety, especially when this pathologic emotion is associated with evidence of autonomic nervous system involvement. In acute psychopathologic reactions, a general sedative action also appears to be an important contributing factor to the effectiveness of the drug. Meprobamate lacks this latter property and hence is of little value in extremely disturbed patients. However, it appears to be equally effective with, and often more effective than, reserpine in reducing anxiety and tension when these features are the leading components of a patient's illness.

ANXIETY IN PSYCHONEUROTIC REACTIONS

The greatest clinical value of meprobamate, therefore, lies in the treatment of psychoneurotic conditions in which anxiety and tension constitute central features. Several patients will be described to illustrate the effectiveness and limitations of meprobamate therapy.

Case 1. A 45-year-old stockbroker was seen in consultation because of a constant feeling of uncertainty, apprehension, and phobias of 3 months' duration. Difficulty falling asleep and frequent interruptions during the night were prominent. He became intensely anxious in crowded places and small rooms. His symptoms were severe enough to force him to curtail his social activities, and at times he was unable to attend important business conferences. The major precipitating factor for his condition, as it later developed, was the onset of puberty in his adolescent son, whom he consciously loved deeply but with whom he was unconsciously competitive.

At the age of 25, shortly after his marriage, he experienced a similar anxiety psychoneurotic reaction. These symptoms did not significantly interfere with his life adjustment until 10 years later. Then, at age 35, he entered psychotherapy. After 18 months of treatment his condition was markedly improved, and he remained relatively free of symptoms until the present illness.

He was readily able to recognize the nature of his current state but was not aware of the unconscious factors contributing to it. He was placed on meprobamate, 400 mg three times daily and 800 mg at bedtime, for 1 week. Thereafter the dose was reduced to 400 mg as needed in situations likely to precipitate anxiety experiences. Within a few days he was practically free of anxiety. His sleep pattern improved markedly. He was able to resume his normal social and business activities. He was seen twice weekly in psychotherapy and in a dozen sessions he had realized and worked through the underlying dynamic conflicts. Within 1 month meprobamate was eliminated entirely, and the patient remained essentially free of his anxiety.

This patient illustrates a psychoneurotic reaction in which generalized anxiety and specific phobias constituted the central psychopathologic features interfering with his life adjustment. Meprobamate strikingly reduced the anxiety, allowing him to resume his normal activities. For many reasons, including his keen analytic mind and his previous psychotherapeutic experiences, he was able to utilize successfully a limited number of sessions to evaluate and resolve the conflicts giving rise to his reaction.

In any patient of this age group, however, one must always be cautious lest a more serious psychopathologic state lies hidden behind the manifest psychoneurotic symptoms. Although it is reported that meprobamate does not induce the type of mood depression seen with reserpine, this drug may prematurely remove anxiety serving a protective function and facilitate the emergence of a more severe reaction. The following case illustrates such a situation.

Case 2. A 39-year-old housewife, in the setting of domestic difficulties with her husband and in-laws, suddenly developed severe tension and anxiety, characterized by headaches and painful rigidity of neck muscles; fears of losing her mind or becoming incapacitated to a degree which would prevent her from caring for her home; and nausea, vomiting, and anorexia with an associated weight loss of 10 lb in only 3 weeks. Occasionally she felt low and sad, but no well-defined alteration in mood could be established in the initial interviews. She would lie in bed for several hours before falling asleep and would awaken frequently during the night, occasionally recalling nightmares.

Prochlorperazine was instituted in doses of 40 mg daily, with no significant alleviation of her symptoms. This medication was terminated after 2 weeks and replaced by meprobamate, 400 mg four times daily. Within 24 hours a striking improvement in her condition occurred. Anxiety and tension decreased. Her headaches, muscular tightness, and gastrointestinal distress were alleviated. During the next month she was seen twice weekly in psychotherapy. Sensitive dynamic material discussed in interviews was rapidly incorporated into a basic self-depreciatory attitude. Feelings of hopelessness and futility became increasingly apparent. Guilt attached to adolescent and early adult sexual indiscretions emerged, and the patient ignored reassurance and attempts to divert the discussions along more constructive avenues. When strong suicidal urges were revealed, hospitalization was arranged to allow the continuation of psychotherapy.

There are two very interesting aspects to this patient's clinical response to meprobamate. First, meprobamate succeeded in reducing anxiety and tension after prochlorperazine had failed to do so. Secondly, it is not uncommon for patients of this age group to present symptoms of anxiety and tension which mask the development of more severe psychopathologic states, such as depressive or paranoid reactions. The abrupt removal of her psychoneurotic symptoms seemed to strip away the outer layer of her illness, allowing the depression to emerge more clearly. Moreover, in order to understand these changes, it is important to recall the complex nature of psychoneurotic anxiety symptoms which not only protect the patient against an awareness of underlying conflicts, but also provide a means for the expression of forbidden emotions and the acquisition of pathologic satisfaction. In this patient, guilt regarding unconscious hostility directed toward her sick and aging mother constituted a leading dynamic factor. In martyrlike fashion, the patient was able to express this hostility to her mother by repeatedly complaining of distress and requesting reassurance which her mother was in no position to give. Furthermore, her symptoms secured for her considerable sympathy and understanding from her husband and children, who had previously paid little attention to her personal needs. The action of the physician in administering meprobamate and robbing the patient of her suffering undoubtedly stirred more unconscious resentment within her, forcing her to seek an even more pathologic level of adjustment. Early recognition of the depressive mood facilitated hospitalization and sound medical management.

In addition to being useful in the control of persistent or phobic anxiety and tension, meprobamate is also effective in the management of acute anxiety attacks. These may last for minutes or hours and are characterized by intense apprehension, ordinarily lacking any specific precipitating object which the patient can recognize and often associated with autonomic physiologic concomitants of anxiety.

Case 3. Six weeks prior to consultation, a 34-year-old electrician suddenly awoke in the middle of the night perspiring profusely, with heart racing, intensely apprehensive but unaware of any disturbing dream or event of the previous day sufficient to account for such a reaction. This attack lasted for 2 hours. As is often the case, the patient was afraid that he might have had a heart attack. However, after his family physician had made a careful examination and had reassured the patient that no organic disease was present, he agreed to seek psychiatric attention. After the first few interviews, he again had a similar reaction. This time it occurred while he was driving to work, and he was forced to stop his car and rest for nearly an hour before the attack subsided and he was able to go on.

He was given 400-mg meprobamate tablets and advised to use them if his anxiety recurred. Several days later, while lunching with his co-workers, he had another attack. He promptly took 800 mg and within 30 minutes was free of the anxiety symptoms. This regimen was continued until, with further psychotherapy aimed at the resolution of pertinent unconscious conflicts, he was freed of his symptoms and the drug was no longer necessary.

Because of the infrequency of this patient's attacks and the fact that he was usually able to control his behavior while experiencing them, he was encouraged to use meprobamate only when required instead of being placed on a regular routine of medication. In another situation, where such attacks were more frequent or disabling, a regular regimen of meprobamate therapy might be more desirable.

In each of the examples thus far presented, anxiety and tension have been manifested in a direct manner. It will be recalled that pathologic anxiety may also be handled by the formation of complex psychoneurotic symptoms, such as dissociative phenomena, obsessions, and compulsions. In such instances, meprobamate is not influential in alleviating the clinical condition. The following case illustrates this point.

Case 4. A 32-year-old physician sought psychiatric help because of severe obsessive ruminations about his career and personal life. During ward rounds, he would be preoccupied with doubts about the adequacy of his clinical judgment, which was, in fact, superior to that of many of his colleagues. When dating women in whom he was interested, he would be besieged by thoughts of being weak and unmanly. This condition first appeared following graduation from college, but it did not seriously interfere with his life until 3 months before the initiation of treatment, during the final year of his residency and shortly after his engagement had been formally announced.

In order to alleviate his anxiety, meprobamate was administered in doses of 400 to 800 mg four times daily. The drug was continued for 4 weeks. Although there may have been a slight decrease in the tension and pressure of speech which the patient manifested in interviews, he obtained little or no freedom from his obsessions. The drug was then terminated and intensive psychotherapy continued.

This patient experienced well-defined obsessions in dynamically significant situations. At other times he was relatively free of symptoms. Neither sleep nor appetite was unduly affected. The administration of meprobamate provided no relief from his psychopathologic state. Meprobamate is also ineffective in dissociative states, such as hysterical paralysis or amnesia, in which conscious anxiety has been largely replaced by physical or psychologic symptoms.

ANXIETY IN OTHER DIAGNOSTIC SETTINGS

In addition to benefiting conditions in which anxiety and tension are central features, meprobamate may also be used in a more limited manner to alleviate these features in schizophrenic or depressive states. Although phenothiazines appear to be much more effective in reducing the agitation which often accompanies depression of mood, particularly when hostile emotions contribute significantly to the patient's restlessness, meprobamate may occasionally be preferred for the control of anxiety-driven overactivity. The following case illustrates such an application of meprobamate.

Case 5. A 48-year-old teacher presented a 3-week history of severe depression of mood with suicidal impulses, early morning awakening, anorexia, and a 10-lb weight loss. He was severely anxious, with marked restlessness, insomnia, profuse perspiration, and many fears regarding his physical and mental health. Tension was experienced as pressure on the back of his skull and continuous tightness in his chest. This psychopathologic reaction, precipitated by the death of a younger brother, occurred in the setting of a 15-year history of moderate anxiety, tension, and hypochondriasis which had not previously interfered with his life adjustment and for which he had never sought treatment.

In the hospital, he was eventually placed on 800 mg meprobamate four times daily. No change in his hopelessness or futility was noted. However, overactivity was reduced. His tension was distinctly relieved, and his concentration and sleep improved substantially. He was able to take part in social and rehabilitative activities. In psychotherapeutic sessions he was less preoccupied with morbid topics. Meprobamate was terminated after 2 months, and his anxiety and tension did not return. It was then necessary to administer eight ECTs to relieve the depression of mood.

In this patient, anxiety and tension significantly complicated a depressive reaction. As a result, concentration was impaired, social activities were disrupted, and the patient was driven to focus his attention on his depressive state. Anxiety intensified his suffering and obstructed psychotherapeutic efforts. There was no evidence of overt pathologic hostility, sexual unrest, or paranoid features, any of which would have been an indication for phenothiazine therapy. The use of meprobamate to alleviate his anxiety and tension allowed dynamic investigations to be carried out before the administration of electroconvulsive therapy.

In a similar manner, meprobamate may be of limited usefulness in the management of patients with chronic alcoholism, in whom anxiety and tension appear to increase the tendency to drink.

Case 6. When first seen for treatment, a 43-year-old married engineer presented a 5-year history of heavy alcohol intake. He would become markedly intoxicated every few weeks. He experienced several black-out reactions. Attempts to reduce the amount of alcohol consumed or to eliminate it completely failed entirely. He was threatened with loss of employment and divorce unless he corrected his condition. During the first few sessions, resistance to therapy was prominent. He continually expressed marked resentment toward his family, his employers, the referring physician, and the psychiatrist. He adamantly refused hospitalization. Prochlorperazine was instituted, the patient receiving 10 mg four times daily. Within 48 hours a striking decrease in resentment occurred. The drug was continued for 2 weeks and then terminated without a return of hostile emotions. However, he continued to appear tense, complaining of "shakiness and nervousness," and he strongly desired to use alcohol to alleviate these symptoms. He was placed on meprobamate, 400 mg four times daily. Within several days, the patient reported a substantial decrease in anxiety and tension. Although the impulse to drink was still present, the patient felt better able to resist this urge when it occurred. He was better able to control his emotions and worked constructively to improve his relationship with his business associates and family. During the ensuing months of treatment several episodes of intoxication occurred. Nonetheless, the patient was encouraged by the signs of progress in his therapy. He finally accepted the fact that he was an alcoholic and agreed to join Alcoholics Anonymous to facilitate his rehabilitation.

This patient illustrates the effective use of meprobamate to reduce anxiety and tension which, in this case, increased the intensity of his desires for alcohol and decreased his ability to resist such urges. The contrast between the influence of prochlorperazine, a phenothiazine derivative, and meprobamate is well exemplified. Prochlorperazine substantially reduced the profound hostility of the patient, but anxiety and tension remained unaffected until meprobamate was instituted.

In certain schizophrenic patients, meprobamate seems to be helpful in reducing anxiety and tension; in others, it produces little clinical change. This observation seems to substantiate the impression that anxiety in many schizophrenic patients is biologically different from psychoneurotic anxiety, although the manifestations may be superficially similar. Meprobamate is often ineffective in relieving anxiety in many schizophrenic patients of the pseudoneurotic type, even though this pathologic emotion appears to be a very prominent feature of the condition.

Meprobamate versus Barbiturates

Meprobamate seems most effective in reducing anxiety when the pathologic emotion is associated with tension. In patients in whom anxiety exists without prominent tension, barbiturates may be superior in relieving the disturbing emotion.

Case 7. A 27-year-old insurance salesman entered psychotherapy for the relief of frequent and often persistent feelings of anxiety. His apprehension was intensified by new situations, such as meeting clients or attending unfamiliar social activities. When anxious, he would perspire freely, develop nausea and anorexia, and have difficulty in concentration. He had no difficulty falling asleep but would awaken often during the night. His pulse was usually elevated, ranging from 90 to 110 beats per minute. In spite of his distress, he presented no subjective complaints of tension and usually assumed a relaxed posture. Only the worried expression of his face betrayed his inner distress. Rather than force himself to face traumatic situations, he tended to withdraw from them until his anxiety decreased. Little effort was made to hide his emotions or disability from his family, his friends, or the physician.

He was begun on meprobamate, 400 mg four times daily. After 1 week, when no significant change was noted, this was increased to 800 mg four times daily. The drug was continued for another 3 weeks, but no substantial improvement occurred. Meprobamate was discontinued, and the patient was given 30 mg phenobarbital three times daily and 60 mg at bedtime. Within 3 days he reported a distinct reduction in the frequency and intensity of his anxiety and the restoration of uninterrupted sleep. His self-confidence was enhanced, and his utilization of psychotherapeutic interviews improved. The regular use of barbiturates was terminated after 3 weeks. Thereafter the medication was used only when indicated by the presence of strong anxiety. With further psychotherapeutic progress, the drug was eventually abandoned altogether.

Although meprobamate and barbiturates may often be used interchangeably, there do seem to be some differences in the actual effects of these drugs in certain patients. The following case also illustrates such differences.

Case 8. A 24-year-old graduate student experienced marked anxiety during the early phases of psychotherapy. This anxiety impaired his ability to associate freely, to communicate his emotions, and to respond to interpretations offered by the therapist. He described an almost constant state of apprehension and uncertainty, lacking any well-defined object. Palpitations and profuse sweating of the forehead and hands were prominent concomitants of his anxiety. In order to facilitate psychotherapy and increase his ability to study, he was placed on phenobarbital, 30 mg three times daily. A striking reduction in anxiety occurred. His concentration improved, and his participation in treatment was enhanced. This regimen was continued for nearly 3 months, at which time it was possible to omit phenobarbital completely.

In spite of the observable improvement, there were still many situations which would produce marked tension in the patient. These were realistically stressful, such as angry telephone calls from his domineering father, unexpected school assignments which could be completed in the required time only with great effort, and learning that his girl friend was contemplating marriage to another suitor. In each instance he would feel muscular tautness and fatigue. His concentration would be impaired, and he would find it difficult to fall asleep at night. Irritability and impatience with himself only tended to aggravate his condition. The maintenance dose of phenobarbital did not protect him from these repeated disturbances. However, the use of 400 mg meprobamate at these times effectively reduced his tension and permitted him to continue his work productively.

In this example, barbiturates were very effective in reducing the patient's generalized feeling of uncertainty and apprehension, but meprobamate was superior in controlling tension resulting from real external conflicting situations.

The question of whether meprobamate possesses any significant advantages over the barbiturates is of more than speculative interest. The cost of the former drug to the patient is many times that of phenobarbital, for example, and there is little justification for putting the patient to such an expense unless it is warranted. Meprobamate appears to be a safer drug in patients who are potentially suicidal, since large amounts can be tolerated without necessarily leading to death. However, a few serious cases of coma and vasomotor collapse have been reported following the ingestion of massive amounts of meprobamate. Moreover, meprobamate, because it can relax voluntary musculature, may indeed be more effective in alleviating tension characterized by muscular rigidity, tightness, or pain. Ordinarily it seems more prudent to use barbiturates for a week or two on a trial basis prior to the initiation of meprobamate therapy, unless specific contraindications exist. The occurrence of barbiturate habituation is well established. There are reports which suggest that pathologic dependency on meprobamate may also occur. The dynamic factors contributing to habituation, after all, exist within the sensitive patient more than within the molecules of the medication.

Meprobamate versus Phenothiazines

When anxiety and tension occur in combination, the indications for meprobamate may be clearly defined. However, when these features are also associated with pathologic hostility or sexual unrest, one must choose between meprobamate and the phenothiazines. It is often difficult to determine the relative prominence of these pathologic emotions. The tense patient may be irritable. The angry patient may be anxious because of the depth and consequences of his hostility. The sexually aroused patient may also manifest anxiety or hostility, or both. The physician may be hard pressed at times to decide what the fundamental changes in emotions actually are. When such a complex picture is present, it is judicious to use phenothiazines first, assuming that pharmacologic therapy is indicated, since these compounds possess a broader spectrum of action in various psychopathologic states. Moreover, the consequences of intense hostility or sexual unrest are often more detrimental to the patient's social adjustment and participation in therapy than those of anxiety and tension. The administration of a phenothiazine derivative may not have to be continued for more than a few weeks. Thereafter, if anxiety and tension are still present and somatic intervention is indicated, barbiturates or meprobamate may be substituted to reduce these features. The following case illustrates this treatment regimen.

Case 9. A 42-year-old married woman began intensive psychotherapy for the relief of acute anxiety attacks and a fear of developing a serious physical disorder which might lead to sudden death. These symptoms occasionally reached great intensity, interfering with concentration, sleep, and appetite. Prior to psychiatric consultation, her internist had placed her on 400 mg meprobamate four times daily, with very slight improvement. In the initial interview, it was apparent that, in addition to her anxiety and tension, the patient manifested sexual unrest in her flirtatious, erotic gestures and expressed marked resentment toward various family members. She angrily proclaimed her doubts about the need for psychotherapy. Prochlorperazine was instituted in doses of 5 mg four times daily, replacing meprobamate. Within 48 hours a definite improvement in her condition occurred. Pathologic hostility and sexual unrest disappeared. Her resistance to treatment decreased, and her motivation for psychotherapy was enhanced. Tension and anxiety were still present but not to a disturbing degree. The phenothiazine derivative was terminated after 3 weeks, with no recurrence of her original state. She was seen 3 times weekly in psychotherapy. During the seventh month of treatment, anxiety and tension increased markedly in the setting of analysis of sensitive dynamic material. Sleep was impaired. It was difficult for her to concentrate and attend to her household responsibilities. No evidence of sexual unrest or hostility was present. Meprobamate was instituted in doses of 400 mg four times daily. Within several hours after the initial dose she began to feel better, and within 2 days her anxiety, tension, and related symptoms had entirely disappeared. This drug was continued for 10 days, then terminated, and no longer required.

In this patient meprobamate was of little value when sexual unrest and pathologic hostility were associated with anxiety and tension. This combination of factors responded well to a phenothiazine derivative. Many months later, the patient again experienced intense anxiety and tension, but without sexual or hostile features. Meprobamate was again instituted, this time with very satisfactory results.

Meprobamate has also been used in the management of tension, anxiety, and overactivity in children, but it does not appear to possess any demonstrable superiority to the barbiturates or diphenhydramine.

SUMMARY

Meprobamate is an effective agent in the reduction of pathologic anxiety, particularly when this emotion is associated with tension. In this regard, its activity resembles that of the barbiturates and rauwolfia derivatives. In many situations it possesses no significant advantage over the less costly barbiturates. Although it lacks the potent sedative effects of reserpine in markedly disturbed patients, it is clearly easier to use, freer of undesirable side effects, and actually more effective than reserpine in the management of anxiety and tension as seen in many psychoneurotic conditions. The phenothiazine drugs reduce sexual unrest, hostility, and associated psychopathologic symptoms. Meprobamate does not. However, it is often superior to phenothiazine derivatives in the treatment of patients with anxiety and tension.

10

ELECTROCONVULSIVE TREATMENT

A score of years has now passed since the introduction of electro-convulsive treatment in the field of psychiatric treatment. During this period, ECT has gained world-wide recognition as an effective means of managing certain psychiatric illnesses. A large body of knowledge has been accumulated on the effectiveness of ECT, and innumerable modifications on the method have been created. Despite all this activity, however, the exact mechanism of action of ECT remains unclear. Perhaps as a result of this lack of understanding, efforts at integrating ECT with psychotherapeutic methods of treatment have been few and far between. All too frequently, the treatment of psychiatric illnesses becomes involved in the question of ECT versus psychotherapy, and the benefits of one of the two approaches are frequently lost in the resulting unilateral decision.

While this lack of clarity is understandable, it is clearly undesirable. In the succeeding pages, an attempt will be made to clarify some of the ways in which ECT can be incorporated into an over-all plan of psychotherapeutic treatment of psychiatric illnesses.

MECHANISM OF ACTION

It is known that about 400 to 500 ma. of current passes through the brain in the course of each ECT. In all probability, this current passes along the major neuronal pathways. Perhaps as a result of this knowledge, the effectiveness of ECT is frequently attributed to damage which it produces in the brain. Despite the fact that electroencephalographic studies indicate the possibility of damage, the evidence for histologic damage is slender. Some findings indicate that the effectiveness of ECT is linked to the susceptibility of the brain to toxic damage, but this possible relationship is far from causal.

On the other hand, there is considerable knowledge which indicates that the therapeutic effectiveness of ECT must be something more specific than just the toxic effect of the electricity. It is, of course, well recognized that simple destruction of brain tissue does not relieve emotional situations. In addition, clinical experience indicates that "missed" convulsions, i.e., those in which a grand mal seizure does not follow the administration of electricity, produce greater amounts of memory difficulty and confusion and greater amounts of electroencephalographic change, but do not produce a therapeutic effect. The convulsive episode appears to be essential if ECT is to benefit the patient.

This suggestion of the specificity of the convulsion for therapeutic effect is supported by several factors. The therapeutic effect, for example, can be produced by Metrazol, which does not produce the electrical damage associated with ECT but does produce the convulsion. Furthermore, psychologic tests indicate that there is marked similarity in specific features between the postconvulsive psychopathologic state in epilepsy and that in electrically induced convulsions. It appears worthwhile, therefore, to seek some specific mechanism for the therapeutic effectiveness of ECT and to consider that this specificity may well lie in its convulsion-producing properties.

METHOD OF ADMINISTRATION

The classical method of administration of ECT is a simple one. The patient is prepared by the subcutaneous injection of 0.0006 Gm atropine sulfate three-quarters of an hour prior to the treatment, in order to control salivation. At the time of treatment, he is placed on a specially constructed table, or on a bed which is supported by bedboards, in a reclining position. His body is placed in dorsal extension by a sandbag placed under the dorsal vertebrae or by the construction of the table. Pillows are placed between the patient's knees to cushion his movements, and attendants are available to modify the movements of the extremities during the treatment. The patient's temples are prepared by the application of suitable electrode jelly, electrodes are attached at the level of the coronal suture, and a rubber mouth gag is placed between the teeth. The physician in charge places his hand firmly under the patient's chin, and the dose of electricity is administered. The usual amount of electricity is 100 to 160 v of alternating (60 cycle) current which is administered for 0.1 to 0.6 second. The amount and duration of the treatment are controlled in a number of standard electroconvulsive machines.

Immediately following the application of the current, the patient enters a state of extreme tonus, frequently with a cry. There is marked sudden dorsal hyperextension, which lasts approximately 10 seconds. Gradually the rigidity and the hyperextension fade off into clonic movements. These are initially mild and rapid, but gradually become slower and more and more profound over the following 40 seconds, at which time they generally cease. During the period of this convulsion, the physician prevents dislocation of the jaw and swallowing of the tongue, and other attendants prevent mechanical injury to the extremities which might result from the patient's uncontrolled movements. Following the cessation of clonic movements, the patient is placed on his side and allowed to recover in a comfortable and quiet situation. There is usually marked confusion and amnesia for a period of 20 to 30 minutes, after which the patient can be allowed to resume normal activities, according to his physical condition.

A number of modifications of this classic routine for the administration of ECT have been suggested. Infrequently, modifications of the basic position have been recommended. More frequently, there have been suggestions for the modification of the current applied to the patient. These modifications have included the administration of subliminal amounts, unidirectional current, brief stimulus therapy, glissando technique, and electrostimulation. Under certain situations, there is undoubtedly a need for many of these modifications. Their application to the general use of ECT, however, appears to be limited.

A second type of modification which has been suggested is the use of sedatives and anesthetics in conjunction with ECT. Many physicians use Sodium Amytal or Pentothal Sodium in order to reduce the patient's fear and anxiety and to control postconvulsive excitement. It seems advisable to hold the use of these drugs to a minimum, in order to prevent the complications which result from the addition of medications to an otherwise straightforward treatment.

A third type of modification which has been developed since 1945 is the use of muscle relaxants in conjunction with ECT. Through the use of these relaxants, the danger of fractures and mechanical injury can be markedly decreased, and the stresses placed on the patient's respiratory and cardiovascular system can be markedly reduced. The use of curare and tubocurarine appears to be effective but fraught with hazard. Since 1955, however, synthetic muscle relaxants have been developed, of which the best appears to be succinylcholine. This rapidly acting muscle relaxant can be administered intravenously immediately prior to treatment and produces muscular relaxation for a period of 1 to 3 minutes; the dosage level can be adjusted to give moderate relaxation or complete immobility. As a result, its use, together with suitable anesthetic agents, is widespread. Muscle relaxants are now generally used in cases in which there is evidence of recent fracture, osteoporosis, coronary artery disease, a history of cardiovascular or respiratory difficulties, or any other indications that the convulsion might injure the patient's physical well-being. When muscle relaxants are used in conjunction with ECT, 90 per cent oxygen is administered by mask prior to the onset of the effective medication, and forced respiration must be carried on while the patient is paralyzed.

The use of 90 per cent oxygen without muscle relaxants has been widely recommended. If oxygen is administered by mask for a period of 4 to 5 minutes prior to the ECT and for another 5 minutes after the convulsion, the oxygen saturation of the blood remains much higher than otherwise and presumable damage to the central nervous system is minimized. In many institutions, the use of oxygen in this fashion is now routine.

Course of Treatment

Three courses of treatment are commonly used at the present time. The most commonly used course of treatment is that involving *standard frequency*. In this frequency pattern, ECT is administered two or three times a week for the duration of a course of treatment. The duration of such a course of treatment would usually average about 8 treatments when depressive illnesses are involved and about 15 to 20 treatments when chronic schizophrenic and paranoid illnesses are involved.

A *rapid course* of treatment involves the administration of ECT once or twice a day for a period of several days. Such a course of treatment usually involves the administration of five to eight ECTs and is commonly used in the therapy of catatonic stupors. *Protracted treatment* is not commonly utilized; it is valuable, however, in the therapy of chronic disorders such as manic-depressive reactions. Under such circumstances, ECT is administered once or twice a month for a period of several years, in order to prevent relapse or recurrence of illness.

SIDE EFFECTS AND COMPLICATIONS

The most frequently observed side effects of ECT are those which are linked with the effect of the treatment on central nervous system function. After four ECTs, given at intervals of 2 or 3 days, it is found that most patients begin to show some memory difficulty. This difficulty involves a recent memory loss and, in early stages, is mild in degree. After 12 ECTs, recent memory loss is usually quite marked, and the patient is often found to have a marked amnesia for the period of treatment and for 1 and 2 months prior to the onset of treatment. At this time, also, confusion may be present, and the patient may have difficulty in understanding simple activity in the environment. By the time 20 ECTs have been administered, memory difficulty and confusion are usually very marked.

These clinical findings, which indicate the presence of physiologic changes, are mirrored by the development of electroencephalographic changes. After four ECTs, it is common to find some degree of cerebral dysrythymia, consisting of occasional bursts of high-voltage 4- to 6-cycles per second activity in the electroencephalogram. These changes become more profound as the number of treatments increases, and by the time 12 treatments have been given, there is usually a definitely abnormal pattern seen on the electroencephalogram. In addition to the high-voltage low activity previously described, there is found an occasional 3-cycles per second wave and some spikes.

Both the clinical and the electroencephalographic indications of physiologic alteration appear to be reversible. They are at their maximum immediately after any ECT and gradually disappear after a course of ECTs has been completed. By 6 months after the last ECT, it is usually impossible to elicit any signs of memory difficulty, and the patient's electroencephalogram has returned to normal. The fact that these changes are linked with the physical effects of ECT is indicated by the fact that they come on more rapidly, and are manifested in a more severe fashion, if the treatments are given more frequently; similarly, the greater the number of ECTs, the more profound the difficulties.

Another kind of side effect, probably psychologic in origin, consists of the appearance of fear and anxiety in connection with treatment. These emotions appear in few persons and are usually linked to personality characteristics. Rigidly organized persons, who depend for their security on excellent memory, meticulous attention to detail, and a constant need for a clear orientation in the environment, are those who experience increasing fear and anxiety as increasing numbers of treatments take place.

The most frequent complications of ECT are mechanical ones (Kalinowsky and Hoch, 1952). These consist, for the most part, of fractures and dislocations. The most common fracture which occurs during ECT is a compression fracture of the bodies of the dorsal vertebrae in the region of D7. Such compression fractures require no special treatment, aside from having the patient rest and sleep on a mattress supported by a bedboard. Other fractures and dislocations which occur in the course of treatment are usually related to injuries sustained in the course of the patient's movements during his convulsive episode.

Fatalities are rare with ECT, the reported incidence being in the neighborhood of 0.05 per cent. Such fatalities are usually linked to myocardial infarction or to respiratory failure; the latter is attributed to the central action of the electric current.

CLINICAL EFFECTIVENESS OF TREATMENT

The indications for ECT must be considered under two distinct headings. Firstly, it is necessary to determine that ECT will be effective in the psychopathologic condition requiring treatment. Secondly, it is imperative that the treatment be timed properly, in accordance with the state of the patient's illness and the stage of his psychotherapeutic progress.

Diagnostic Considerations

DEPRESSIVE REACTIONS

It is clear that there are several psychopathologic situations in which ECT will work effectively. From the most superficial standpoint, it is possible to approach this problem on a diagnostic basis. Considered in this fashion, it has long been known that ECT is most effective in the treatment of affective illnesses, such as depressions in middle or late life and manic-depressive depressions. In these conditions, if ECT is administered at the correct time, one may expect to produce improvement in 90 to 100 per cent of the patients treated. The usual course of treatment in such an illness consists of six to eight ECTs, with the maximal degree of improvement usually appearing after the third or fourth treatment and little or no improvement occurring after eight treatments. It is well recognized that the uniformity of responses in this group of illnesses is a highly specific one; in no other group of illnesses does ECT produce its effects as reliably and with as little evidence of organic damage. The following patient illustrates this very well.

Case 1. A 59-year-old white housewife was admitted to the hospital with a 3-month history of increasing depression with retardation, suspiciousness, fearfulness, fatigue, anorexia, insomnia, and a 10-lb weight loss. On admission, the patient demonstrated marked retardation and was occasionally unresponsive. She was fearful of all activities, with paranoid delusions about the behavior of other patients and staff. There was a fluctuating amount of suicidal ideation.

Two weeks after admission, the patient received eight ECTs, given two times per week. After the fourth ECT, there was a marked improvement in her mood and a disappearance of the paranoid ideation. By the eighth ECT, the depression had completely cleared, and the patient had returned to her previous level of adjustment.

This patient had a previous good life adjustment, and her depression had come on in the setting of aging and the departure of her children from the home. Given ECT, she recovered to her preillness state of adjustment and was able to see the stresses under which she had fallen ill and to adapt to the realistic situation in which she found herself. Psychotherapy was limited to efforts of a supportive nature in this instance. The patient has done well for 3 years subsequent to her hospitalization, without any further psychotherapy.

Even within the group of depressions, the results achieved with ECT will be only temporary if the dynamic situation is unfavorable. This is dramatically illustrated in the following example of a patient with a manic-depressive reaction.

Case 2. A 56-year-old white writer was admitted to the hospital with a 2-year history of increasing depression associated with feelings of guilt and fatigue, mounting feelings of inadequacy, and a 6-month inability to work. During the 6 months immediately preceding admission, the patient had suicidal ideation, anorexia, with a 20-lb weight loss, and almost total insomnia.

This patient was born in Iowa, completed a university education with honors, and had achieved a considerable reputation as an editor of literary magazines. In his work and in his social and family relationships, he had always been an aggressive, unyielding, demanding, and authoritative figure. His depression occurred in the setting of his increasing awareness of the resentment that those close to him felt toward his domineering attitudes, on which his success had always hinged.

On admission to the hospital, the patient displayed marked depression, with feelings of hopelessness and suicidal ideation. He had intense resentment toward all the persons in his environment, and this soon became a central focus of the therapeutic relationship. His attitude toward therapy was sardonic, critical, and sarcastic. A great deal of dynamic material of an infantile nature was explored, and although the patient saw the reflections of his need to win approval in his active striving for success in life, he remained unable to use any approach other than an aggressive one in dealings with other persons. Similarly, in interviews, new material was used to fan the flames of the patient's hostility. After 8 months of hospitalization, the depression continued unabated, with continuing suicidal drive. Because of the long duration of the illness and the failure of psychotherapy, ECT was administered. The patient received eight ECTs, administered two times per week. His depression cleared rapidly after the fourth ECT and was completely dissipated by the time he had received eight ECTs. Within 2 weeks after the termination of the treatment, however, his symptoms returned in full force, and he resumed his severe, suicidal depression. Continuing analysis over the next 5 months did nothing to relieve the depression or the persistent hostility, and it was necessary to transfer him for chronic hospitalization, after 13 months in the hospital.

Case 2, with a diagnosis of a manic-depressive reaction, illustrates two factors which mitigate against the success of ECT in the treatment of depressive reactions. The first of these is the presence of marked hostility associated with the depression. When ECT is given in the presence of such a combination, the depressive elements in the picture will usually be relieved but will frequently return. The relationship between the hostility and this return is unclear, but it is a common clinical phenomenon. The second factor which Case 2 illustrates is that, when the patient's personality is a tightly integrated one and when it has contributed to the onset of the illness, changes in the personality adaptation must be achieved if the benefits of treatment are to be lasting. When such personality change has not been achieved, the symptomatic improvement achieved by ECT is likely to be lost, as the patient resumes his life. In Case 2, both these unfavorable factors were present, and the patient displayed a classical, almost immediate, return to his severest level of symptomatology.

MANIC AND CATATONIC EXCITEMENTS

The second diagnostic indication for ECT is in the treatment of excitements, both manic and catatonic. In these conditions, rapid administration of ECT is usually necessary, with ECTs being administered at the rate of one or two a day. After three to five such treatments, the excitement will have subsided. One may expect an initial improvement rate of 95 to 100 per cent in these conditions; such results, however, are temporary in nature. If the course of the illness is a chronic one or a recurrent one and if psychotherapeutic progress is not considerable, these illnesses will frequently recur. The effectiveness of treatment diminishes markedly with each recurrence of illness; with the second, third, and succeeding episodes of excitement, it becomes necessary to use larger and larger numbers of ECTs in order to bring the excitement under control, and the amount of control becomes increasingly smaller. Case 3 illustrates the effectiveness of ECT in the treatment of a manic excitement.

Case 3. A 30-year-old white secretary was admitted to the hospital with a 5-week history of increasing overactivity, overeating, restlessness, irritability, sexual unrest, hostility, eroticism, sexual delusions, and assaultiveness. Born to a poor family, she had attended parochial schools and had then entered secretarial work. Married at age 24, she had had a satisfactory marital adjustment, but no children. The over-all pattern of her personality adjustment had been one of activity and moderate aggressiveness until the onset of the present illness.

On admission, the patient remained erotic and markedly excited. Her behavior was characterized by exposure, masturbation, and sexual approaches to both male and female patients and staff. She did not sleep, was continually moving, and displayed flight of ideas. Two weeks after admission, she was given a course of ECTs, receiving three ECTs on successive days and three more ECTs at 3-day intervals. By the third ECT, the patient was markedly less excited and erotic, and she had returned to a normal behavioral pattern by the completion of the sixth ECT. Subsequently, she talked of the origin of her sexual outburst, revealing many details of her unsatisfactory sexual life. She felt marked guilt about her lack of children and maintained an ambivalent relationship with her husband, condemning him for his passivity and yet dominating him in all their interrelationships. As this material was analyzed, the patient was able to achieve a more open relationship with her husband and was discharged to continue psychotherapy on an ambulatory basis. She has continued to do well for 3 years following discharge from the hospital.

CATATONIC STUPORS

The same pattern of improvement applies in the treatment of catatonic stupors. In these conditions, the initial stuporous condition may be relieved by three to five ECTs. Such ECTs may be administered at the usual rate of two or three times a week or may be administered daily. Almost all such patients show rapid improvement as the immediate effect of treatment. Once more, however, recurrences of the stuporous condition augur for less effective treatment with each succeeding recurrence.

SCHIZOPHRENIC REACTIONS

Schizophrenic reactions, apart from the catatonic type of reaction, do not usually respond well to ECT. Moderate or mild improvement is usually seen in approximately 70 per cent of these illnesses, but such results may be obtained by many other forms of treatment. Moreover, it is characteristic that the reactions which respond most favorably are those with strong affective components. The usual course of treatment in these illnesses is 12 to 20 ECTs. There is much to suggest that the therapeutic effectiveness of ECT in these disorders is not the result of a specific action, as it is in the treatment of affective disorders. Instead, it would appear that the therapeutic effectiveness of ECT in schizophrenic reactions is secondary to its destructive effect in breaking up fixed patterns of behavior and thinking. Through this destructive effect, the fixed pathologic situation of the patient becomes more amenable to psychotherapeutic intervention and modification. The eventual outcome, therefore, appears to depend on how successful the psychotherapeutic management is; if the psychotherapy can alter the patient's patterns after ECT has broken them up, the eventual outcome is likely to be good. The following case illustrates its effectiveness in breaking up patterns of thinking and behavior.

Case 4. A 25-year-old female editorial assistant was admitted to the hospital with a 1-month history of withdrawal from her normal social environment, deteriorated life in the Greenwich Village section of New York, inability to concentrate or carry on in her work, increasing delusional thinking, and increasing depression, culminating in a suicidal attempt 4 days prior to admission.

Born to an Indian family, the patient had been raised as the only Indian in an all-white community. She was very close to her quiet but fiery father and had adopted a tomboy role to win her battle for his affections with her sister. She did well in public school and college, graduating with a bachelor's degree at age 22. Subsequently, she had worked for a number of magazines in editorial positions and, 2 years prior to admission, had left home to live in New York City. Eighteen months prior to admission, she had entered into a complex sexual relationship with a dependent young man and had become increasingly ambivalent about the moral and sexual elements in this relationship. In the hospital, she remained markedly withdrawn and negativistic, curling up on her bed, speaking only in a low voice, and demanding an infantile type of attention from the staff and from other patients. She was continually preoccupied with suicide and made many feeble gestures, by slashing her wrists. On the occasions when she would enter into social activities and begin to be active with other persons, she rapidly entered into close relationships with young female patients, in which relationships she consistently displayed a strong homosexual drive. Periodically, she would become very hostile and negativistic toward the therapist, refusing to speak for four to five interviews at a stretch. Over a period of 5 months, the interview material yielded a large amount of exploratory and explanatory material, with the patient readily seeing the dynamic origins of her present behavior. There was no alteration in the pattern of her dealing with this behavior, however, which remained ruminative and autistic and which was associated with depressive affect. Because of the rut formation and the persistence of the autistic withdrawal, in addition to the depression, the patient was started on ECT in the sixth month of her hospitalization. Over the subsequent weeks, she received 14 ECTs given twice a week. Gradually her mood improved, and suicidal drive diminished. By the administration of the tenth ECT, there was a marked interruption of her previously consistent pattern of withdrawal. She became active and energetic, entering into a wide variety of social relationships. Her activity was not ideally organized, but she saw it as an exploration of new means of adjusting to other persons. Following the conclusion of ECT, she remained in the hospital for 2 months, gradually accepting the need to adopt a coherent pattern of existence. She was discharged from the hospital at that time and has remained well, while continuing in psychotherapy, for 1½ years after discharge.

This case, as has been indicated, illustrates a dual use of ECT in the setting of a simple schizophrenic reaction. Firstly, the disruptive effects of large amounts of ECT were used to break up the patient's rutlike pattern of behavior. This aim was accomplished satisfactorily, so that the psychotherapist was able to lead the patient to new and better methods of organizing her behavior. Secondly, ECT was given to terminate the depressive elements of the illness. This aim was accomplished with the first 7 or 8 ECTs, but its effect was not completely beneficial until the disruptive effect of ECT had taken place, after 10 ECTs.

PARANOID STATES

Paranoid states and paranoid reactions, like schizophrenic reactions, tend to respond well only to large numbers of ECTs, between 12 and 20. Improvement does not occur at the early stages of the course of treatment but rather tends to appear gradually after 10 treatments, and the permanence of good results depends on the efficacy of the psychotherapy which is being carried out. The following case material illustrates the utilization of ECT in the paranoid situation and once more illustrates the associated relief of depressive elements which can be produced by ECT.

Case 5. A 39-year-old white married housewife was admitted to the hospital with a 10-year history of anxiety, tension, and feelings of inadequacy. Over the year immediately prior to her admission to the hospital, the anxiety had grown much worse, with paranoid delusions of persecution by various members of her family, suicidal ideation associated with depression, and delusional body concern. In the hospital, her suffering was relieved with the use of chlorpromazine, and she proceeded to describe her feelings of sexual confusion, doubts about her parenthood, hostility and ambivalence with regard to both parents, her paranoid feeling of responsibility for deaths in her family, and her grandiose delusions of responsibility for all evil in the world. On the termination of chlorpromazine treatment, 4 months later, the patient had satisfactory amounts of understanding of her illness, but was unable to change her previous methods of adjustment. An analysis of associated features revealed depression, fear, anxiety, and agitation. Accordingly, the patient was begun on ECT and received a total of 12 ECTs, at a frequency of two per week. Just as in Case 4, the depressive elements in the illness were relieved after 8 ECTs, and the patient began to experiment with new methods of adaptation after she had completed 12 ECTs. She remained in the hospital for 1½ months following the completion of ECT and was discharged at that time. She has continued to do well for 2 years.

In this chronic schizophrenic illness, paranoid type, we see an effect of ECT which parallels that in a chronic simple schizophrenic illness in Case 4. Once more, the primary effectiveness of ECT was demonstrated in its relief of depression. Again, the disruptive effects of ECT were used to alter the patient's habitual pattern of adaptation and were successful in achieving this end.

PSYCHONEUROTIC REACTIONS

Most psychoneurotic reactions do not respond favorably to ECT. Patients with such reactions usually respond with considerable anxiety and fear and frequently with an exaggeration of the psychoneurotic defense mechanisms which they characteristically use. Psychoneurotic depressive reactions, on the other hand, frequently respond favorably, so far as their depression is concerned. It is common to obtain an improvement in 90 per cent of such patients. This improvement, however, is localized to the area of their depressive affect. The result of treatment is usually that the psychoneurotic patient feels more hopeful and less depressed and is therefore more capable of handling the underlying psychoneurotic illness than he was prior to the administration of ECT.

The following case material illustrates the use of ECT in a long-standing psychoneurotic illness. It also illustrates the over-all ineffectiveness of ECT if it is not used on the basis of satisfactory psychotherapeutic progress.

Case 6. A 50-year-old white married housewife, with no children, was admitted to the hospital with a 25-year history of intermittent depression. Born of Russian immigrant parents, she had attended public school and teacher's school and then had continued teaching until 2 years prior to admission. In her adolescence and early adulthood, she was lonely and compulsive in behavior and had very few social relationships. She married a passive lawyer at age 29 in order to satisfy an urgent desire for married life and respectability, but she had a totally unsatisfactory sexual relationship, marked feelings of contempt for her husband, and anxiety in his presence. She had experienced four periods of depression, each lasting a year, over the preceding 25 years. In the intervals of relative well-being, her adjustment had been tenuous at best and marked by anxiety and compulsive mechanisms of defense. In the year immediately prior to her admission to the hospital, she had had nine ECTs in one course, six ECTs in a second course, and six ECTs in a third course, each producing a temporary improvement in spirits but followed within a week or two by a recurrence of her illness at its worst. In the hospital, she manifested anxiety, tension, compulsive concern about body and cleanliness, obsessive rumination about feelings of inadequacy and sexual difficulties with her husband, and suicidal ideation. She was placed in psychotherapeutic management for a period of 6 months in the hospital and successfully analyzed her lifelong masculine drives, relating them to her early parental relationships and to sibling rivalry. She saw clearly the reflections of this in her marital situation. Her depression remained intense, however, and it was necessary to administer ECT in the sixth month of hospitalization. The patient received seven ECTs at this time and was completely relieved of depression. She remained in the hospital 2 more months, applying the previously learned elements of psychodynamics, and had no recurrence of depression. She was discharged from the hospital at that time and has continued to do well for 1 year.

From a diagnostic viewpoint, therefore, it may be seen that ECT works most effectively in affective disorders, which include depressive reactions, manic-depressive reactions, and manic excitements. Its effectiveness is also marked in schizophrenic reactions of a catatonic type and in psychoneurotic reactions of a depressive type. Its effectiveness appears to be minimal in the treatment of other schizophrenic reactions and paranoid states, in which beneficial results are usually linked with the destructive action of ECT.

Associated Psychopathologic Situation

It is possible to go beyond diagnostic considerations in determining the indications for ECT. Apart from the diagnostic category into which a patient has been placed, the dynamic psychopathology which the patient displays can offer clues as to the possible effectiveness of the treatment. These dynamic psychopathologic features consist of the predominant emotions and symptomatology which the patient displays. Such dynamic features extend across diagnostic categories and offer a supplementary aid in determining the indications for the use of ECT (Regan, 1957). It has been found, for example, that patients whose predominant psychopathologic features consist of paranoid ideation, anxiety or agitation, fear, or marked sexual unrest are apt to respond well to ECT, 95 to 100 per cent of patients with these characteristics obtaining good results. Conversely, patients whose most prominent pathology consists of hostility, guilt, or marked body concern tend to respond unfavorably to ECT.

It is possible to improve the accuracy of indications for ECT by combining these two approaches, the diagnostic and the psychopathologic. By the use of such a method, it is found that affective illnesses which are associated with marked paranoid features, anxiety or agitation, fear, or sexual content tend to respond most favorably to the administration of ECT. On the contrary, any illness will tend to respond unfavorably if it is associated with hostility, guilt, or body concern. The percentage of patients with affective illnesses who are treated with ECT and who improve is virtually 100 per cent, if patients with unfavorable psychopathologic characteristics are excluded from such treatment. In the same fashion, significance of an unfavorable diagnostic category can be mitigated by the presence of associated favorable psychopathologic characteristics. Even simple schizophrenic reactions, which ordinarily have a favorable response in only 69 per cent of cases, respond with excellent results if fear is present. On the other hand, simple schizophrenic illnesses which are associated with anxiety respond much less favorably than the average of 69 per cent for the group.

The effectiveness of ECT in relieving depression which occurs in the setting of a schizophrenic reaction is illustrated well in the following case.

Case 7. A 21-year-old white student was admitted to the hospital with a 3-month history of increasing feelings of inadequacy, depression, preoccupation with his body, suicidal ideation, diminished concentration, withdrawal, and inability to continue with his college work. Born of a successful, domineering father and a kind, overprotective mother, the patient had always been active and popular until the completion of high school, at age 18. At that time, it was necessary for him to leave his native country and come to the United States for his college education. In this setting, he became increasingly shy, with feelings of strangeness, which would be relieved on his summer vacations at home. During the last of these summer vacations, however, 6 months before his admission to the hospital, he had felt himself to be rejected by his fiancée and had experienced feelings of sexual inadequacy; in this setting his illness began.

On admission to the hospital the patient was cooperative but markedly depressed. His speech was retarded, and he carried on a pattern of repetitive compulsive activity. Affect was inappropriate, and speech was wandering, with ideas of reference and delusions of persecution. He denied hallucinatory experiences but had periods of unresponsiveness during which observers believed him to be hallucinating.

The patient's fear and anxiety were controlled, during the first 3 months of hospitalization, with the administration of chlorpromazine. On this medication, he discussed his past sexual difficulties and confusion, his close relationship with his mother and brothers, sibling rivalry, and difficult relationship with his father and other authority figures. Psychotherapy produced a marked increase in the patient's awareness of himself and in his ability to handle his environment. As his dynamic conflicts were explored, his thinking difficulty became much less severe and paranoid ideation also disappeared. The same exploration, however, was associated with marked feelings of futility about ever resolving these conflicts, and depression increased, with exacerbations of suicidal ideation. Accordingly, in the third month of hospitalization chlorpromazine was stopped, and ECT was administered. The patient received seven ECT's, given two times per week. By the fifth treatment his depression was markedly relieved, and by the seventh treatment there were no more traces of depression. The course of treatment was terminated at this time, and the patient was able to deal with the previously analyzed material from an optimistic point of view. He was moved to an open floor in the hospital, made a satisfactory adjustment there for 2 more months of hospitalization, and was then discharged. He has continued to do well for 3 years following discharge, without further psychotherapy.

This history indicates the value of associated psychopathologic findings in determining the use of ECT. Beyond this, it provides an interesting illustration of the way in which the properly timed use of ECT can be integrated into the course of treatment of many illnesses. In this instance, the patient's illness was marked by depression, with some suicidal ideation, from the first. If, however, the ECT had been administered early in treatment, its effect would merely have been temporary because the underlying illness would have remained, and the patient would have once more become involved in the difficulties which produced the depression. Instead, however, the therapeutic plan enabled a considerable resolution of the underlying schizophrenic difficulties and a marked improvement of thinking prior to the administration of ECT. At that point, when the symptoms were cleared with the course of ECT, the patient was able to go on in a constructive fashion, thus minimizing the possibility of a return of symptoms.

Personality Factors

Two additional helps are available in selecting patients for the administration of ECT. Both these methods depend on laboratory procedures and have been used only under limited clinical situations. These are the methods of Funkenstein (1957) and Shagass (1956). Both these methods depend on finding the individual's tolerance to the administration of certain drugs, in one case Mecholyl and in the other case Sodium Amytal. It would appear that these methods are closely linked with the personality characteristics and characteristic defense mechanisms of the patients involved. When they are fully worked out, therefore, they will provide a third avenue of approach to the problem of selecting patients for ECT. When it is possible to join these personality-evaluating mechanisms to the previously defined diagnostic and psychopathologic criteria, predicting the effectiveness of ECT should be much more accurate.

Combined Physical Treatments

In certain types of schizophrenic reactions, particularly those which occur in adolescence, there is marked anxiety, which requires treatment by means other than ECT. In such illness, it is common to incorporate ECT, as a secondary feature, with the primary physical measure. The following case illustrates the combined use of insulin subcoma and ECT.

Case 8. A 17-year-old white female, a single high school student, was admitted to the hospital with an 11-year history of bizarre sexual activity, obesity, isolation, depression, suicidal thoughts, and feelings of inadequacy and strangeness. She came from a highly educated and cultivated family and had felt alienated from her peers since age 7. For the 11 years of her present illness, she followed a continuing pattern of close, dependent, sexually loaded relationships with adults of both sexes. In the hospital, she displayed a continuing pattern of confusion, anxiety, and dissociation from responsibility for her activities. She formed an ambivalent relationship with her therapist, pleading for his care and kindness but refusing to talk in interviews and expecting that he know intuitively what she desired. She remained in the hospital for a period of 10 months without improvement. At this time, she was begun on subcoma insulin treatment and received 63 treatments, 50 of which produced a precoma state. She also received 15 ECTs, which were given twice a week, on days she did not receive insulin. During the course of her therapy, there was a marked alleviation of anxiety as the insulin treatments began to take effect. The patient's behavior and thinking became better organized. Gradually, she was able to talk more openly in the interviews, to organize the pattern of her activity, to recognize the positive elements in her relationships with her parents, and to depend in a less autistic fashion on the therapist. At the same time, the depressive mood disappeared within the first eight ECTs. At the conclusion of treatment, the patient remained well and was discharged from the hospital in a moderately improved state. At the time of discharge, she still displayed a tendency toward dissociation, vagueness and rambling of speech, and slight flattening of affect. She had reasonable plans for a life adjustment, however, and planned to continue in psychotherapy.

Case 8 illustrates the combined use of a medication which promotes a synthesis of thinking—insulin—and a treatment which disrupts thinking—ECT. In such an instance, the two treatments can work synergistically. The ECT broke up the fixed pattern of the patient's behavior, while the anxiety-relieving and synthesizing aspects of the insulin helped her distinctly in formulating new methods of adaptation and new plans for the future.

Timing of ECT Administration

Two aspects are important in the timing of the administration of ECT. The first is the natural history of the illness being treated. Characteristically, most illnesses have a gradual period of onset, followed by a period of stability. Following the stable phase, there may be a spontaneous remission or a gradual deterioration into a fixed chronic condition. It would appear that ECT can give only temporary relief from the course of illness if it is administered during the phase of onset. Clinical experience indicates over and over again that patients who receive ECT during the period of onset of a depressive illness follow a characteristic pattern. There is immediate relief following the administration of treatment, with the patient returning to a state of apparent well-being. Within a matter of weeks, however, the illness recurs, and the downhill course of illness is resumed. Futile attempts to interrupt such an onset frequently result in the administration of enormous numbers of ECTs to patients who have not yet entered the stable phase of illness. Similar processes occur in schizophrenic reactions and paranoid states. It is therefore most important to make certain that a patient's illness has entered the stable phase before the administration of ECT is recommended. The importance of proper timing of ECT is illustrated by the following case.

Case 9. A 70-year-old white housewife, with two children, was admitted to the hospital with a 2-year history of anxiety and tension surrounding her husband's retirement. For 2 months prior to admission, after a vacation, she had become increasingly depressed, fearful, and anorexic, with many physical complaints. On admission to the hospital, she was disheveled and frequently exposed herself. She was agitated, pacing the halls and banging her head against the walls. There was intermittent loss of bladder and bowel control. Because of the gross disturbance of behavior, she was given a course of ECT shortly after admission, when her psychopathologic picture included depression, paranoid features, anxiety, agitation, and some hysterical exaggeration of symptoms. She was given three ECTs at daily intervals and three more ECTs at intervals of twice per week. At the end of the six ECTs, she was in a normal behavioral state but denied the existence of any illness. As she began once more to face the realistic problems of return to her home life, however, depression recurred. She manifested increasing ambivalence and hostility toward her daughter and her husband and could not conceive of any solution to the realistic problems which confronted her. Gradually, in the face of depression, she was able to analyze her feelings of aggressiveness throughout life, her need to be independent and to dominate, and the relationship of these needs with her parental relationships. By the time this material had been successfully analyzed, over a course of 3 months, the patient had returned to her previous depressed state. She was once more staggering, pacing halls, banging her head against the walls, and making suicidal gestures. She was placed once more on ECT and given a series of 10 ECTs, 2 per week. By the fourth treatment, the gross symptomatology was markedly diminished; by the tenth treatment, the patient had returned to her preillness state. Over the course of several more weeks of hospitalization, she was able to formulate plans for dealing constructively with her husband and the rest of her family and had no evidences of return of depression. In the 6 months subsequent to discharge from the hospital, she has continued to do well.

In this depressive illness in late life, it is not absolutely clear whether the first course of ECT was administered too early in the downhill course of a depressive illness or whether it was administered too early in the psychotherapeutic course of the patient. The use of ECT was indicated by the dangerous activity of the patient, and action could not be postponed. Joined with cases similar to Case 10, this material provides us with an indication that, no matter how clear the immediate psychopathologic indications are for the use of ECT, its use does not have optimal justification unless it is timed properly from an over-all point of view.

The second significant aspect of timing in the use of ECT involves the basic personality and the psychotherapeutic state of the patient. In illnesses which are self-limiting and in which the personality of the individual is a well-organized and healthy one, it may be expected that restitution of well-being and elimination of the illness will enable the patient to resume the normal pattern of his life. Such instances are very common in depressive illnesses in middle or late life. It has been found frequently that patients with such illnesses, once they are restored to health by ECT, can go on for the remainder of their lives without ever having a recurrence of illness and without the benefit of anything but the most superficial forms of psychotherapy (see Case 1). Many depressions, however, and most schizophrenic illnesses may be seen to originate in basic defects in the individual's personality. It is apparent that many patients who enter depressive illnesses in the forties, fifties, or sixties do so as a result of deeply ingrained personality characteristics. The restitution of such persons to momentarily healthy function is fruitless unless some measures are taken to enable them to lead a life which is organized along healthier lines; if this is not done, illness is virtually certain to recur. In view of the fact that psychotherapeutic change is necessary in a number of these illnesses, therefore, the goals of treatment must be taken into consideration in determining the proper time for the administration of ECT. It is characteristic of ECT that patients who have responded favorably to the treatment tend to deny the existence of illness and to avoid continuing psychotherapeutic measures until their next episode of illness. Any psychotherapeutic progress that is desired, therefore, must be accomplished prior to the administration of ECT. From the psychotherapeutic point of view, therefore, it is necessary firmly to establish a goal for the treatment. If an alteration in personality function is desirable, all effort should be concentrated on intensive exploratory psychotherapy prior to the administration of ECT. Only when sufficient progress has been made that the psychotherapist believes the patient can indeed form a better life adjustment in the future may ECT be given with any hope that its effect will be a permanently beneficial one.

The following case, and several earlier ones, illustrate an initially unsuccessful use of ECT, in a patient in whom the psychopathologic situation was favorable from a descriptive point of view, but where intensive work had to be done with personality integration before the symptomatic effects of ECT could be permanent.

Case 10. A 58-year-old white dentist was admitted to the hospital with a 1-year history of severe depression associated with anxiety, tension, and body concern. Eight months prior to admission, he had received six ECTs, with relief of symptomatology. On his return to his home situation, 5 months prior to hospitalization, symptoms had gradually returned, and for the 2 months immediately preceding his admission he had been unable to work. For 2 weeks prior to his admission, he had experienced marked indecisiveness, phobias, and suicidal ideation; for 1 week prior to his admission, he had been unable to leave his bed.

A review of this man's past life indicated a marked inadequacy of personality adjustment. Born of a passive father and a domineering mother, he had managed to achieve a satisfactory school adjustment, graduating from professional school. He entered professional life, but always maintained himself in a passive, meticulous, nonaggressive type of role. He continued to live with his mother, had no active social life, married a domineering woman while in his forties, and was widowed at the age of 50. Subsequently, he had returned to live with his mother, who bitterly condemned his efforts to engage in a social life of his own and who succeeded in breaking up an engagement which he had entered 2 years prior to his admission.

In the hospital, the patient revealed depression, with paranoid ideation and body concern. In psychotherapy, he discussed past patterns of dealing with his mother and with other social figures, analyzed his need for dependency and his failure to assert his own feelings, and finally revealed his resentment at lack of support from his father and from later male authority figures. At this point, after 4 months of hospitalization, ECT was administered. The patient received seven ECTs at this time and was completely free of depression by the sixth. He remained in the hospital 1 more month, reviewing the course of his psychotherapy and putting the insights accumulated during psychotherapy into action. He established himself in an independent apartment, resumed his relationship with his fiancée, and worked out a satisfactory, mutually agreeable relationship with his mother. He continued in psychotherapy on an ambulatory basis after discharge; there has been no recurrence of his illness for the past 2 years.

Case 10, with a depressive reaction in middle life, reveals the futility of administering ECT in the hope of producing a permanent symptomatic cure, if the underlying personality dysfunction has not been corrected. There was no appreciable difference between the effectiveness of ECT given in the early stages of the illness and that of ECT given during the course described above. In the earlier situation, however, the basic personality disability had not been analyzed; although the patient had returned immediately to a satisfactory life adjustment in appearance, he was soon back in the old pattern of neurotic dependence and his illness recurred. With the second course of ECT, however, a change had been made in personality function, and his improvement was a permanent one.

SUMMARY

It may be seen that electroconvulsive therapy may play a number of roles effectively in psychiatric treatment. In the treatment of affective disorders, six to eight ECTs may be expected to relieve most depressive illnesses, when given at the regular rate of administration. In the treatment of catatonic and manic excitements, three to five ECTs, given rapidly, will usually terminate the excitement. In the treatment of certain schizophrenic illnesses and paranoid states, 12 to 20 ECTs will reduce the stability of the illness and make the patient more amenable to psychotherapeutic measures. In the first two of these fields of operation,

ECT may be seen to work with a certain degree of specificity. In the third, however, it appears that the effectiveness of electric shock depends, for the most part, on its disruptive effect on the central nervous system.

It is not enough, however, simply to link the use of ECT with gross diagnostic categories. The facts indicate that ECT is not effective in an across-the-board fashion. Instead, with each of the diagnostic entities described, ECT works in a variable fashion, depending on the associated psychopathologic situation and on the basic personality of the individual. If the selection of patients for ECT is made carefully and the psychopathologic and personality situations are favorable, excellent results may be anticipated in the diagnostic categories described above. If the selection is not adequate and the associated features form an unfavorable constellation, the results will be unfavorable, even within the most favored diagnostic categories.

Furthermore, it must be remembered that the effective utilization of ECT depends also on its timing in the course of therapy. Like other physical treatments in use today, ECT remains an ancillary form of treatment. If it is administered during the wrong phase of illness—either too early or too late—the results obtained can be expected to be temporary, not altering the long-term course of the illness. If it is not given in conjunction with the psychotherapeutic needs of the situation, relapse may be expected. Maximal effectiveness may be obtained only when the physician keeps in mind two basic rules with respect to the administration of ECT:

1. Use ECT under optimal diagnostic, psychopathologic, and personality situations.

2. Administer ECT at a time when its temporary effect in relieving symptoms may be expected to produce results which the patient's state of illness and therapy are prepared to maintain.

11

STIMULANTS AND ANTIDEPRESSIVE AGENTS

The value of electroconvulsive therapy as a means of alleviating depression of mood has already been described. There are a number of situations, however, in which this treatment cannot or should not be administered. It is not usually desirable in depression of mood occurring in psychoneurotic settings. It is contraindicated in the presence of certain serious physical disorders, such as extensive cardiovascular disease. Many patients refuse the treatments. Many physicians hesitate to recommend them if the intensity of the patient's depression is not sufficiently great. Therefore, the need for pharmacologic agents which will reduce pathologic depression is very real.

There are four groups of compounds currently in use or being investigated for the treatment of depression. These include amphetamine and its derivatives; methylphenidate; monoamine oxidase inhibitors; and imipramine. The compounds of the amphetamine group have been employed for many years, allowing the accumulation of extensive knowledge of their effectiveness, limitations, and complications. On the other hand, methylphenidate, monoamine oxidase inhibitors, and imipramine must be considered to be in an experimental phase of development, no matter how promising the initial results seem.

Amphetamine

Amphetamine (Benzedrine, Amphetamine, Raphetamine) was used effectively in the treatment of narcolepsy as early as 1935. Its chemical structure readily demonstrates its resemblance to ephedrine and norepinephrine.

162

It is a potent stimulant of central nervous system activity, but only about half as potent, dose for dose, as the dextrorotatory form of amphetamine, called dextro amphetamine (Dexedrine, Dextro Amphetamine, d-Amfetasul). The mechanisms whereby these compounds produce central stimulation are essentially unknown. Clinically, this activation results in an increased level of alertness, decreased fatiguability, and at times a slight elevation of mood. In spite of the enhanced ability to carry out mental and physical activity, the actual performance itself does not change. For example, under the influence of one of these drugs, a student may be able to work past his usual point of fatigue and perhaps at a greater rate. However, there is no improvement in his capacity to learn or solve specific problems. The diminished sense of fatigue appears to be the result of central changes, that is, a decreased awareness of fatigue, since no metabolic alterations have been observed in various muscle groups. There does not appear to be any direct effect on the

Amphetamine   Ephedrine   Norepinephrine

metabolic rate. When tissue destruction and weight loss are observed in patients using amphetamine, this seems to be the result of anorexia and reduced food intake. The termination of these drugs, especially if large doses have been administered, is often followed by extreme exhaustion and depression of mood.

METHOD OF ADMINISTRATION

The average daily dosage of amphetamine or dextro amphetamine ranges from 5 to 20 mg, administered orally in tablet or elixir form. Its effects can be noted within 30 to 60 minutes after ingestion. It is customary to give the desired amounts in divided doses in the morning and early afternoon to prevent undue stimulation at night which might interfere with the patient's sleep. Dextro amphetamine is available in combination with amobarbital. The latter drug is added to reduce the tension, anxiety, and agitation which can complicate use of this stimulant. Because of the potentially serious side effects described and the danger of habituation, the administration of these drugs must be carefully supervised. Prolonged use, over many weeks or months, is to be assiduously avoided.

SIDE EFFECTS AND COMPLICATIONS

Side effects resulting from the use of amphetamine or dextro amphetamine are common and occasionally may be very serious. These drugs may intensify anxiety and hostility and produce tension, restlessness, overactivity, and insomnia. At times, severe psychopathologic reactions may occur, characterized by intense fear or panic, severe depression with suicidal drives, delusions, or hallucinations. These emotional and psychopathologic complications may be partly due to toxic effects on the central nervous system, but they also seem to depend upon the presence of potentially disturbing features within the recipient.

The cardiovascular system may be affected. Palpitations, increased or decreased blood pressure, pallor or flushing, anginal pain, and syncope have been observed. Hence, these compounds are contraindicated in patients with hypertension, cardiovascular disease, or hyperthyroidism. The gastrointestinal tract may also be adversely influenced, with anorexia, nausea, vomiting, and diarrhea occurring. These drugs, therefore, should be avoided in patients with serious disorders of this system, such as peptic ulcers and mucous or ulcerative colitis.

The presence of severe brain damage or epilepsy also must be considered a contraindication to their use. Toxic doses may lead to convulsions or coma. Such reactions have been observed in patients receiving a dose as low as 30 mg. Deaths have been reported as a result of excessive amphetamine ingestion; hence, its administration may be dangerous in suicidal patients.

One of the most insidious complications of the prolonged use of amphetamine or dextro amphetamine is habituation. Addiction to these drugs, with the characteristic development of tolerance and withdrawal symptoms, has been reported but does not appear to be common. Habituation, however, can readily occur and constitutes a serious problem in many poorly organized or psychopathic persons.

CLINICAL EFFECTIVENESS OF TREATMENT

The influence which these stimulants have on the emotional and psychopathologic states of patients appears to depend largely on the nature of the pretreatment condition and the personality of the patient receiving the drugs. Their direct effect is to increase alertness and decrease the recognition of fatigue. In certain patients, particularly those who have been under pressure to carry out complex work but are handicapped by some degree of retardation and exhaustion resulting from mild depression, such a change may lead to a renewed sense of well-being. On the other hand, overt manifestations of anxiety, fear, or hostility may be intensified by the administration of these stimulants. In sensitive patients, this may lead to the formation of more complex psychopathologic states, with paranoid misinterpretations, delusions, and hallucinations. One depressed patient may feel some relief with these drugs. Another may only become more painfully aware of his inner suffering and hopelessness. Many intensely depressed patients, such as those in the depressed phase of a manic-depressive reaction, may demonstrate little or no response to amphetamine.

Amphetamine and dextro amphetamine may be used primarily in the management of psychoneurotic reactions in which mild depression of mood, associated with fatigue and retardation, significantly impairs the function of the patient or impedes psychotherapy. In such instances, these drugs should be used for a limited time and periodically interrupted to avoid dependency upon the medication. The following case illustrates the successful use of dextro amphetamine combined with amobarbital in the treatment of a psychoneurotic patient in whom these symptoms threatened to disrupt life adjustment.

Case 1. During a 6-month period, this 29-year-old university history instructor developed a psychoneurotic illness, characterized by loss of interest in his work, difficulty in remaining attentive in the classroom, and procrastination in the preparation of his lecture material. He was unable to fall asleep for several hours at night and would frequently oversleep in the mornings. His self-confidence was diminished. He felt that his ability to understand and apply imagination to his work was severely limited in comparison with that of his contemporaries. He was often discouraged and moderately depressed. Anxiety was occasionally present, but it was not a prominent feature of his condition. No well-defined precipitating factors could be elicited to account for his state, and only after many months of psychotherapy did it become apparent that unconscious guilt over his ambitions and competitive drives and the repression of heterosexual instincts contributed to the production of his illness.

During the initial examination he appeared tired. His speech was somewhat retarded, and his flow of ideas was limited. He was absorbed in his self-doubts and morbid fantasies. Suicidal tendencies were not apparent.

He was seen three times weekly in psychotherapy. After the first few sessions, it was clear that his procrastination, fatigue, and mild depressive feelings threatened his capacity to continue with his work. Accordingly, he was placed on 5 mg dextro amphetamine with amobarbital, to be taken on rising in the morning and repeated at lunch time. Within 2 days he noted renewed energy, greater freedom from his depressing preoccupations, more self-confidence, and less procrastination. He continued on this medication for the next 3 weeks. No important change in the structure of his psychopathologic state was observed, but the increased alertness and tolerance of fatigue gave him real encouragement and allowed him to carry on his work.

Following termination of the regular use of dextro amphetamine, the patient maintained his improvement. From time to time, during the next 6 months, in the setting of environmental stresses or during the analysis of disturbing material, fatigue, depression, and mild retardation were noted. Dextro amphetamine was given for a few days at these times if the symptoms were sufficiently intense to warrant somatic intervention.

In more intense depressive reactions, regardless of the diagnostic setting and particularly if the danger of suicide is present, it is injudicious to consider the use of amphetamine or dextro amphetamine. They may occasionally intensify the patient's mood disturbance. More often, no clinical change is seen, and correct treatment measures are considerably delayed while the patient and physician decide whether the drug will or will not prove beneficial. It is not uncommon to hospitalize a seriously depressed patient who has been unsuccessfully treated with these stimulants for months before obtaining adequate therapy.

These stimulants were, and still are to some degree, used in obese patients to encourage weight reduction. They do possess the power to suppress the appetite for food. The use of these drugs for the control of overeating, however, has serious limitations. Besides the general complications inherent in their administration, the anorexia which these drugs induce usually decreases after several weeks. It may then be necessary to increase the dose in order to sustain the desired effects. Moreover, the dynamic basis of obesity is extremely complex. This phenomenon can occur in any diagnostic setting. It may, at times, be the direct consequence of pathologic anxiety or hostility. It may be determined by unconscious motivations. The pharmacologic induction of anorexia is a relatively superficial attack on the problem of obesity, although, no doubt, there are certain patients in whom anorexigenic drugs are useful adjuncts in therapy.

Methamphetamine

Closely related to amphetamine is the central nervous system stimulant methamphetamine (Methedrine, Desoxyephedrine, Desoxyn). It has been used in large intravenous doses of 100 mg to induce "model psychoses." In more modest amounts, ranging from 20 to 40 mg intravenously, this compound exaggerates previously hidden psychopathologic features in patients. For example, a well-controlled paranoid schizophrenic patient may demonstrate delusions for the first time while receiving the drug. Because of this property, it has been employed by some investigators as an aid to diagnosis. The drug also seems to enhance verbal facility and the revelation of dynamically important material. Emotions may be released from dissociation, and clinical improvement may follow in certain patients as a result of this catharsis. Its complications resemble those of amphetamine. The clinical use of methamphetamine in the treatment of psychiatric disorders is largely exploratory and extremely limited. Therefore, it does not deserve extensive consideration here.

Methylphenidate

Methylphenidate (Ritalin) was developed in an attempt to find a drug which would possess the stimulating properties of amphetamine and its derivatives but lack some of the side effects of these compounds. It proved to be a mild cerebral cortical stimulant; the chemical structure is illustrated.

$$CH_3OOC-\underset{\underset{H}{|}}{C}-\underset{\underset{H}{|}}{N}$$

The average daily dosage is 10 mg two or three times daily. It is usually administered in the morning and early afternoon to avoid over-stimulation at bedtime and consequent insomnia. Higher dosage may occasionally be used, reaching a maximum of 60 mg in 24 hours.

Side effects have not been pronounced. The complications include insomnia, intensification of anxiety, headaches, palpitations, occasionally a rise in blood pressure, nausea, and anorexia. In epileptic patients, the frequency of grand mal convulsions has occasionally been increased.

The indications for the use of this drug are essentially the same as for amphetamine and its derivatives. It is therefore used to combat mild retardation and fatigue associated with depression of mood in certain psychoneurotic patients. The medication increases alertness and reduces lethargy and fatigue. Because of these effects, it has been successfully used to alleviate drowsiness and retardation resulting from the administration of phenothiazines or rauwolfia derivatives.

Many investigators feel that methylphenidate possesses certain advantages over amphetamine. It does not seem to exert so strong an influence on the cardiovascular system, and it lacks anorexigenic properties. Nonetheless, caution should be used if the drug is given to patients with heart disease or psychiatric illnesses complicated by severe anorexia. Habituation has not been reported, but it is too early to assume that such a danger does not exist. As with amphetamine, this compound has no place in the treatment of severe mood disorders.

Monoamine Oxidase Inhibitors

In 1952, a major advance was made in the treatment of tuberculosis. Two hydrazine derivatives of isonicotinic acid, isoniazid and iproniazid, were strikingly effective in destroying the tubercle bacillus. Many patients who received these drugs experienced a marked elevation in mood. Iproniazid, in particular, was demonstrated to be a potent inhibitor of monoamine oxidase, an enzyme which facilitates the degradation of epinephrine, norepinephrine, and serotonin. Interference with its activity allows potentiation of these compounds which may be involved in the transmission of neural impulses across synaptic junctions. Encouraged by the mood changes observed in tuberculous patients receiving iproniazid, investigators began to study the effects of this monoamine oxidase inhibitor in psychiatric patients, particularly those in whom apathy, depression of mood, and withdrawal were prominent features. The initial reports were most encouraging, with beneficial results being obtained in more than 50 per cent of patients diagnosed as schizophrenic reactions or depressive mood disorders. Many of these patients had failed to respond satisfactorily to phenothiazines, electroconvulsive therapy, or psychotherapy. Subsequent studies were less enthusiastic. Good responses to the medication were reported among certain depressed patients, but the characteristics which would indicate the type of depressed patient expected to improve on iproniazid were not identified. By the time more elaborate and careful investigations could be established, this drug was proved to be very toxic in the doses required to induce mood changes. Therefore, it was abandoned as a psychopharmacologic agent. However, because of the recent introduction of monoamine oxidase inhibitors which presumably lack the serious side effects of iproniazid, it is important to review the nature of the clinical effects of this drug in patients.

The chemical formula of iproniazid (Marsilid), which is the phosphate derivative of 1-isonicotinyl-2-isopropylhydrazide, is given, for comparison with the structures of the more recently developed monoamine oxidase inhibitors. These include phenelzine (Nardil), β-phenylisopropylhydrazine (Catron), nialamide (Niamid), and isocarboxazid (Marplan).

Like amphetamine, these compounds are central nervous system stimulants. Therefore, they increase alertness and awareness of inner emotions and environmental stimuli. The nature of the stimulation, however, appears to be somewhat different from that of amphetamine. For example, rather than producing anorexia, these drugs appear to increase appetite, weight accumulation, and perhaps even the retention of nitrogen and other dietary substances. Moreover, clinical reports strongly suggest that these drugs produce a definite elevation of mood which transcends mere excitation in certain depressed patients.

The clinical effects of iproniazid do not appear for 2 to 3 weeks after the initiation of treatment. The newer monoamine oxidase inhibitors appear to influence the psychopathologic condition of patients somewhat earlier, perhaps in 1 or 2 weeks. The original dosage recommended for iproniazid was 150 mg daily, orally, in three divided doses. This was later recognized as a hazardous level, and the recommended dosage was lowered to 50 mg in 24 hours. Such a dose, however, was found to be clinically ineffective in producing sufficient stimulation to alleviate depression of mood. Unfortunately, even in so-called adequate doses, many conflicting reports about iproniazid appeared. In some series of patients, it appeared to be dramatically efficacious; in others, it seemed impotent. These difficulties were never satisfactorily resolved.

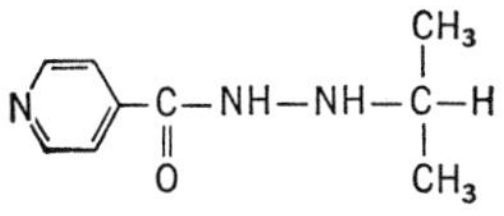

Iproniazid

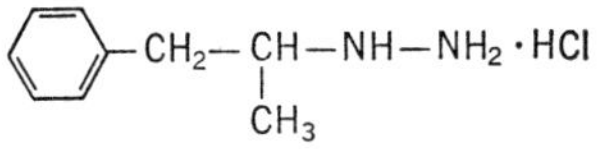

Beta-phenylisopropylhydrazine

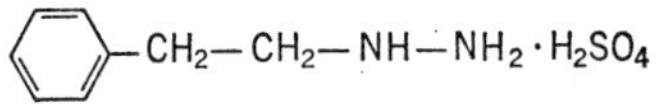

Phenelzine

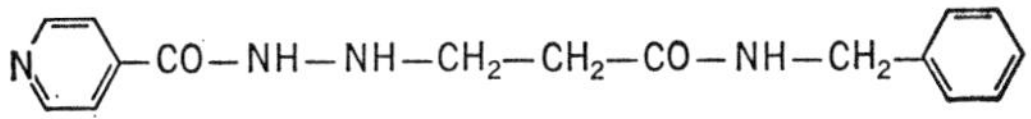

Nialamide

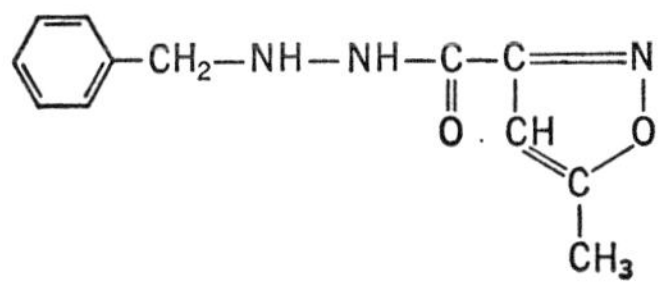

Isocarboxazid

The side effects and complications associated with the administration of iproniazid were frequent and occasionally serious. The most significant of these included headaches, dizziness, agitation, and insomnia; gastrointestinal distress, in particular constipation; allergic reactions, such as dermatitis; and liver damage, at times resulting in death. Presumably the newer monoamine oxidase inhibitors are not associated with the same incidence and intensity of these side effects. However, confirmation of this impression must await more extensive clinical investigation. Meanwhile, these drugs should not be used in patients with liver disease or whose cardiovascular status would be seriously jeopardized by a sharp reduction in blood pressure. Before, during, and for a time after the administration of these drugs, liver function should be regularly checked.

The desirable dosage of iproniazid is 25 mg twice daily, but this will probably be insufficient to induce clinical changes. The dosage ranges of other monoamine oxidase inhibitors are as follows: phenelzine, 15 mg three to four times daily; β-phenylisopropylhydrazine, 12 mg once daily for 2 weeks, thereafter a maintenance dose of 3 mg daily or 6 mg every other day, with periodic interruptions to avoid complications; nialamide, 30 to 100 mg daily in divided doses; isocarboxazid, 30 mg daily in single or divided doses, to be reduced to a maintenance level of 10 to 20 mg daily as soon as the desired clinical effects are secured.

At the present time no conclusions can be drawn concerning the efficacy of any of these drugs. Preliminary reports indicate that they can induce relief from depression of mood, with its subjective feelings of hopelessness, difficulty in sleeping, and loss of motivation and drive. This improvement seems to be more pronounced when these drugs are given to patients with psychoneurotic or primary mood disturbances than to those in other diagnostic categories. These drugs may be used when other somatic therapeutic measures, such as electroconvulsive treatments or imipramine, have not proved successful or are contraindicated.

Imipramine

Imipramine (Tofranil) is a compound which structurally resembles the phenothiazines. Its formula is presented for comparison with that of chlorpromazine. There are two significant differences between these drugs. Imipramine hydrochloride lacks the chlorine (Cl) group seen in

Imipramine   Chlorpromazine

chlorpromazine, and, most importantly, the sulfur (S) has been replaced by CH_2-CH_2. In contrast with chlorpromazine, imipramine often alleviates depression of mood. Imipramine appears to be more effective in patients with affective disorders, particularly of the endogenous type, than in those diagnosed as psychoneurotic or schizophrenic. The mode of action of imipramine is essentially unknown.

METHOD OF ADMINISTRATION

The usual oral dosage of imipramine is 25 mg four times daily. When indicated, the dosage may be increased to 150 or 200 mg per day. Clinical changes may be seen within a few days, although it may require 2 or 3 weeks of drug administration before improvement is clearly discernible. The drug is usually continued for at least 10 to 12 weeks to reduce the likelihood of relapse following its termination. The average maintenance dosage is about 75 to 100 mg daily.

SIDE EFFECTS AND COMPLICATIONS

The most common side effects of imipramine administration are profuse perspiration, fatigue, and interrupted sleep. These usually subside if the dose is decreased or after the medication has been given for several weeks. Tremors may occur. Extrapyramidal symptoms may occur. In a small number of patients, the seizure threshold is lowered, and grand mal convulsions may be precipitated. A lowering of blood pressure and syncope are occasionally seen. Interference with liver function has been reported infrequently. Care should be used in giving the drug to patients with cardiovascular disease.

CLINICAL EFFECTIVENESS OF TREATMENT

The emotional and psychopathologic effects of imipramine appear to differ from those of chlorpromazine. Phenothiazines tend to reduce pathologic emotions of fear and hostility, sexual unrest, elation of mood, and associated psychopathologic features, such as delusions, paranoid features, and hallucinations. By contrast, imipramine does not seem to influence these factors. In fact, it may infrequently lead to a serious intensification of agitation and excitement. The major action of imipramine seems to be the reduction of certain features of depression, in particular sadness, hopelessness, loss of energy and drive, and preoccupations with morbid topics, such as guilt or personal inadequacies. In some patients, the degree of improvement during imipramine therapy is very limited. The intensity of the patient's suffering may be lightened, but no fundamental change in his condition takes place. In others, the improvement is striking and extensive. The following case illustrates a good response to imipramine.

Case 2. A 59-year-old housewife, diagnosed as having a depression of middle life, presented a 6-month history of tension, depression of mood, inability to carry out her daily responsibilities, social withdrawal, anorexia, weight loss, and early morning awakening. Her illness began several months after the death of her husband. During the first 2 months of psychotherapy, significant dynamic

factors, such as loneliness, concern about aging, and her reactions to her husband's death and her children's marriages, were explored. Symptomatic improvement was minimal.

Imipramine was then instituted, in daily oral dosage of 150 mg. Within 1
week, a reduction in the severity of her depression was noted. By the middle of
the third week of treatment, her spirits were good. She was genuinely optimistic
about the future. She renewed her former social activities. She slept well. Her
appetite returned, and she gained weight. During the sixth week of therapy, the
dosage was reduced to 75 mg daily and continued at that level until its termination 3 months later.

The depression which this patient exhibited was uncomplicated by
pathologic emotions. It is unlikely that phenothiazines would have significantly altered her clinical state. When fear, hostility, or paranoid
features are prominently associated with depression, imipramine alone
appears less likely to induce satisfactory clinical improvement. The following case illustrates this point and indicates the desirability of combining imipramine with a phenothiazine compound in certain psychopathologic settings.

Case 3. A 47-year-old accountant presented a 4-month history of depression,
with anorexia, weight loss, early morning awakening, and concentration difficulty. This reaction began in the setting of a series of quarrels with his wife,
during which she threatened to divorce him. Five years earlier, he had suffered
a similar depression after failing to be promoted to a much desired post. At that
time he received seven ECTs, rapidly improved, and refused psychotherapy.

During the initial consultation, the patient was preoccupied with regret over
past misjudgments in his work and failures in his human relationships. Hostility
was apparent. He became intensely angry when speaking of his wife or business
associates. When psychotherapy was recommended, he resentfully accused the
physician of failing to comprehend the extent of his suffering.

Imipramine was instituted, in daily oral dosage of 150 mg. By the fourth
week of treatment, a slight diminution in the intensity of his sadness and hopelessness was observed. His sleep and appetite improved. One week later, because of his persistent hostility, prochlorperazine was added in daily oral dosage
of 40 mg. Within 48 hours a marked improvement occurred. Anger and resentment disappeared. For the first time the patient experienced a sense of well-
being. He was able to concentrate effectively. Shortly thereafter, he was able
to resume many of his responsibilities. His attitude toward psychotherapy improved. He willingly continued in treatment in order to reduce the likelihood of
a recurrence of his condition.

In this patient, imipramine produced a limited degree of symptomatic
improvement. A substantial decrease in depression of mood and hostile
emotions did not occur until prochlorperazine was added to the medication regimen. It seems desirable, therefore, to administer imipramine in
combination with a phenothiazine compound in the treatment of de-

pressed patients who also manifest fear, hostility, sexual unrest, or paranoid features.

When somatic intervention is urgently needed in the treatment of a depressed patient, as in the presence of a serious suicidal risk, electroconvulsive therapy is the treatment of choice. It is still a more reliable method of relieving depression and requires less time to take effect. Nonetheless, there are certain situations in which imipramine therapy may be considered first. If the depression is relatively mild, the physician may hesitate to recommend a course of ECT. He may be unable to administer the treatments if the patient and his family are opposed to them. In certain patients, ECT is contraindicated by a concomitant physical disorder, such as severe cardiovascular disease. In such settings, imipramine may be a useful adjunct in the total treatment program.

SUMMARY

There are several groups of drugs which are available for use in the treatment of depression of mood. These include stimulants, such as amphetamine, dextro amphetamine, and methylphenidate; monoamine oxidase inhibitors; and imipramine. The stimulants act directly on the cerebral cortex to increase alertness and diminish the subjective awareness of fatigue. They may be effective in alleviating lethargy and mild retardation in certain depressive states, such as those seen in psychoneurotic patients. This may produce a renewed sense of confidence and well-being. In addition to physiologic complications, the use of amphetamines may lead to habituation if not correctly supervised. They are of little or no value in the management of severe depression of mood, regardless of the diagnostic setting.

Monoamine oxidase inhibitors appear to reduce the subjective and objective signs of pathologic depression in certain patients with psychoneurotic or primary mood disorders. They may also be effective in some depressed, apathetic schizophrenic patients. Reports of their efficacy are conflicting. Experience with these agents is too limited to distinguish those depressed patients who will respond well to them from those who will not. Side effects of iproniazid have proved sufficiently serious to discourage its use in psychiatric patients. The newer drugs in this group will require further testing to determine when their therapeutic value outweighs their complications.

Imipramine is structually similar to, but not identical with, phenothiazine derivatives. It seems to lack their effectiveness in reducing pathologic emotions of fear and hostility, sexual unrest, and associated delusions, paranoid features, or hallucinations. It is of limited value in schizophrenic or psychoneurotic reactions. Imipramine alone appears to be effective in alleviating depression of mood in patients with primary mood disorders when these conditions are not associated with prominent pathologic emotions. In some patients the drug produces a marked degree of improvement; in others, it seems to decrease subjective suffering and facilitate greater tolerance of the depressive mood. It can be used in conjunction wih phenothiazines in depressed patients who also demonstrate fear, hostility, sexual unrest, or paranoid features. Imipramine may be a useful adjunct in the treatment of depressed patients who require somatic therapy but in whom electroconvulsive therapy is undesirable or contraindicated.

12

INSULIN TREATMENT AND LOBOTOMY

INSULIN TREATMENT

Although insulin treatment has only been in use since about 1935, it is nonetheless one of the oldest major physical treatments currently used in psychiatry. Until the advent of electroconvulsive treatment, it was virtually the only major physical treatment approach that appeared to have a specific value in the treatment of psychiatric illnesses. As will be seen, however, insulin treatment is prolonged, expensive, and sometimes dangerous. It can only be administered effectively with a large, competent, and highly trained staff. With the advent of tranquilizing drugs, during the last several years, there has been a marked decrease in the use of insulin treatment in the United States. Currently, insulin finds its chief use in large state hospitals and in a few smaller psychiatric hospitals. It must be recognized, however, that insulin treatment has specific usefulness and is virtually the only known form of treatment which may be used effectively in certain psychopathologic situations.

Mechanism of Action

Explanations for the effectiveness of insulin treatment have varied and must still be regarded as hypothetical. Certainly there is abundant evidence that both coma and subcoma insulin treatment produce profound alteration in cerebral function. This evidence includes the fact that blood sugars are reduced below 30 mg per 100 cc for several hours of each treatment, the existence of pathologic reflexes, and the alterations of the individual's electroencephalographic pattern. There can be little doubt, therefore, of the impact of insulin treatment on central nervous system physiology.

To go beyond this stage in explaining the effect of insulin is difficult. Perhaps the most comprehensive explanation has come from Himwich and his co-workers. They point out that the clinical course of the individual insulin treatment follows a characteristic pattern, with progressive inhibition of cortical and higher centers and concomitant release of basal ganglia and midbrain activity. This explanation is supported by the electroencephalographic sequence during the treatment. It focuses attention on the ability of the insulin to cause basic shifts in the supposed regulatory mechanisms of the brain. The final explanation for the effectiveness of insulin treatment, however, must remain in doubt.

Method of Administration

There are two major forms of insulin treatment, subcoma and coma. The difference in the two methods lies largely in the desired depth of hypoglycemic stupor, or coma, to which the patient is taken. In insulin coma treatment, the goal is explicit: the desired depth is a state of unconsciousness, as manifested by a total unresponsiveness to stimuli. Subcoma insulin treatment does not have this same clarity in defining its end stages. In general, however, it may be said to involve taking the patient to that depth of hypoglycemic stupor in which he responds only minimally to no more than one or two strong applied stimuli. In such a state, obviously, the patient is on the verge of coma. The depth of the reaction to these two kinds of treatment, therefore, is separated only by a hairbreadth. In many instances, hospitals use the term *coma insulin treatment* to apply to *deep subcoma insulin treatment*.

A third, and less important, form of insulin treatment is ambulatory insulin treatment. In this therapeutic program, a patient is given 5 to 15 units of insulin two to three times per day. This amount of insulin does not lower his blood sugar to the extent that his behavior is markedly impaired, but it does provide some mild soporific action and stimulates appetite. It is said to have some therapeutic usefulness in relieving anxiety, but adequate psychopathologic studies have not been reported.

The details of treatment in coma and subcoma insulin treatment are very similar. Following the administration of a test dose of 1 to 5 units of insulin subcutaneously, a regular treatment progression begins. Each morning, at approximately 7 A.M., the patient is given an injection of intramuscular or subcutaneous insulin. On the first treatment day, the dosage given is 25 units of regular insulin. Some therapists prefer to double the previously administered dose on each successive treatment day, while other therapists prefer to increase the dosage by 25 units on each treatment day. In either case, the result is the same. The dosage is increased daily, according to the therapist's preference, until the patient has reached the desired depth of response for the desired length of time. The dosage is then stabilized in such a way as to maintain this depth on each treatment day. Treatments are administered 6 days a week. A therapeutic course of insulin treatment will usually be measured by the number of hours of coma or precoma which the patient has had or by the number of successful treatments administered. In coma insulin treatment, a satisfactory single treatment will usually involve one-quarter to one-half hour of insulin coma; a satisfactory course of treatment will include 30 to 90 such successful treatments. In subcoma insulin treatment, a satisfactory single treatment will usually involve three-quarters of an hour to one hour of a precoma state; a satisfactory course of treatment will include 30 to 90 such successful single treatments.

The course of a single treatment, when the desired dosage level has been achieved, is a fairly standardized one. Following the administration of insulin, at 7 A.M., the patient shows no obvious alteration in behavior for 30 to 45 minutes. At that time, he gradually experiences increasing weakness, perspiration, and lassitude. He remains in bed while becoming increasingly stuporous, occasionally with feelings of marked fear. During the second hour of treatment, the patient is usually markedly drowsy, occasionally demonstrating a burst of hostile excitement or panic. By the third hour, the patient is in a deeply stuporous state and may thereafter enter a precoma or coma condition at any time. During coma or precoma, it is common to find that a Babinski reaction is present, and an occasional patient will have grand mal seizures. If epileptiform seizures do occur during the course of treatment, they may be controlled by the administration of 30 to 60 mg phenobarbital, orally, four times per day. It is common to administer 0.004 Gm atropine sulfate subcutaneously, some time during the second hour of treatment, in order to minimize nausea and vomiting which occasionally occur during the treatment.

Termination of the daily treatment is brought about at 11 A.M. or earlier, when the patient has already experienced the desired duration of precoma or coma or in the event that any complications appear. The day's treatment is terminated by the administration of glucose. This may be done through the intravenous administration of glucose solutions, which may vary in concentration from 10 to 50 per cent, or by the administration of glucose by gavage, in 20 per cent solution. In either case, the patient rapidly regains consciousness. At this time, he should be given several glasses of orange juice, which has been fortified with glucose, and crackers. After bathing or showering, the patient may have a light breakfast and is then ready to engage in the regular activities of the day. He must be under continual observation, however, lest he have a delayed reaction to the insulin and experience a hypoglycemic reaction in the late afternoon or evening. Care must also be taken that the patient eats his meals, in order to guard against this same possibility. If a delayed hypoglycemic reaction does occur, prompt administration of orange juice fortified with glucose will terminate the reaction.

Accompanying this daily routine, a consistent pattern of medical and nursing care is recognized. At all times during the insulin treatment, the patient must be under continual and direct observation of registered nurses, assisted by specially trained aides. The patient's pulse, respirations, and blood pressure must be checked every 15 minutes. At the same time, the nursing staff observes the patient's responsiveness to various standardized stimuli (Regan, et al., 1956). Under ideal circumstances, a physician should remain continually in the room with patients who are undergoing insulin treatment, but it is permissible for him to be on call if he can be available within 1 minute. Treatment should be terminated immediately in the event of abnormal changes in pulse, respiration, or blood pressure or in the event that the patient shows severe excitement, excessive myoclonic twitching, or convulsive episodes.

Side Effects and Complications

Complications which accompany insulin treatment may be divided into two types, acute and chronic. The acute complications are, for the most part, secondary to the stuporous or comatose state of the patient. Intercurrent infections may flare up in the course of treatment, for example; these include pneumonia, which may be of the aspiratory or regular infectious type. There is also the possibility of physical injury which may result from the patient thrashing around during his stuporous state; it is not uncommon for patients to sustain marked bruises or fractures in this situation.

Another type of acute complication is more specific for the administration of insulin. This is the condition known as *prolonged coma*. Prolonged coma is characterized by a failure to respond to the administration of glucose at the time for termination of treatment. A prolonged coma may persist for as long as several days and *frequently* terminates in death. When the administration of sufficient amounts of glucose has not terminated a prolonged coma, it should be treated by the administration of parenteral fluids which contain physiologic amounts of potassium or by the administration of whole blood.

The chronic complications of insulin treatment include those which are secondary to the mode of treatment and those which are specific for the treatment itself. The complications which are secondary to the mode of treatment include infections at the various sites of injection of insulin and the formation of thrombi and thrombophlebitis at the sites of intravenous injection of glucose. The last-named complications are especially frequent when 30 to 50 per cent glucose solutions are routinely used for termination of treatment. The specific chronic complications which follow the administration of insulin treatment include electroencephalographic damage to the brain and obesity. Obesity is secondary to the increased intake of carbohydrates and fats which is necessary to compensate for the large amount of insulin being administered to the patient. If treatment is successful from a psychopathologic point of view, it is usually not too difficult for the patient to go on a reducing diet following the termination of treatment and to resume his base-line weight. The electroencephalographic changes are manifested by slow 4- to 6-cycles per second activity, with occasional spikes. Such a disturbance in the usual pattern of the electroencephalogram is more common when the patient is subjected to coma than to subcoma insulin treatment, but it appears, to some extent, with both kinds of treatment. It commonly disappears over the course of several months, following completion of the course of insulin treatment.

Other nonspecific complications are sometimes seen in the course of insulin treatment. These include cerebral vascular accidents and myocardial infarction. These are probably related to the strain which the hypoglycemia places on the physiology of the body and to the physical activity in which excited patients sometimes engage during the course of treatment. It is also possible that the fear which some patients experience while undergoing treatment may accentuate previously present cardiovascular abnormalities.

Clinical Effectiveness of Treatment

The manner in which insulin produces its beneficial effects is a characteristic one. During the first few treatments, as the insulin dosage is gradually increased, there is little change in the patient except that he is involved, socially, in a complex treatment program. Once the dosage begins to produce 15 minutes of coma or precoma, however, changes in psychopathology and behavior usually begin to appear. In most instances, if the course of treatment is going to be effective, these changes will be noticeable within the first 15 treatments which produce coma or precoma.

The psychopathologic changes which result from insulin treatment are found chiefly at basic emotional and intellectual levels. On the emotional side, the most noticeable alteration is a marked reduction of anxiety. The tremulous, apprehensive patient with almost no span of attention gradually becomes calm, and the level of anxiety comes within normal limits. Fear will also subside. To less extent, sexual unrest, anger, and resentment will be reduced. As the extent of emotional turmoil is reduced, the patient does not usually show the unresponsiveness found in conjunction with chlorpromazine treatment; instead he remains much more natural in his emotional responsiveness.

The intellectual changes which accompany insulin treatment are also basic and appear early in the course of successful treatment. The first sign, which usually accompanies the reduction of emotions, is an increased organization of thinking. Thoughts and sentences become better formed, and the pattern of speech becomes more coherent. More and more, the patient speaks of the realities of his life and becomes less and less involved in ruminative preoccupations. Only after this pattern of increased organization has persisted for several weeks does one find a change in secondary pathology, such as delusions and hallucinations. As the better organization increases, these secondary signs gradually fade away; one does not look for their disappearance during early stages.

Behaviorally, the patient shows clear reflections of his diminished emotional turmoil and increased organization of thinking. As he comes to deal more and more with reality, he pays more attention to grooming, appearance, and social behavior; his increasing intellectual ability will allow him to do all this more efficiently and more independently. With the diminished emotions, there will be less interference from the pressures of anxiety or the outbursts of sexual or hostile feelings. As the treatment proceeds, the therapist sees the gradual transformation of an individual. The trembling, crouching, mute girl becomes warm, confident, and outgoing; the exposing, masturbating, destructive man becomes a polite, organized participant in group activities.

Several facts about this improvement must be recognized. Obviously, the first of these is that such good improvement may be expected only when the psychopathologic situation is one which will respond to the insulin treatment. The second fact which must be recognized is that the effect is a gradual one. Early in treatment, the improvement will show itself only briefly, during the hour or two immediately following termination of the daily treatment; later it will become stronger and more pervasive. The third factor that must be borne constantly in mind is that improvement is based on the continuation of treatment. When the support of the daily insulin regimen is withdrawn, the patient will rapidly return to his pretreatment status, unless adequate psychotherapeutic progress has allowed him to find new and better ways of dealing with his internal or external problems. The fourth factor is one which has been well illustrated by Whitehorn and Betz (1957): insulin alone will not produce optimal results. Only if the therapist has a thorough knowledge of his patient and can link the physiologic effectiveness of the insulin treatment to good, well-organized, intensive psychotherapy can the described results be attained.

With these factors in mind, it is possible to explore the favorable and unfavorable psychopathologic constellations which influence the effectiveness of the insulin treatment (Greaves, et al., 1955).

The most prominent area of usefulness for coma and subcoma insulin treatment is schizophrenic reactions. A course of treatment will commonly last a minimum of 40 effective treatments and frequently should not be discontinued until the patient has had 90 effective treatments. While proceeding through a course of treatment, it is characteristic that the patient will show increasingly organized thinking as his anxiety becomes less and less prominent. During the afternoons and evenings on days in which he receives treatment, it is possible for the patient to discuss dynamic material which had previously precipitated overwhelming anxiety and fear. Furthermore, he will be able to utilize his understanding of dynamic material in better organizing his behavior and other activities in the environment. During the course of insulin treatment, the patient is best able to make reasonable and appropriate plans for the future, as his effective insight is turned in that direction. It is of crucial importance that these insights be obtained and plans for the future be made while the insulin treatment is still in effect. It is a serious error to allow the postponement of important dynamic discussions until after the conclusion of insulin treatment; such a procedure frequently results in anxiety recurring when the material is finally brought up, and the patient, unable to handle the anxiety without the insulin, has a major recurrence.

Among the schizophrenic reactions, it is found that those reactions which are associated with the highest chronological level of personality integration are the ones which profit best from the administration of the insulin treatment. These, obviously, are the paranoid schizophrenic reactions, which occur latest in life; the catatonic schizophrenic reactions; and the pseudoneurotic schizophrenic reactions. Those illnesses which are acute in onset and short in duration have a considerably better prognosis for rapid response than do more chronic and insidious illnesses. Although it does not have an absolute statistical validity, it is frequently found that the patients who respond favorably to insulin treatment show some degree of response, however minimal, during the first 15 successful treatments; those who fail to show any response to the first 15 treatments usually show no response during the entire course of treatment.

The following case illustrates the beneficial value of subcoma insulin treatment in a severe simple schizophrenic reaction, where considerable affect was available.

Case 1. A 15-year-old schoolgirl was admitted to the hospital with a 2-year history of mounting anxiety and depression, which had resulted in a behavioral pattern of slovenliness, seclusiveness, and poor scholastic performance. During the 4 months prior to admission, paranoid delusions had become evident and were associated with rage outbursts at her family.

On admission to the hospital, the patient was withdrawn and apathetic, with bursts of intense anxiety and inappropriate giggling. She had a spiking pulse, ranging from 70 to 120 beats per minute. During the first 4 months of hospitalization, psychotherapeutic interviews were characterized by muteness and negativism, as were social activities. With little change in the pathologic picture, subcoma insulin treatment was begun in the fifth month of hospitalization. The patient received 54 treatments, precoma being achieved first during the fifth treatment and regularly after the fourteenth treatment. The patient received a total of 40 hours of precoma; daily dose of insulin averaged 200 units.

During therapy, slight improvement was noted after the thirteenth treatment and dramatic improvement after the nineteenth treatment (the ninth in which the patient reached a precoma state). There was marked reduction in anxiety, tension, and depression. The patient's affect became more appropriate, and after 1 month of therapy delusional experiences had ceased. Her relationships with her therapist and with other patients became warmer, and she began to discuss previously hidden anxieties in interviews. She analyzed her body image, her loneliness and secondary dislike of others, and her inability to resolve her conflicts with her immigrant, overprotective parents.

The clinical and interview behavior continued when insulin treatment was terminated. The major topics of discussion were explored more extensively and applied to everyday living. Gradually, over the succeeding 6 months, the patient attended school outside the hospital and resumed relationships with her family. She was discharged after 13 months of hospitalization, markedly improved.

The patient, with a simple schizophrenic reaction, illustrates the effectiveness of insulin subcoma treatment in dealing with the extreme anxiety found in a schizophrenic reaction. After the anxiety had been alleviated with insulin, the therapist and the hospital were able to establish realistic and meaningful relationships with the patient. These relationships, in turn, were built up securely while insulin treatments continued. When treatment was terminated, therefore, the basic groundwork had been prepared for continuing psychotherapeutic efforts.

Experience indicates that coma insulin treatment is more effective in dealing with the very serious, fixed, chronic paranoid schizophrenic reactions. Subcoma, on the other hand, is as effective as coma insulin treatment in dealing with less severe paranoid illnesses and with other kinds of schizophrenic reactions.

Under some conditions, patients with affective illnesses may be treated by the use of subcoma insulin treatment. Manic excitements usually respond favorably to the administration of insulin treatments, but it is a matter of several days or weeks before the excitement is brought under control with the subcoma insulin treatment. Therefore, although this is an effective treatment procedure, it must be viewed less favorably than electroconvulsive treatment and the phenothiazines. Depressions also respond occasionally to subcoma insulin treatment. Considering the high degree of specificity which ECT treatment has for these conditions, however, it is doubtful that there are many instances where subcoma insulin treatment is indeed a treatment of choice.

PSYCHOPATHOLOGIC CONSIDERATIONS

In all diagnostic groups, the presence of marked anxiety or fear greatly enhances the chance that subcoma insulin treatment will be effective. It is worthy of note that the rates at which schizophrenic reactions tend to respond favorably to subcoma and coma insulin treatment are parallel to the amount of affect, and particularly to the amount of anxiety and fear, which are associated with the subgroups of schizophrenic reactions. The pseudoneurotic, the catatonic, and the paranoid schizophrenic reactions are commonly associated with large amounts of anxiety and readily mobilized affect. They respond better to insulin treatment than do the simple and hebephrenic schizophrenic reactions, which are not associated with much affective display.

An illustrated example of the anxiety-relieving potential of subcoma insulin treatment may be seen in the following case.

Case 2. A 35-year-old professional worker was admitted to the hospital with a 16-year history of intermittent bouts of anxiety and depression. Over the 10 years prior to admission, he had received five ECTs during a brief hospitalization and 16 months of continuous psychotherapy, as well as frequent brief episodes of psychotherapy from various therapists. Six months prior to admission, in an ambiguous work situation, the patient's long-term borderline adjustment began to crumble. Anxiety and tension gradually increased until they were almost intolerable and were associated with ruminativeness, insomnia, inability to work, delusions of persecution, and homicidal ideas.

On admission, the patient displayed marked anxiety, tension, and depression, and was preoccupied with thoughts of destruction. After $3\frac{1}{2}$ weeks, he was placed on subcoma insulin treatment. He received a total of 67 treatments, precoma being achieved first during the eighteenth treatment and regularly after the twenty-seventh treatment. The patient received a total of 40 hours of precoma; the daily dose of insulin averaged 310 units.

With the initiation of precoma during treatment, a distinct change took place in the patient's therapy and in his behavior. Anxiety and tension diminished, and the interviews became more productive, the patient discussing the privations in his early life and his long-established doubts of his own ability. As this insecurity was explored, more and more direct hostility appeared in interviews and social behavior. He was able to see some of the reasons for the hostility and gradually to learn methods of handling it which were better than his previous total suppression. After the termination of insulin treatment, the patient returned to part-time activity outside the hospital, dealt successfully with an extremely difficult home situation, and was discharged, improved, after 5½ months of hospitalization. Although he has had occasional difficulty since discharge, he remains a productive professional worker 5 years after discharge.

This paranoid schizophrenic reaction offered little grounds for optimism at the time of the patient's admission to the hospital. The illness had a 16-year duration, with a previous hospitalization and chronic partial incapacity, despite a large amount of good psychotherapy. The most striking factor in the success of therapy was the fact that the man had never come to grips with his anger and resentment because of his anxiety. This anxiety appeared to function as a protective barrier, blocking the emergence of the hostile feelings. When the anxiety was controlled with insulin, the hostility emerged directly and the patient was then able to handle it in a more efficient manner than previously.

The presence of extreme fear, especially when it has achieved the state of panic, is an indication that insulin treatment will be highly effective. If panic occurs, even in the setting of a depressive illness, insulin treatment will usually be very effective. It may be expected that the insulin treatment will work far more rapidly than usual. Instead of the 60 to 90 treatments which are commonly necessary before results are obtained, a series of 30 treatments will frequently achieve the desired results in the presence of a panic. Furthermore, patients with panic usually respond very early in the course of treatment, and it is unusual for a patient to have as many as 10 successful treatments without having already shown marked signs of improvement.

The presence of the mood of depression is not a favorable sign for the administration of insulin treatment. Patients with simple schizophrenic reactions, for example, who have depression or elation as major features in their illness have a much lower response rate to treatment than do the simple schizophrenic patients who show anxiety or fear. Usually, when depression is present in a schizophrenic illness, it is necessary to use electroconvulsive treatment, if it is desired that a depression be handled by means of physical treatment.

The presence of resentment and anger, like depression, does not indicate a favorable response to insulin treatment. In catatonic excitements, for example, virtually 100 per cent improvement may be found in patients who have leading symptoms of fear and anxiety. On the other hand, a response in the neighborhood of 40 per cent improvement is found in similar patients who have anger as their outstanding emotional characteristic.

Frequently, however, an appreciation of the reason behind overt hostility may indicate that anxiety is the fundamental problem. In such an instance, subcoma insulin will produce beneficial results, as illustrated in the following case.

Case 3. A 24-year-old housewife was admitted to the hospital with a 2-month history of severe anxiety and depression following a hysterectomy. As anxiety mounted, she became increasingly hostile, overactive, and demanding, with auditory and visual hallucinations.

This patient's past history is significant in that she had long experienced difficulty in her dealings with parents, siblings, and peers. Her marriage was chaotic, and a separation was contemplated at the time of onset of the symptoms leading to admission. She had had 6 months of psychoanalytic psychotherapy at age 17 and had received eight ECTs at age 18 for a depressive reaction.

On admission, the patient was in a catatonic excitement, with marked hostility, erotic behavior and talk, destructiveness, delusions, and hallucinations. During the early period of hospitalization, efforts were directed primarily at controlling the excitement. The patient received two courses of ECT, for a total of 13 ECTs; she then had one course of chlorpromazine, for a total of 35 days, discontinued because of severe rash; finally, a third course of 3 ECTs was given. Each of these programs gave temporary help in controlling the excited state of the patient, but therapeutic efforts were largely expended in this controlling fashion and little exploratory work took place.

After 6 weeks of hospitalization, the patient was begun on subcoma insulin treatment. She received 54 treatments, precoma being achieved during the seventh treatment. The patient received a total of 38 hours of precoma; the daily dose of insulin averaged 175 units.

During treatment, there was little alteration in the patient's excited behavior until the eleventh episode of precoma. At that time, the overactivity rapidly subsided; there remained severe anxiety which, over the succeeding 10 treatments, also subsided. Her social ability became excellent, while interviews came to be intensely active, with productive exploration of infantile conflicts and their application to current problems.

After the termination of insulin treatment, exploratory therapy became less active. The patient gradually resumed activities outside the hospital. She was discharged after $4\frac{1}{2}$ months of hospitalization, markedly improved; she has remained well for 5 years following discharge.

This acute catatonic schizophrenic reaction provides a good illustration of the symptomatic nature of several physical treatments. As might be expected, the excitement could be controlled by ECT and chlorpromazine; in addition, ECT could help alleviate depression, and the chlorpromazine could help alleviate hostility. Neither treatment, however, could assuage this patient's anxiety, which had developed as her marriage was threatened and her self concept threatened by the hysterectomy. Insulin could alleviate this anxiety; when it did so, the excitement subsided and psychotherapeutic efforts could progress.

Conduct of Psychotherapy during Insulin Treatment

There are two ways in which interview psychotherapy may be conducted during the course of insulin treatment. The first, and more typical, of these methods involves the use of the organizing and symptom-reducing qualities of insulin to allow for improved psychotherapy of the classical type. In this approach, the insulin treatment improves, albeit temporarily, the patient's state. It thereby provides the psychotherapist with a more stable and receptive patient, allowing him to conduct much more vigorous interviews than he would otherwise be able to do. When insulin is used in this way, the therapeutic interviews are carried out in the 2 hours immediately after the completion of the daily insulin treatment, when the patient may be expected to be functioning at his optimal intellectual level. While the course of 30 to 90 treatments is being carried out, the therapist makes every attempt to discuss problematic and conflictual material, with the assurance that the anxiety and fears which are stirred up by discussions will be handled by the sedative and controlling action of the insulin. In essence, this approach is similar to carrying on psychotherapy with the help of the phenothiazines. It differs in that there is a possibility that insulin has a much more specific effect on anxiety, particularly the anxiety of schizophrenic patients.

A second type of utilization of the insulin treatments with psychotherapy, a much less common one, is somewhat similar to the use of Sodium Amytal interviews. Very frequently, it is helpful for the psychotherapist to interview the patient during the second or third hour of his daily insulin treatments. At this time there is considerable inhibition of higher cerebral integrative functions, but the patient is still able to talk and remember and to respond emotionally. As a consequence, it is frequently possible for the therapist to attain progress in one of two directions. First, he may use this opportunity to obtain historical material which has previously been concealed, consciously or unconsciously. He thereby gains in his understanding of his patient's conflicts and problems, which he may then discuss or handle in some other way in his posttreatment interviews with the patient. Second, the therapist may use an interview during the second and third hour of daily insulin treatments as a means of establishing a closer relationship to the patient, and giving strong help and support. During this time, when the patient's integrative functions are less efficient, he may implant strong suggestions of therapeutic benefit. Certainly, in any event, it is important for the therapist occasionally to visit the patient during the course of the insulin treatments in order to manifest his genuine concern for the traumatic and serious treatment which the patient is undergoing.

SUMMARY

Subcoma and coma insulin treatment may be regarded as effective means of treating patients with schizophrenic illnesses, especially those who have fairly well-organized personalities. These treatments produce a relief from anxiety and allow a long-term psychotherapeutic program to be initiated. The usual course involves 30 to 90 daily treatments. During these days, the stabilizing effect of the insulin will allow the patient to accomplish a great deal of dynamic exploration and to make appropriate plans in his psychotherapeutic interviews. The treatments are most effective in helping patients who have anxiety and fear as their leading emotional characteristics. The response of patients who are in panic states, regardless of the basic diagnostic category, is usually excellent. This treatment, therefore, must be regarded as effective, but limited in application because of its expense, the associated dangers, and the necessarily long duration of treatment.

LOBOTOMY

Prefrontal lobotomy, which was described by Moniz, in 1936, is a drastic physical treatment which can serve a useful purpose in certain therapeutic situations.

Method of Treatment

There are a number of varieties of lobotomy currently being used. The usual operation consists of a standard incision which is made in the superior portion of each frontal lobe. These incisions are made by means of a special scalpel, which is introduced through bilateral burr holes placed at lower ends of the coronal sutures. The external guideposts in making the cortical incision are the burr holes, with the sphenoidal ridges as internal landmarks. By means of the incision, connecting fibers between the frontal lobes and the posterior portions of the brain (including the thalamus, hypothalamus, and posterior lobes of the cortex) are severed.

There are a number of variations on this basic operation. These include the original technique of leukotomy described by Moniz, as well as so-called milder operations: operations performed through the orbit, chemical lobotomy, lobectomy, topectomy, and paramedian lobotomy. It is difficult to discern any significant difference in the effectiveness of the various operative procedures. It is quite clear, however, that unilateral lobotomies are, on the whole, much less effective than bilateral lobotomies in achieving the desired goals of treatment.

Complications

The complications which are associated with lobotomy are those which might be associated with any operation on the brain. They include, most prominently, hemorrhage and infection at the time of operation. On the whole, the operation is remarkably benign, with a very low operative mortality and a low incidence of complications.

Psychologic Effects of Lobotomy

The chief psychologic effect of a prefrontal lobotomy is a rather specific dulling of emotional responsiveness. Usually there is little or no alteration in the disordered thought content and the disordered perceptions of the patient. The patient with a schizophrenic reaction, for example, will continue to have his previous characteristic thought disorder, which may include delusions and hallucinations. Postoperatively, however, he will not show the same degree of anger, fear, or anxiety which he previously experienced in relation to this disordered thought content. Instead, his affective response will be bland, almost absent. This blandness will be found in relation to the disorders of intellectual content already noted and also will be shown in response to the events of everyday life and to the demands of society. The patient, therefore, cannot be expected to show the same amount of love, concern, and relatedness to persons who are close to him that he showed preoperatively. The epitome of emotional blandness may be seen in patients who are given a prefrontal lobotomy for the relief of intractable pain, as, for example, in the case of carcinomatosis. Such persons will continue to have the carcinomatous condition, and they will continue to report pain, which will vary in no degree from the pain which they experienced previously. They will *not*, however, show the same degree of suffering or disturbance which they previously showed from the pain.

Linked to this emotional blandness and lack of relatedness are many behavioral characteristics which are seen in patients who have received prefrontal lobotomies. These patients frequently cause disturbance in their environment, because they lack the emotional drive to cooperate with environmental rules and regulations. It is common for postlobotomy patients to lose their previous concern about appearance and behavior; frequently they will urinate in public or appear socially in states of undress. Similarly, they frequently fail to follow the usual pattern of living; their eating and sleeping habits may become chaotic. Since their emotional responsiveness is lacking, it is very difficult for any measures to lead these persons to follow the demands of the environment. The only approach which can be used effectively is an intellectual one; the patients will not respond to emotional pull and therefore must be led to see that meeting social demands will produce for them the most effective way of living. It is this need for intellect to control behavior, obviously, that is one of the reasons why a well-integrated preoperative personality is one of the most essential criteria for good results after a lobotomy.

It should be mentioned that one of the characteristic behavioral features associated with the majority of patients who have had prefrontal lobotomies is moderate to extreme obesity. This may be connected to the lack of emotional relatedness noted previously or to an unknown physiologic abnormality. It *is* known, however, that most patients who have had lobotomies gain upward of 30 lb in the postoperative period. They are beset with a need to eat almost continually and have an apparently insatiable craving for food. If left alone, they may well be content to eat almost continually. Very frequently, in the immediate postoperative period, the problem of controlling excessive eating is one of the most serious ones that the staff of the hospital or the patient's family needs to face.

Associated with the other psychologic manifestations which follow lobotomy, there is some intellectual impairment, probably the result of damage to the brain incurred at the time of operation. This is usually slight in relation to previously learned abilities; the language capacities, the habit capacities, and the understanding of previously known phenomena remain relatively intact. It is in understanding and solving new problems that the patient with a lobotomy shows most marked impairment. This deficit may, of course, be related to motivation, but it is apparently a very consistent postoperative finding.

Indications for Lobotomy

There is some difference of opinion, at the present time, about the specific indications for the use of a prefrontal lobotomy. There is general agreement that this operation should be restricted to severely ill patients and that it is most effective in schizophrenic reactions and severe psychoneurotic reactions which occur in persons with previously integrated personalities. There is disagreement, however, on when the operation should be performed. Many persons with extensive experience with lobotomy have deplored the hesitancy which is shown toward the use of lobotomy and the delays which take place before administering the operation. According to these authorities, the operation should be used, if possible, within the first year of illness for markedly better results. Other authorities, including Kalinowsky and Hoch (1952), believe that the lobotomy should not be administered until the patient has had an adequate trial of other physical treatments, including electroconvulsive treatment.

Prefrontal lobotomy has also been recommended for the treatment of severe and recurrent manic-depressive illness. It appears to be more effective in the treatment of the manic-depressive illnesses which are manifested by recurrent depressions. It is somewhat doubtful whether or not the prefrontal lobotomy in such a situation is more effective than long-term prophylactic administration of electroconvulsive treatment, which does not have nearly the same drastic effect on the personality.

In addition to arguments about the timing of lobotomy, there is considerable uncertainty as to the specific indications for lobotomy within the diagnostic categories in which it is indicated. It must be recognized, for example, that lobotomy is a permanent procedure and that the effects of its administration will be lifelong for the patient receiving it. Quite clearly, lobotomy should not be given to every psychoneurotic or schizophrenic patient. When should it be given?

To this question, the physician will find few answers. Perhaps the best has recently been formulated by Slocum, et al. (1959), who restrict its use to those patients who have failed to respond to other treatment and who have intractable distress from long-standing anxiety. Certainly, many physicians believe that lobotomy, within the diagnostic categories recognized, should be reserved for those patients who are in extreme and unrelievable suffering.

On another level, it seems false to use lobotomy as a means of getting a patient out of a hospital. There are several objections to such a use. The first objection is one of simple safety. For example, it has been emphasized that patients who have had lobotomies continue to have all the basic difficulties of their illnesses. It is, therefore, extremely dangerous to perform a lobotomy on a patient who might then be released from the hospital with continuing delusions and homicidal ideation. In such a situation the delusions and homicidal ideation might easily motivate, on an intellectual basis, homicidal activity which the patient's lack of emotional relationship with the environment would not hinder in any way.

The second objection to using lobotomy to get a patient out of a hospital is on the basis of the human aspect of medical treatment. It can easily be recognized that patients who have severe schizophrenic or psychoneurotic illnesses need not *always* be released from a hospital, or returned to a previous work situation, in order to lead comfortable lives. On the contrary, many of these persons can achieve the best life adjustment possible for them by working within a protective setting. By performing a prefrontal lobotomy on such patients, it may be possible to push them out of the protective setting and allow them to perform acceptably in outside society. Such pushing is done, however, at the cost of the person's emotional intactness. They might easily be far more comfortable and happy, without a lobotomy and without loss of ability to relate emotionally, if they are allowed comfortably to exist within a protective setting.

These several points should therefore be kept in mind by the physician who contemplates recommending a lobotomy. The operation is associated with some social risk and with marked personal loss. It is a drastic and permanent procedure, which not only affects the illness but also affects the whole life of the human being to whom it is done. Great caution must be used, therefore, especially in the light of new advances in medications which have recently been achieved in the field of psychiatric treatment. Its use should probably be limited to those patients with well-organized personalities who need its benefits for the relief of intractable emotional suffering.

Relationship to Psychotherapy

It is difficult to describe how prefrontal lobotomy may be linked with psychotherapy. On the one hand, it is quite obvious that intensive psychotherapeutic efforts of a directive and reeducational type are absolutely essential for a prolonged period of time following lobotomy. Whether this be done in a hospital, as most workers recommend, or whether the patient be returned rapidly to his family, it is clear that prolonged rehabilitation efforts should extend over a period of 1 to 5 years postoperatively with these patients. Such rehabilitation measures require the work of physicians, nurses, social workers, family members, and every available resource which can be called on in the community. The patient must be given constant guidance and instruction, and great care must be taken to use patience and tolerance in dealing with the behavioral difficulties which the patient shows. With this intensive effort, it is usually possible, if the patient has had a previously well-integrated personality, to help him achieve a satisfactory living and work adjustment outside the hospital situation. There is a great need after lobotomy for a concerted psychotherapeutic treatment plan.

On the other hand, in patients who have had a prefrontal lobotomy, there is very little effective opportunity to utilize exploratory psychotherapy. These patients have little or none of the emotional relationships, the emotional disturbance and suffering, or the motivation that is so essential to the execution of exploratory psychotherapy. In consequence, they will easily shrug off the attempts of the therapist to establish a rapport or a transference relationship, and interview psychotherapy is most likely to be sterile. The authors have seen attempts at exploratory psychotherapy carried out by zealous persons, but the results have always been of the same discouraging nature. It must be recognized, however, that the failure to carry out successful exploratory psychotherapy in patients who have had prefrontal lobotomy may be related to the inherent distrust with which psychotherapists regard the prefrontal lobotomy.

SUMMARY

Prefrontal lobotomy, which involves severing a major portion of the connections between the patient's frontal lobes and posterior portions of his brain, is a drastic procedure. Although the operation is relatively safe, it makes a permanent alteration in the individual's relationship to himself and to the world. He loses his emotional responsiveness and his human relatedness. In the process of losing emotional responsiveness, he suffers much less from the effects of such illnesses as schizophrenic, psychoneurotic, and recurrent manic-depressive reactions, as well as from intractable physical pain. As a result of this diminution of suffering, the patient may well be able to improve his adjustment to society following the operation. This improved adjustment to society requires intensive, cooperative treatment, of a directive and reeducational nature, to help a poorly motivated patient make progress. A great deal depends on the previous integration of the patient's personality and on the duration of the illness prior to the administration of the treatment. This operation, while unquestionably effective, must be used cautiously at the present time, because of the great advances currently being made in the field of pharmacologic treatment of psychiatric illnesses. It should probably be limited to relief of severe and intractable suffering.

13

ENDOCRINE THERAPY

Prior to the introduction of the newer tranquilizing agents, many clinicians and investigators were actively probing the possibility that endocrine factors contributed to the development of certain psychopathologic disturbances and that hormones might be valuable in the treatment of psychiatric patients. Interesting leads were uncovered, but no findings of general importance were detected with the laboratory methods then available. Studies of the effectiveness of various endocrine substances in the treatment of psychopathologic disorders were often contradictory and usually inconclusive, largely because of a lack of adequate biological and psychologic controls and because of difficulties in establishing adequate methods of evaluation. The impressive results obtained in psychiatric patients with the phenothiazine derivatives temporarily diminished interest and activity in the field of psychoendocrinology. With the discovery of new and important facts about hormone function, the development of more refined techniques of chemical analysis, and the synthesis of products of intermediary endocrine metabolism, investigations in this area have received new impetus. Moreover, many physicians administer various endocrine products for the management of relatively mild metabolic disturbances reflected in such symptoms as tension, fatigue, menstrual irregularities, or sexual difficulties in which psychodynamic factors play significant roles. It therefore seems desirable to review briefly what is known about the influence of these substances on pathologic emotions and psychopathologic features. However, their use in the treatment of psychiatric patients must be considered largely exploratory.

Endocrine diseases are often associated with psychopathologic symptoms. For instance, patients with hyperparathyroidism frequently manifest marked depression of mood. Hyperthyroid patients are often anxious and irritable, prone to temper outbursts and, occasionally, to paranoid suspiciousness. Myxedematous patients, on the other hand, may be physically and mentally retarded, apathetic, depressed, irritable, bewildered, and confused. Similarly, psychopathologic changes may often be seen in untreated cases of pituitary or adrenal dysfunction.

Endocrine studies have been carried out in a number of patients with well-defined psychopathologic states. However, results have often been inconclusive or applicable only to a very restricted group of illnesses. For example, one investigator will report decreased production of adrenal steroids in chronic schizophrenic patients. Then, another will report adequate adrenal steroid function in similarly diagnosed patients. Such typical disagreements frequently may be due to a lack of adequate biological controls, such as dietary intake and specimen collection. They may also reflect undue dependency upon general diagnostic terminology and failure to consider the particular emotions and dynamic factors of importance in the patient's condition at the time of study. When prolonged investigations, such as those of Gjessing in patients with periodic catatonia, have been carried out, each phase of the patient's illness was compared with the preceding and subsequent one. In this way, definite patterns have emerged which may be pertinent to the understanding of endocrinologic correlates of pathologic emotions.

In certain settings, endocrine factors may combine with psychodynamic considerations to produce psychiatric illnesses. This may be particularly true of diseases occurring at puberty, during the puerperium, and in the early aging period. Certain forms of schizophrenia, for example, are most likely to appear in early adolescence. Some of these patients reveal delayed sexual maturation and maintain a physical appearance which seems much younger than their chronological ages. Schizophrenic, depressive, and paranoid reactions developing in the postpartum period are often extremely resistant to ordinary psychotherapeutic and somatic modes of treatment. Mood disorders in women not infrequently begin at the time of menopause. The central role ascribed to sexuality in the development of various psychopathologic conditions has been repeatedly emphasized, and it is important to recall that an intimate relationship exists between normal sexual drive and the integrity of hormonal function.

Unfortunately, studies of the emotional and psychopathologic changes occurring in patients receiving various endocrine substances, either as part of treatment for endocrine diseases or in the setting of psychiatric therapy, are limited in number and scope. In very few have these compounds been given to a sufficiently large group of patients to permit statistical analysis. Moreover, psychologic studies accompanying hormone administration have often been very superficial, emphasizing general diagnostic considerations and failing to consider adequately the complex personality structure of the individual patient. For example, one investigator may obtain significant improvement in schizophrenic patients by the administration of cortisone; another may report complete failure in a second group of schizophrenic patients similarly treated. Perusal of the case histories included in such studies may often reveal that the two groups were not necessarily comparable or that the physicians did not agree on the definition of improvement. Moreover, the actual emotional changes occurring in the patients during hormone administration were often remarkably similar, regardless of whether any symptomatic benefit was derived.

The field of endocrinology is so vast and complex, and the practical results of hormonal studies in psychiatric patients thus far are so limited, that this discussion will be restricted to a description of those endocrine products which have been most extensively applied in the treatment of psychopathologic conditions. Isolated reports of the beneficial effects of such glandular material as pineal extract are most stimulating but unsubstantiated. Pituitary hormones, such as the adrenocorticotropic and gonadotropic hormones, have been used in a limited number of patients with variable consequences. The two groups of endocrine products which have been most widely studied in psychopathologic states are the thyroid hormones and the sex and adrenal steroids.

Thyroid Hormones

Undoubtedly, thyroid hormones have been administered to more psychiatric patients than any other endocrine preparation. In addition to their use in the treatment of myxedema, they have been given to many adolescents and adults with normal protein-bound iodine levels, normal uptakes of radioactive iodine, somewhat reduced basal metabolic rates, and mild or moderate symptoms of depression, tension, fatigue, and obesity. They have also been evaluated as therapeutic agents in patients with disturbances which are primarily psychopathologic in nature.

Thyroxine   3-5-3'-Triiodothyronine

Desiccated thyroid, thyroxine, and 3-5-3'-triiodothyronine are the most commonly employed thyroid hormones. The chemical structures of thyroxine and triiodothyronine are illustrated for comparison. Triiodothyronine is much more potent, milligram for milligram, than thyroxine.

Unlike the latter, which may require about 7 days to influence metabolism, the effects of triiodothyronine can be observed within 24 to 48 hours after the initial administration. The usual daily oral therapeutic dosage of desiccated thyroid ranges from 0.1 to 5 grains, that of thyroxine from 0.1 to 0.5 mg, and that of triiodothyronine from 25 to 100 μg. In many psychiatric patients, much larger doses have been used at times. Side effects and complications to the administration of thyroid hormones are well known. These include headaches, palpitations, increased appetite, weight loss, and tremulousness; in severe cases, debilitation may result and, occasionally, the marked toxic crisis known as thyroid storm. It has been reported that certain psychiatric patients, particularly those diagnosed as chronic schizophrenic reactions, seem to tolerate very high doses of thyroid hormones without undue side effects. Certainly, these hormones are contraindicated in patients with significant cardiovascular disease or certain endocrine disorders.

CLINICAL EFFECTIVENESS OF TREATMENT

In certain patients, diagnosed as having periodic catatonic reactions, in whom cyclic variations in nitrogen retention and excretion seem to correspond to the onset of acutely disturbed episodes, the administration of very large doses of desiccated thyroid or thyroxine has reportedly led to the prevention of recurrences of these anticipated psychopathologic phases. These thyroid preparations have also been employed in the treatment of several large series of chronically ill schizophrenic patients, apparently with some observable but poorly defined improvement in function. The following cases will illustrate the type of emotional changes seen in patients receiving various thyroid hormones, possible therapeutic benefits derived from their use, and the complexities and risks inherent in their administration.

Case 1. A 28-year-old woman was hospitalized for treatment of a severe obsessive-compulsive psychoneurotic reaction of 2 years' duration which had failed to respond to intensive psychotherapy, phenothiazine treatment, and electroconvulsive therapy. The patient's ability to function was markedly impaired by the persistent need to wash her hands every 15 minutes, avoid touching any objects which were even slightly soiled, and reset her hair several times each day. Concentration was seriously disturbed. She was preoccupied with ideas of guilt and worthlessness. She described feelings of hopelessness, although her depression of mood was not evident in her countenance.

After evaluation of her thyroid function, which was well within normal limits, she was placed on triiodothyronine, in daily oral dosage of 200 μg for 4 weeks. By the end of the first week of drug administration, she was manifestly hostile, becoming intensely angry when slightly provoked and expressing previously hidden resentment toward her husband and mother. Hostility remained prominent as long as the thyroid hormone was continued. Her compulsive symptoms were somewhat intensified.

Ten days after termination of triiodothyronine, her anger and resentment had disappeared, and a remarkable improvement in her clinical condition was noted. She was relatively free of her compulsive activity. Concentration was improved. Her spirits were cheerful and optimistic for the first time in more than a year. This state of well-being continued for nearly 6 months, when, in the setting of a dynamically disturbing environmental situation, mild evidence of her obsessive-compulsive symptoms temporarily returned.

In this patient, the administration of triiodothyronine was associated with the appearance of intense hostility which had previously been repressed or suppressed. Whether the drug directly stimulated these pathologic emotions or only served to increase the patient's awareness and expression of her inner feelings is unclear. Considering the frequency of irritability, resentment, and anger as manifestations of hyperthyroidism, it is not surprising that the administration of large doses of thyroid hormones would induce similar emotional changes in sensitive persons. However, not all patients seem to react to triiodothyronine in this way. Apathetic, deteriorated chronic schizophrenic patients, for example, often show little or no affective change when given these thyroid hormones. The alleviation of the obsessive-compulsive features in this patient, which took place following the termination of the hormone, was probably the consequence of the cathartic release of her pathologic hostility. It is also possible, however, that unknown rebound physiologic changes may have occurred, but such considerations remain largely speculative.

In addition to facilitating the appearance of hostile emotions, the administration of triiodothyronine has also been associated with the emergence of previously hidden sexual drives. The following case illustrates this effect.

Case 2. A 30-year-old physicist began psychotherapy at age 27 for the relief of depression of mood, loss of interest in his work, concentration difficulty, and a marked lack of sexual desire. Although his presenting symptoms were largely psychoneurotic in character, rigidity of personality structure and the occasional development of a distinct disorder in logical thought processes substantiated the impression that schizophrenic features were also present. After 6 months of psychotherapy, with little significant improvement in his condition, the intensity of his state was such that he could no longer work effectively. Eighteen ECTs were administered to alleviate his depression of mood and apathy. Following the sixth treatment, rage outbursts appeared. These subsided only after the end of the series of treatments. Depression diminished substantially. However, he continued to complain of lack of interest, absence of sexual drives, and depersonalization, described as "my body is dead, my soul is missing." Triiodothyronine was instituted in a daily dosage of 100 μg, and this regimen was then continued for 6 weeks. Within 7 days, depersonalization had nearly disappeared. The patient was aware of renewed desire to return to work. For the first time in 3 years he experienced erections and nocturnal emissions. This improvement continued for 8 months after termination of the thyroid hormone. Although periods of depression and anxiety returned from time to time, his sexual drives remained strong and unaffected.

In this patient, therefore, the administration of triiodothyronine was associated with the return of sexual drive, erections, and nocturnal emissions. Again, this effect may be due to an increase in the level of consciousness, allowing suppressed and repressed feelings to emerge. It may also be due to an influence of the thyroid hormone on the metabolism of adrenal or testicular hormones. All patients who receive triiodothyronine do not manifest increased sexual tension. In some, the induction of mild or moderate sexual excitement while receiving thyroid hormones may actually be detrimental to their well-being and life adjustment. The following case illustrates such a situation.

Case 3. An 18-year-old girl was seen in consultation in a state of marked depression. She revealed severe anxiety, inability to concentrate, social withdrawal, and intense guilt regarding sexual promiscuity. A well-defined thinking disorder was apparent, and the diagnosis of schizophrenic reaction, undifferentiated type, was readily established.

At age 16 she had first noted the onset of strong sexual urges, experienced as exciting genital sensations which occurred frequently even in the absence of environmental stimulation. Her dreams were filled with sexual content. Her behavior, as described by her parents, had become strikingly erotic, although she herself was unaware of the extent to which she invited male attention. Eventually, she became involved in a sexual intercourse experience with a man in his early thirties. Immediately thereafter, guilt, worthlessness, and futility combined with heightened sexual desires had led her into a series of intimate relationships and the eventual development of her psychopathologic state.

For 6 months prior to the onset of her intense sexual urges, the patient had been receiving 4 grains of desiccated thyroid daily for the management of menstrual irregularity. She was maintained on this hormone for the entire 2-year period during which her sexual activity increased and her psychopathologic condition was developing. After psychiatric hospitalization, thyroid was terminated. Sexual unrest continued for about 4 weeks, then subsided, and did not recur.

In this patient the administration of the thyroid hormone was associated with the appearance of strong sexual urges. Because of the dynamic personality structure of this particular patient, these drives facilitated behavioral difficulties and eventually may have colored her serious psychopathologic reaction.

The administration of thyroid hormones may modify the effectiveness of other somatic therapies. The following case is an example of a clinical situation in which the results of electroconvulsive therapy may have been enhanced by the previous administration of triiodothyronine.

Case 4. A 48-year-old unmarried secretary was hospitalized because of a 1-year history of severe obsessions and compulsions. Morbid thoughts of sickness and death recurred to her frequently. She felt forced to repeat words and questions in an attempt to be accurate to a degree which she herself recognized as pathologic. At times she was unable to speak at all, lest she say something which did not correctly correspond to her original ideas or feelings. Depression was not evident, although such a prevailing mood was suspected because of her age, the content of her thinking, and the nature of contributing dynamic factors, such as the recent death of her brother.

Intensive psychotherapy was carried out for 8 months, without any significant improvement. After her thyroid function had been evaluated and found to be normal, she was placed on triiodothyronine, in daily oral dosage of 200 μg for 3 weeks. Within 5 days, depression of mood was obvious, with tearfulness and complaints of feeling discouraged and hopeless. Resentment was expressed openly for the first time. Simultaneously, her obsessive ideas and compulsive activity were intensified. Following termination of the hormone, her depressive mood continued, but her obsessive-compulsive features subsided markedly. Seven ECTs were then administered, with a rapid clearing of her depressive state. She was then able to leave the hospital and resume her usual life.

In this patient, the administration of triiodothyronine was associated with the appearance of previously hidden depression of mood and hostility. Severe obsessive-compulsive symptoms subsided after the termination of the hormone. It seems likely, in view of the vast experience with this method of treatment, that the administration of ECT to this patient at the time when only her obsessions and compulsions were prominent would not have led to a favorable clinical change. The use of triiodothyronine, with the alleviation of psychoneurotic features and the increase in overt depression of mood, may have influenced the biological milieu so as to facilitate the efficacy of ECT.

Steroid Hormones

Steroid hormones are produced by the ovaries, testes, and adrenal glands. The particular steroids which have received attention in the management of psychiatric patients include estrogens, progesterone, testosterone, cortisone, and dehydroisoandrosterone. The basic chemical structures of each of these groups are illustrated. Many synthetic preparations based on these compounds have been developed, resembling them closely with regard to certain metabolic activities but lacking others which would be undesirable when the hormones are used for very specific clinical purposes. Inasmuch as none of these steroids has yet come to occupy a significant role in the treatment of psychopathologic conditions, it seems sufficient to discuss them in a general way, without elaborating on dose schedules; side effects, which sometimes can be quite severe, such as the induction of adrenal insufficiency; or the complex differences between one synthetic hormone and another.

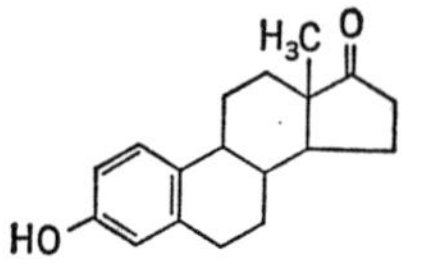

Estrone (an estrogen)

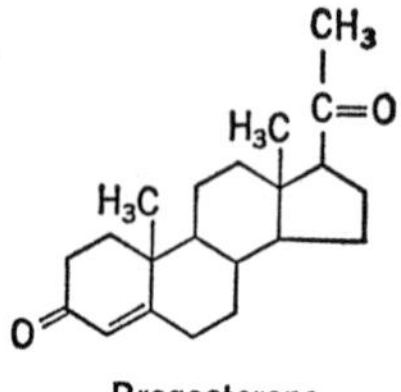

Progesterone

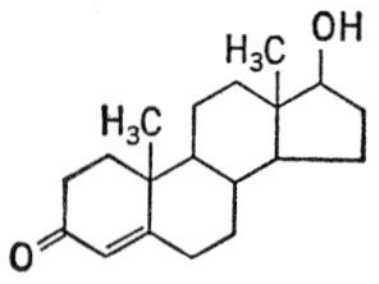

Testosterone

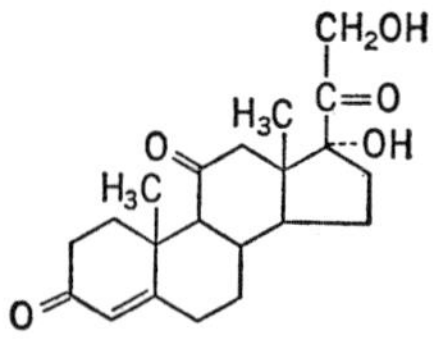

Cortisone

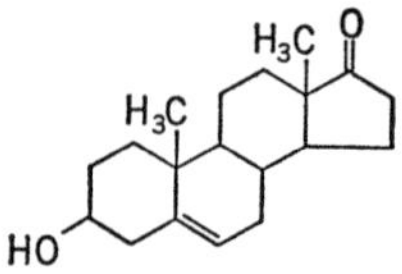

Dehydroisoandrosterone

ESTROGENS

Estrogens have been used in the treatment of many menopausal women who manifest anxiety, tension, and mild depression of mood. Although they appear to be effective in alleviating physical symptoms such as hot flashes, chills, perspiration, weakness, and fatigue, they do not significantly influence pathologic emotions, moods, or associated psychopathologic symptoms. Therefore, they are of little or no value in the management of mood disorders or serious psychoneurotic conditions occurring in middle life or the early aging period. It has been reported that estrogenic substances are capable of intensifying or restoring sexual drive in certain female patients, but some degree of ovarian insufficiency may be a requirement for such activity.

PROGESTERONE

Progesterone, as well as estrogens, has been used to reduce pathologic sexual unrest in male patients, particularly when this factor promotes undesirable behavior. The value of such a procedure is debatable.

It is unclear whether the administration of these hormones actually decreases sexual tension or alleviates pathologic emotions, such as anxiety, which intensify behavioral difficulties. No direct influence on homosexual orientation has been observed.

In the discussion of thyroid hormones, a case was presented in which triiodothyronine may have facilitated the response of a patient to electroconvulsive therapy. In similar fashion, progesterone has been administered in association with ECT in the treatment of intensely depressed postpartum patients. The results of this combination appear encouraging, but further investigations are necessary to clarify the value of such a procedure.

TESTOSTERONE

As estrogens are widely used in aging women, testosterone is often administered to men in their middle years for the purpose of restoring energy and sexual drive. Whether this hormone is capable of producing any such effects in the absence of some degree of testicular insufficiency is extremely debatable. Attempts to employ testosterone in the treatment of impotence have been singularly unsuccessful, since the basis of this symptom is more often psychologic than organic; rarely has hormone treatment been combined with psychotherapy. Certainly testosterone, like estrogen, is of no value in the management of mood disorders or severe psychoneurotic disturbances.

CORTISONE

Severe psychopathologic reactions were described in a number of patients receiving cortisone when this adrenal steroid was first introduced for the relief of symptoms of various physical diseases such as rheumatoid arthritis. Several attempts to clarify the therapeutic potentials of cortisone in psychiatric patients were carried out. Some investigators concluded that its administration would produce clinical improvement in schizophrenic patients. Others failed to demonstrate any beneficial effects. Unfortunately, this hormone was studied primarily with regard to its value as a method of treatment rather than for the purpose of determining emotional and psychopathologic changes occurring in patients receiving it, regardless of whether or not they showed improvement. When detailed case histories of patients treated with cortisone are reviewed, certain interesting trends appear. Some of the patients demonstrated an intensification of pathologic moods of elation or depression, hostility, and paranoid delusions. Others manifested strong sexual unrest. Still others showed no emotional changes whatsoever while receiving cortisone. The differences in responsiveness to this adrenal steroid were attributed to existing pretreatment personality factors, but an equally meaningful physiologic explanation may well have escaped detection.

Cortisone was also used in the management of delirium tremens, but its application in this condition has largely been supplanted by the phenothiazine drugs. Some investigators have described an enhancement of the efficacy of electroconvulsive therapy when it is combined with cortisone, but these observations still require substantiation.

In contrast to cortisone, which seems to increase the level of consciousness, certain adrenal steroids possess anaesthetic properties. Some of these compounds, such as hydroxypregnanedione, have been used experimentally to reduce pathologic emotions.

DEHYDROISOANDROSTERONE

Dehydroisoandrosterone is an adrenal steroid which has been employed in the treatment of a limited number of schizophrenic patients who demonstrated abnormal urinary excretions of 17 ketosteroids, in particular, an elevation of beta fractions. This hormone seems to reduce pathologic hostility and restore sexual drives in some patients but to facilitate aggressive behavior and rage outbursts in others. Although it is of no current practical clinical value, it deserves mention, since its application is one of the few examples of endocrine treatment in schizophrenia based on an observable biological deviation in the function of the parent gland.

SUMMARY

Many endocrine substances have been evaluated as therapeutic agents in the management of psychiatric conditions. Thus far, none have produced indisputable clinical improvement in any well-defined diagnostic or psychopathologic setting. Thyroid hormones and sex and adrenal steroids have been more widely used than any other hormonal preparations for this purpose. Although some favorable results have been obtained, more detailed and controlled investigations of the specific emotional changes occurring in patients during the administration of various endocrine substances are urgently needed. It is most likely that abnormalities in the intermediary metabolism of hormones will have to be demonstrated in psychiatric patients before endocrine therapy can be established on a sound and predictable basis.

14

MISCELLANEOUS DRUGS

There are a number of pharmacologic agents which have been used in the treatment of psychiatric patients which cannot be grouped with the major somatic therapies described thus far. This miscellaneous classification of drugs includes anticonvulsants, disulfiram, anti-Parkinson compounds, diphenylmethane derivatives, para-acetamidobenzoate, and methaminodiazepoxide.

Anticonvulsant medications, such as diphenylhydantoin sodium, have been developed primarily for the control of various forms of epilepsy. However, they also may be valuable in the alleviation of pathologic emotions and associated psychopathologic features occurring in epileptic patients and in patients who, although lacking clinical evidence of epilepsy, demonstrate abnormal electroencephalographic patterns.

Disulfiram has no direct influence on pathologic emotions. It is a drug which arrests the metabolism of alcohol at the acetaldehyde phase, thereby inducing severe physiologic distress in patients who combine it with alcohol. Because of this action, it may be a useful adjunct in the management of certain carefully selected alcoholic patients.

Anti-Parkinson drugs are effective in alleviating the motor and coordination impairment associated with the use of phenothiazine derivatives or reserpine. Diphenylmethane derivatives, such as azacyclonol, benactyzine, and hydroxyzine, may be effective in modifying pathologic anxiety. Para-acetamidobenzoate is a mild stimulant recommended by some clinicians for the relief of depressive moods or apathetic states in psychoneurotic and schizophrenic patients. Methaminodiazepoxide is a new compound which appears to reduce pathologic anxiety and tension in various diagnostic settings.

In this chapter, the nature and effectiveness of each of these drugs will be discussed.

Anticonvulsant Drugs

There are six major groups of drugs which have been employed successfully in the management of epileptic disorders. These groups are pharmacologically, chemically, and clinically distinct. They include barbiturates, hydantoinates, oxazolidines, acetylureas, pyrimidines, and succinimides. Some of these compounds are useful in more than one kind of epilepsy. Many of them are potentially toxic and hence require careful supervision.

The most useful and generally effective anticonvulsant barbiturate is phenobarbital (Luminal). This drug can be utilized in the treatment of patients with grand mal seizures, petit mal attacks, or psychomotor episodes. Moreover, it reduces pathologic anxiety and tension. The effective adult dosage ranges from 50 to 400 mg daily, in divided doses. Side effects are usually mild, consisting of drowsiness and diminished mental activity. Allergic reactions are rare.

The most important members of the hydantoinate series are diphenylhydantoin sodium (Dilantin, Diphenylhydantoin) and methantoin (Mesantoin). Both are valuable in the treatment of grand mal and psychomotor seizures and undesirable in petit mal states. The usual daily dosage of each ranges from 0.3 to 0.6 Gm, administered in three or four divided doses. The side effects of diphenylhydantoin treatment include rashes of the cutaneous tissues or mucous membranes, occurring about the middle of the second week of administration, lasting 4 days, and then disappearing. Serious skin lesions are rare. Hypertrichosis of the face and extremities may occur. The gums occasionally become swollen. Neurologic complications, which often may be alleviated by a temporary reduction in dosage, include nystagmus, ataxia, tremors, slurred speech, diplopia, and blurred vision. Gastrointestinal distress, such as nausea, anorexia, and abdominal pain, may occur. The complications of methantoin therapy are similar, although neurologic side effects are somewhat less frequent. Several fatalities have been attributed to aplastic anemia, leukopenia, and agranulocytosis in patients receiving this drug.

The most important members of the oxazolidine series are trimethadione (Tridione) and paramethadione (Paradione). These drugs are used only in the treatment of petit mal epilepsy. Their usual dosage range varies from 0.3 to 2.7 Gm per day, in three divided doses. Complications include blood dyscrasias, rashes, nephrosis, and blurring of vision. These seem to be more prevalent with trimethadione than with paramethadione.

Phenacemide (Phenurone) is the only member of the acetylurea group which is effective without being too dangerously toxic. Its complications are sufficiently frequent and severe, however, for it to be reserved until all other reasonable measures to control psychomotor epilepsy, the only form of this disease in which the drug is effective, have been tried. It is contraindicated in patients with histories of significant allergic reactions or liver disease, since fatal cases of hepatic damage and aplastic anemia have been reported in patients receiving this medication. Severe psychopathologic symptoms, such as depression, insomnia, and suicidal attempts, have been reported during its administration. The usual daily dosage is 1.5 to 4 Gm, in three divided doses.

Primidone (Mysoline) is the only member of the pyrimidine group which is useful in the treatment of epilepsy of the grand mal or psychomotor type. The daily dosage ranges from 0.5 to 2 Gm per day, in two or three divided doses. Side effects include nausea, vomiting, dizziness, sleepiness, and psychopathologic symptoms in particular paranoid reactions.

Phensuximide (Milontin) is the only succinimide in clinical use in the treatment of epilepsy. It is indicated in the management of petit mal attacks. Side effects are occasionally seen, including rashes, drowsiness, and renal changes. The usual daily dosage is 500 mg 4 times daily.

Phenobarbital and diphenylhydantoin are the two medications most commonly used in the management of grand mal epilepsy. In the treatment of petit mal seizures, phenobarbital, trimethadione, or paramethadione are most often employed. Primidone, diphenylhydantoin, or phenobarbital is most often used to treat patients with psychomotor disturbances. Not infrequently, combinations of these drugs produce results which are superior to those obtained by the use of only one of them.

Many patients with epilepsy also demonstrate pathologic emotions and associated psychopathologic features. These factors may influence markedly the frequency or intensity of the epileptic attacks. Moreover, the underlying neurologic disorder contributes greatly to the personality disturbance—directly, through changes in cerebral function, and indirectly, because of the personal and social complications of being epileptic. In many epileptic patients, adequate therapeutic control of seizures is accompanied by an improvement in their emotional states. Conversely, therapeutic alleviation of psychopathologic features often leads to a decrease in the incidence of seizures.

The administration of a suitable anticonvulsant, such as phenobarbital or diphenylhydantoin, to a patient with psychomotor epilepsy will frequently alleviate emotional and behavioral difficulties. Phenacemide may be used judiciously in these states. In some patients with psychopathologic changes such as recurrent, intense, unprovoked rage outbursts, who cannot be satisfactorily classified as epileptic but who demonstrate unusual electroencephalographic patterns, the use of anticonvulsants will also lead to improvement in their emotional states.

Pathologic emotions, such as anxiety or hostility, often tend to aggravate an underlying epileptic condition. Occasionally, the administration of anticonvulsants and psychotherapy prove insufficient to control the clinical state. In such situations, other pharmacologic agents may be used to relieve distressing psychopathologic features. For example, phenothiazines can be employed to reduce fear, hostility, or sexual unrest if these factors are present in an epileptic patient. Phenothiazines, it will be recalled, lower the seizure threshold and therefore are ordinarily undesirable in the treatment of patients who are prone to epileptic attacks. On the other hand, these emotions can also precipitate undue neurophysiologic reactions. Therefore, when used carefully and with adequate medical supervision for a well-defined purpose and for a limited time period, phenothiazines can successfully reduce pathologic emotions and facilitate improvement in epileptic patients. It is essential to continue anticonvulsant medication, such as diphenylhydantoin or phenobarbital, along with the phenothiazines and to terminate the tranquilizing agent as soon as the desired clinical effect has been established. Meprobamate and reserpine have also been used successfully in conjunction with anticonvulsants for the control of pathologic anxiety and tension in epileptic patients.

Disulfiram

Disulfiram (Antabuse) is useful in the treatment of certain patients with chronic alcoholism. Its formula is given. This drug does not produce any well-defined emotional or psychopathologic changes, nor does it directly influence the need for alcohol experienced by the patient. However, it does create a biological milieu in which ingestion of alcohol re-

$$C_2H_5 \diagdown N-C-S-S-C-N \diagup C_2H_5$$
$$C_2H_5 \diagup \; \underset{S}{\overset{\|}{}} \qquad \underset{S}{\overset{\|}{}} \; \diagdown C_2H_5$$

sults in severe physiologic disturbances, causing the patient extreme discomfort. In certain alcoholic patients, the knowledge that drinking will produce such a reaction will be sufficient to deter them from using alcohol. This toxic reaction is characterized by widespread vasodilation, leading to flushing, nausea, a fall in blood pressure, anxiousness, and, occasionally, general collapse. In rare instances, alcohol and disulfiram combine to produce severe psychopathologic states characterized by confusion, elation or depression, or paranoid delusions. Side effects of disulfiram administration include fatigue, lethargy, and, at times, impotence.

Disulfiram acts by inhibiting the metabolism of alcohol at the acetaldehyde stage, allowing an accumulation of this toxic substance. Its actions continue for 48 to 96 hours after the administration of the last dose.

The usual daily dose of disulfiram is established in the following manner. On each of the first 2 days of treatment the patient is given 1 Gm orally. On the third day the dose is reduced to 0.75 Gm. Thereafter he is maintained on 0.25 to 0.50 Gm daily. In order to convince the patient of the consequences of drinking while receiving disulfiram, he may be encouraged to take about 40 cc of whisky on the fourth day of drug administration to produce typical physiologic distress.

Because of its toxic nature, particularly its influence on the cardiovascular system, disulfiram should not be administered to patients in poor physical health. Severe cardiac or hepatic diseases and profound metabolic disturbances are probably contraindications to its use. Moreover, this medication should not be administered to alcoholic patients who are very depressed or who reveal suicidal trends, since it can be successfully employed, especially in combination with alcohol, as a means of self-destruction.

As already described, chronic alcoholism can occur in many personality and diagnostic settings. Disulfiram is most effective in those patients who are relatively well-integrated, motivated to pursue a program of therapy, aware of the need to terminate their use of alcohol, and reliable with regard to the self-administration of medicines. The following case illustrates the effective utilization of this drug in a carefully selected patient.

Case 1. A 43-year-old business executive presented a history of excessive alcohol intake for 5 years. During the 6 months prior to consultation he had been drinking to the point of intoxication at least once weekly and, consequently, had missed several days of work each month. His tolerance for alcohol had diminished. Under the influence of alcohol he manifested intense hostility, becoming easily enraged and occasionally destructive. Analysis of his drinking habits revealed that he was more likely to drink when he was alone in the evenings. He was a bachelor and for nearly a year had been regularly dating an attractive, personable woman several years his junior. She disapproved of his drinking and tried to help him in constructive ways. Because of her attitude, he refrained from drinking in her presence. Hence, it was possible for him to spend many evenings with her without taking a drink or even desiring one.

When first seen by the psychiatrist, he was acutely intoxicated and required immediate hospitalization. He remained in the hospital for 3 weeks. At this time resentment and tension were prominent features. He demonstrated some suspiciousness but no paranoid delusions. Prochlorperazine was instituted, and he received 10 mg four times daily for nearly 1 month, leading to a striking reduction of his pathologic hostility. At the time of his discharge, he was placed on 0.5 Gm of disulfiram daily and warned of the complications which would result if he drank while taking this medication. He returned to work and was seen regularly in psychotherapy. He faithfully adhered to the disulfiram regimen and refrained from alcohol.

This patient was intelligent and ordinarily possessed good judgment. He had developed an alcoholic problem in the setting of a complex psychoneurotic illness and was clearly aware of the real and potential difficulties surrounding his drinking. He was unusually well motivated to pursue treatment. The fact that his association with another person had successfully deterred him from drinking encouraged the physician to provide the patient with another support in the form of disulfiram.

Phenothiazines, meprobamate, phenobarbital, or antidepressive drugs can be used, when indicated, in association with disulfiram. The phenothiazines in particular may be of considerable value in the control of hostile emotions, which in certain alcoholic patients seem to precipitate drinking episodes.

Diphenylmethane Derivatives

There are three important diphenylmethane derivatives which have been used in the treatment of psychiatric patients. These are benactyzine, azacyclonol, and hydroxyzine. The chemical structure of each is given. Although these drugs have received considerable attention and some enthusiastic support, it is unlikely that any of them will prove to be significant pharmacologic agents. The effects which they seem to produce on pathologic emotions and associated psychopathologic features appear to be more reliably achieved by other agents which possess fewer unpleasant complications.

The first member of this series is azacyclonol (Frenquel) which is a gamma isomer of pipradrol hydrochloride, a stimulant. Azacyclonol has been tested in a very limited number of patients. It appears to reduce hallucinations and delusions resulting from the administration of lysergic acid diethylamide as well as hallucinations and delusions occurring in patients experiencing acute schizophrenic reactions. The effective dosage varies widely, ranging from 20 to 400 mg daily. Because azacyclonol is clearly less reliable and less effective than the phenothiazine derivatives in the management of severely disturbed patients and possesses little or no significant effect on psychoneurotic symptoms, its use has been largely discontinued.

Benactyzine (Suavitil, Phobex) was originally reported to be effective in alleviating anxiety and phobic symptoms in psychoneurotic patients.

In combination with meprobamate it was employed with some measure of success in the treatment of patients with mild and moderate degrees of depression of mood. However, these observations have not been sufficiently substantiated to warrant its use as an antidepressive drug.

The usual dose of benactyzine is 1 mg orally three times daily. This may be gradually increased to 3 mg three times daily, the maximum daily dosage being 10 mg.

Unfortunately, psychopathologic complications occur frequently in the course of benactyzine therapy. It is unclear whether these are directly

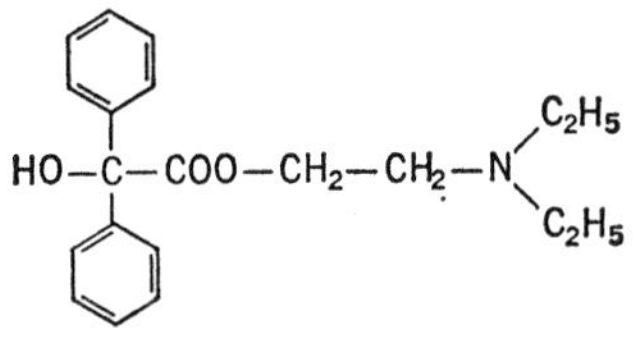

HO—C—COO—CH₂—CH₂—N⟨C₂H₅/C₂H₅

Benactyzine

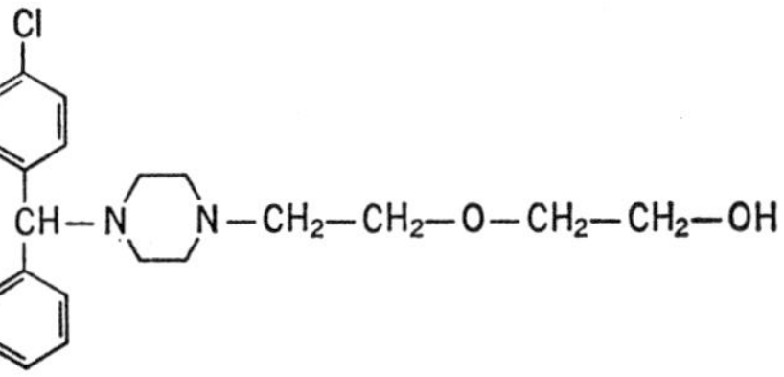

CH—N⟨ ⟩N—CH₂—CH₂—O—CH₂—CH₂—OH

Hydroxyzine

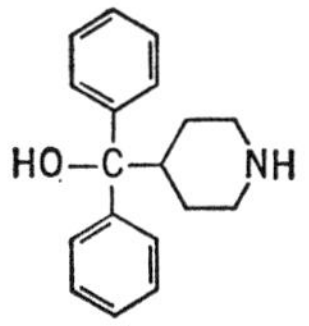

HO—C—⟨ ⟩NH

Azacyclonol

produced by the drug or whether they result from the emotional alterations taking place in the patients receiving the drug. Nonetheless, they are often severe enough to interfere with function and well-being, thereby offsetting any beneficial influence of the medication. These side effects include severe preoccupation and absent-mindedness, concentration difficulty, depersonalization, apathy, and, occasionally, transient disorientation. Physical side effects of benactyzine administration include paresthesias, dryness of mouth, nausea or diarrhea, dizziness, palpitations, and diminished motor coordination. The nature, extent, and frequency of these side effects combined with the limited influence which this drug has on psychopathologic states cast doubt on its clinical usefulness.

Hydroxyzine (Atarax) appears to be the most useful member of this series. It seems to be effective, in doses of 25 mg two to four times daily, in reducing pathologic anxiety and tension in mild psychoneurotic states. Pharmacologically, it inhibits certain effects of epinephrine, serotonin, acetylcholine, reserpine, histamine, and the posterior pituitary hormone. No serious side effects have been reported. However, it does not clearly possess any superiority to meprobamate or barbiturates and certainly has not been as extensively investigated as these agents.

Para-acetamidobenzoate

Deanol (Deaner) is a precursor of acetylcholine. In a limited number of studies it has been described as producing increased energy and decreased depression in chronic psychoneurotic and schizophrenic patients. It is administered in daily oral dosage ranging from 10 to 50 mg. The clinical effects do not usually appear until the medication has been given for 2 or 3 weeks. It is contraindicated in patients with grand mal epilepsy, inasmuch as it has been known to precipitate convulsions. The most prominent side effects are headache and insomnia. Clinical and experimental evidence for the therapeutic effectiveness of deanol is limited and as yet unconvincing.

Anti-Parkinson Drugs

The administration of phenothiazines or reserpine is frequently complicated by the development of mild or severe disturbances in motor function and coordination which resemble the neuromuscular symptoms of Parkinson's disease. These side effects, when encountered, can often be relieved by a reduction in the dosage of the pharmacologic agent being used. When such a reduction is contraindicated because of the danger of losing control over the emotional state of the patient, drugs which are used in the clinical management of parkinsonism can be employed to counteract these symptoms. The two most widely used drugs of this type are trihexyphenidyl hydrochloride (Artane) and benztropine methanesulfonate (Cogentin). Both possess parasympatholytic activity. The usual dose of each is 2 mg orally once or twice daily. Side effects include dryness of the mouth and blurring of vision.

Methaminodiazepoxide

Methaminodiazepoxide (Librium) has recently been introduced as an agent capable of reducing pathologic anxiety and tension. It has anticonvulsant properties and appears to be a more potent muscle relaxant than meprobamate. The most satisfactory results of treatment with this drug have been observed in patients with psychoneurotic illnesses, although certain patients with schizophrenic or depressive mood disorders also appear to have benefited from its administration. The side effects noted include lightheadedness, drowsiness, and ataxia. Dissociative symptoms and hostile outbursts have been seen in several patients receiving this drug. The usual oral dose ranges from 10 mg twice daily to 25 mg four times daily. It is as yet unclear whether methaminodiazepoxide possesses qualities making it different from or superior to meprobamate or barbiturates. This compound will require further clinical investigation before final conclusions about its usefulness can be drawn.

SUMMARY

There are a number of pharmacologic agents which have been used in the treatment of psychiatric patients and which do not fall into one of the major groups already described. These include anticonvulsants, disulfiram, diphenylmethane derivatives, para-acetamidobenzoate, and anti-Parkinson compounds. The anticonvulsant drugs, such as phenobarbital and diphenylhydantoin, are used primarily to control symptoms of epilepsy. Since emotional and psychopathologic disturbances are commonly found in epileptic patients, the control of seizures frequently alleviates certain disturbing psychologic features. Psychopathologic reactions in certain patients, associated with abnormal electroencephalograms but without epileptic diagnoses, may also respond to the administration of these compounds. Disulfiram, which combines with alcohol to inhibit its metabolism at the acetaldehyde phase, thereby producing distressing toxic symptoms, can be used to assist certain alcoholic patients in resisting their urge to drink.

Diphenylmethane derivatives have been reportedly effective in reducing anxiety when it occurs in psychoneurotic patients. Benactyzine and hydroxyzine are the most widely used members of this group. While they appear to relieve pathologic anxiety, they demonstrate no clear superiority to the barbiturates or meprobamate. Benactyzine, in particular, may be associated with unpleasant side effects. Para-acetamidobenzoate is a mild stimulant which has been reported to be useful in the treatment of depression of mood. The evidence for its therapeutic effectiveness is extremely limited. Anti-Parkinson drugs, such as trihexyphenidyl and benztropine methanesulfonate, can be successfully used to counteract the motor and coordination dysfunction often seen in patients receiving phenothiazine derivatives or reserpine when this complication cannot be handled satisfactorily through a reduction in the dosage of these drugs. Methaminodiazepoxide is a newly introduced drug which may be effective in reducing anxiety and tension in various diagnostic settings.

Part Three

THE INTEGRATION OF TREATMENT METHODS

15

THE TREATMENT OF PSYCHONEUROTIC
REACTIONS

Psychoneurotic reactions are psychopathologic states characterized by the presence of abnormal anxiety manifested directly or through the formation of complex symptom patterns. These patterns are used to subdivide psychoneuroses into five basic types: anxiety reactions, dissociative reactions, obsessive-compulsive reactions, depressive reactions, and psychophysiologic reactions. Rarely does one manifestation of anxiety occur in isolation; ordinarily a psychoneurotic patient reveals anxiety in several forms; a phobic patient may also be depressed; an obsessive-compulsive patient may also demonstrate dissociative features. In contrast to schizophrenic and mood disorders, the prevailing mood of the patient, his logical thought processes, and his contact with reality are essentially unaffected.

Psychodynamic factors are of central importance in the etiology of psychoneurotic reactions. A disturbing stimulus arising from within the patient, such as a sexual urge, or from the environment, such as rejection by a beloved person, provokes conflict between the patient's ego and superego and his turbulent unconscious. The result is anxiety. This pathologic emotion not only warns the patient of impending danger, but also fosters the forces of repression which protect him against awareness of the central conflicts. His symptoms, distressing as they may be, often gain desirable ends, such as sympathy or control over other human beings; hence he is frequently reluctant to part with them until the conflicts have been resolved and he has learned a healthier mode of living.

Inasmuch as the most significant causal factors in psychoneurotic ill-

215

nesses are psychologic, the primary method of treatment for all these conditions is psychotherapy. Certain somatic therapies may be valuable adjuncts in the management of such patients. However, they should not be administered indiscriminately. They should be given only for clear and specific purposes. In order to utilize these somatic therapies effectively, it is essential to understand the fundamental aspects of psychotherapy as applied in the treatment of psychoneurotic reactions.

Dynamic Psychotherapy

There are several important forms of dynamic psychotherapy. The selection of the particular method to use in a particular patient depends on factors which will be described here in detail.

PSYCHOANALYSIS

The most extensive and intensive form of psychotherapy is psychoanalysis. The goal of this technique transcends symptomatic relief. An attempt is made to resolve those conflicts and modify those character traits of the patient which rendered him sensitive to the development of his psychoneurosis. A new balance between ego, superego, and id is sought. Previously hidden or undeveloped personality assets frequently emerge. Emphasis is placed on the revelation and working through of dynamic forces in the patient's unconscious. In order to achieve these aims, two technical measures of fundamental importance are employed. The first is free association, whereby the patient is expected to express at once all thoughts, feelings, sensations, and perceptions of which he becomes aware. In this way, resistances can be constructively recognized and eliminated, with the consequent appearance of previously repressed dynamic material. The second important aspect of psychoanalytic technique is the creation of transference neurosis. In the relationship with his therapist the patient literally and repeatedly reexperiences dynamically disturbing situations which ordinarily transpired in his earlier life, especially during childhood. In order to foster this distortion of reality, the analyst conceals many features of his own personality. The use of the couch, with the therapist sitting behind the patient and out of view, enhances the formation of transference. Through silence and through carefully timed and selected interpretations and responses, the analyst helps the patient correct his misinterpretations, release disturbing emotions, and find a new and higher plateau for his human relationships.

Psychoanalysis, as a method of treatment, is costly in terms of time and money. The usual course of treatment extends over at least a 2- or 3-year period, at the rate of four or five sessions per week. When it is indicated, there is no substitute for this far-reaching therapeutic method. However, there are many patients in whom such a procedure is unnecessary, impractical, or contraindicated. Therefore, many of the principles and much of the dynamic knowledge acquired through psychoanalytic experience have been modified and adapted to suit other forms of treatment, namely, intensive, brief, or supportive psychotherapy.

INTENSIVE PSYCHOTHERAPY

Intensive psychotherapy, like psychoanalysis, attempts to do more than alleviate psychopathologic distress. Modification of character structure and resolution of conscious and unconscious conflicts are attempted in order to help the patient recover from his psychoneurotic state and to protect him, as much as possible, against a recurrence of his illness. Transference factors and free association may be employed but do not necessarily constitute the central procedures. The patient is ordinarily face to face with the therapist, who introduces himself more actively into the therapeutic process, offering direction through questions, interpretations, and suggestions. When indicated, he may attempt to correct detrimental environmental factors in the patient's life: for instance, he may interview significant relatives and offer advice regarding their relationships with the patient. The usual frequency of sessions ranges from two to four times weekly, and the length of treatment averages from 6 to 18 months. Somatic therapies are more likely to be used in the course of intensive psychotherapy than during psychoanalysis.

BRIEF PSYCHOTHERAPY

Psychotherapeutic techniques may be used in more abbreviated fashion. Brief psychotherapy is aimed at the alleviation of those factors within the environment and within the patient which contribute to his immediate psychopathologic reaction. Little attempt is made to investigate unrelated personality factors, probe extensively into unconscious dynamic considerations, or influence the character structure of the patient. Therapy is concluded when symptomatic relief is obtained and maintained for a reasonable period of time. The degree of activity on the part of the therapist will depend largely on the nature of the problems and on the ability of the patient to recognize spontaneously and cope with immediate conflicts. Such therapeutic endeavors may be completed after six interviews or even less, although they may extend over several months at a rate of once or twice weekly. This short form of psychotherapy is often associated with the use of somatic methods of alleviating pathologic emotions.

SUPPORTIVE PSYCHOTHERAPY

In certain settings, where the primary purpose of treatment is symptomatic relief and assistance in dealing with real and enduring environmental difficulties, psychotherapy may be largely supportive. The patient may be encouraged to ventilate his current emotions and instructed with regard to external and internal factors causing his distress. Strong reassurance and suggestion may be complemented by drug therapy. This approach is commonly employed by the family physician, who assumes the responsibility of treating psychoneurotic patients with limited therapeutic expectations.

SELECTION OF PSYCHOTHERAPEUTIC METHOD

One may consider four basic therapeutic approaches to the treatment of a patient diagnosed as psychoneurotic: psychoanalysis, intensive dynamic psychotherapy, brief psychotherapy, and supportive therapy. The selection of the particular method of treatment for a particular patient depends upon the type of psychoneurotic reaction, the nature of prevailing pathologic emotions and associated psychopathologic features, the extent of impairment of the patient's ability to function, and the dynamic setting of the illness.

Differentiation of psychoneurotic illnesses on the basis of the leading manifestations of anxiety is of limited help in selecting the correct therapeutic approach. Psychoanalysis and intensive dynamic psychotherapy may be indicated in any form of psychoneurotic reaction, acute or chronic, although these methods are usually reserved for illnesses which have been evident for some period of time. Brief psychotherapy is more often used in the treatment of acute reactions, characterized by the presence of anxiety, tension, dissociative symptoms, depression, or psychophysiologic disturbances, particularly when the illness develops in the setting of a circumscribed, well-defined precipitating factor. Phobic or obsessive-compulsive psychoneurotic reactions are less likely to respond to brief methods. Somatic treatment may be used in any type of psychoneurotic state, acute or chronic, to relieve anxiety, tension, phobic or conversion symptoms, and mild depression of mood. Physiologic agents are not currently available which will reliably alleviate obsessive-compulsive symptoms.

The nature and degree of pathologic emotions and associated psychopathologic features play significant roles in the decision to employ somatic therapies and in the selection of the particular pharmacologic agent to be used. However, these do not usually influence the decision regarding the type of psychotherapy to be carried out.

From a practical viewpoint, the dynamic setting of the illness, more than diagnostic or psychopathologic considerations, will determine the method of psychotherapy to be employed. Those factors which constitute the dynamic setting include the degree to which the patient's function is impaired by symptoms, the environment in which he exists, his age and physical condition, his personality assets and liabilities, previous treatment for the same or related conditions, the available treatment resources at the current time, his motivation for treatment, and the attitude of his immediate family toward his illness and therapy.

The degree of impairment of function caused by the illness will influence the selection of the psychotherapeutic method. If a patient's concentration is poor and his attention limited so that he cannot continue his career effectively and if these complications do not respond within the first weeks of treatment, it will be very difficult to obtain the necessary freedom from the pressure of immediate disturbing factors to probe into the unconscious and work constructively with such material as dreams. Therefore, psychoanalysis would not be desirable as long as the impairment continues at such a level. In intensive psychotherapy, the physician would be in a somewhat better position to offer direction and use somatic methods of treatment to alleviate the symptoms. Psychoanalysis requires a somewhat more stable environmental situation than does intensive psychotherapy. The working through of resistances and the evolution of character changes attempted in psychoanalysis would often be hopelessly blocked if, throughout the course of treatment, the patient's wife repeatedly demanded divorce, his employer threatened him with dismissal, and unexpected business trips forced him to interrupt the continuity of the sessions. In intensive psychotherapy, the physician is in a much stronger position to take action to reduce disturbing environmental factors and shift from the analysis of complex fantasies to the discussion of everyday difficulties. If these considerations are sufficiently intense, however, even the goals of intensive psychotherapy may be temporarily or permanently defeated.

It is often desirable to employ psychoanalysis or intensive psychotherapy in young men or women in their twenties and thirties, who have reached a level of personality integration but still look forward to many years of productive living. It would be unwise and imprudent to embark upon either of these therapeutic courses in a 75-year-old man with a limited life expectancy or a patient with the diagnosis of metastatic gastric carcinoma. In such instances, more abbreviated measures would clearly be indicated.

The personality of the patient must be suited to psychoanalysis. An adequate degree of intelligence, imagination, and verbal facility is essential. The patient should be able to recognize inner feelings, appreciate psychologic experiences, and synthesize dynamic material spontaneously. The same may be said for intensive psychotherapy, although in this technique the psychiatrist is more prepared to compensate for deficiencies in the patient, helping him to recognize simple emotional experiences, coordinating the flow of sensitive material to help him understand what is taking place, and allowing for a patient's natural lack of spontaneity or verbal ability. Brief psychotherapeutic methods are often more desirable, however, for patients who are generally quite limited with regard to most of these considerations. When hidden or undeveloped abilities are present within the patient, psychoanalysis is probably the most effective method of helping a patient grow to fulfill his innate stature.

The motivation of the patient is perhaps one of the most important determinants in the selection of treatment methods. Some patients incorrectly believe that psychoanalysis is an expensive, wasteful luxury. Others are convinced that it is the only effective method of treatment. Still others may fear the possibility of dependency on the physician developing in the course of analysis or intensive psychotherapy. Some are eager and willing to seek a solution to their difficulties. Others resist the idea that psychologic factors are important, demand immediate relief through medication, and will dismiss their physicians if they do not acquiesce. Therefore, although intensive measures may be desirable, brief psychotherapy may be the only method which the patient will allow—occasionally, only when it is associated with the use of drugs. Sometimes the physician must stand his ground in hopes that his suggestion for therapy will be heard by the patient months or even years later. At other times, the extent of the disturbance or the complications in the life of the patient and his family are such that the physician will decide to give in to the patient's resistance, offer symptomatic relief, and anticipate another opportunity to recommend more extensive measures.

Intensive psychotherapy or psychoanalysis is ordinarily required when the psychoneurotic illness occurs in the absence of one well-defined precipitating factor and when the personality difficulties of the patient are complex. If, for example, a dissociative reaction occurs in the setting of a serious automobile accident, brief psychotherapy may be sufficient to restore the patient's emotional well-being. A few sessions may help a college student whose excellent scholastic performance has rapidly deteriorated following the death of his father. If he possesses strong recuperative powers and is able to secure insight rapidly, he may quickly see the connection between his guilt and his disability and work out the dynamic conflict. On the other hand, if anxiety symptoms develop slowly and insidiously in an apparently benign environmental situation and the sources of the disturbance lie deeply hidden within the patient's unconscious, extensive therapeutic measures will be required.

The final considerations in the selection of the mode of psychotherapy are the nature of any previous treatment which the patient may have received and the availability of current therapeutic resources. If a psychoneurotic patient has previously been treated with drugs alone, with brief psychotherapy, or with a combination of both methods and has secured only temporary relief of symptoms or no relief at all, the decision to recommend psychoanalysis or intensive psychotherapy will be enhanced. If, on the other hand, he has previously been treated intensively and his present condition has been precipitated by new dynamic factors, a short-term psychotherapeutic approach may be sufficient to relieve his present state and restimulate the insights which he had formerly secured. When a patient has received psychoanalysis or intensive psychotherapy and is still beset by anxiety symptoms, supportive therapy may be the only course available.

Even when the indications for psychoanalysis or intensive psychotherapy are clear, it is important to realize that such resources may not be available to the patient. It has been said that unless one half of the nation was caring for the other half, there would not be enough therapists to care for all the patients with psychoneurotic illnesses. On the other hand, the demand for the services of the well-trained psychiatrist is offset by the remnants of the social stigma of being psychologically ill, the failure of many clinicians to recognize the presence of psychiatric disorders unless they are flamboyant, and the complex resistance of many patients and cultural groups to psychotherapy. Where financial resources are limited and outpatient facilities overcrowded, it may frequently be necessary to handle many psychoneurotic patients in brief psychotherapy in the office of the internist or the general practitioner, with the benefit of psychiatric consultation when desired. It is often wise to offer a patient a trial of brief psychotherapy or intensive dynamic psychotherapy before recommending psychoanalysis if there is any doubt about the necessity of the latter procedure, as it is inherently a lengthy and costly method of therapy. However, when intensive therapy or psychoanalysis is indicated and the patient can obtain the treatment even though it may mean some inconvenience, one cannot justify offering him less.

Somatic Therapy

Somatic therapies may often be employed in the treatment of psychoneurotic conditions. Their use may be of incidental or paramount importance. For example, they may be used rarely, and then only for short periods of time, in well-organized, functioning patients engaged in psychoanalysis or intensive psychotherapy, because drugs which would prematurely or extensively eliminate pathologic anxiety and associated symptoms might reduce a patient's motivation for treatment, discouraging and preventing him from working through crucial dynamic conflicts. On the other hand, somatic methods may occasionally be very valuable adjuncts in the course of brief or supportive psychotherapy.

Certain treatments are commonly used in the control of pathologic emotions and associated psychopathologic features occurring in psycho-neurotic settings. These include the barbiturates, meprobamate, certain members of the phenothiazine series, and stimulants, in particular amphetamine and dextro amphetamine. Diphenylmethane derivatives have been widely employed, but thus far demonstrate no clear superiority to barbiturates or meprobamate and may be associated with unpleasant side effects. When depression of mood is prominent and persistent feature of a psychoneurotic condition and does not respond in a reasonable period of time to psychotherapy or mild stimulants, monoamine oxidase inhibitors or imipramine may be tried, although they are usually reserved for depressive states occurring as part of primary mood disorders. There is ordinarily no place for electroconvulsive or insulin therapies, rauwolfia derivatives, steroids, lobotomy, or carbon dioxide treatment in psychoneurotic patients. Rarely, in a state of marked panic or excitement, a psychoneurotic patient may be given electroconvulsive therapy or a course of insulin coma therapy to alleviate his intense psycho-pathologic state, but ordinarily phenothiazines are equally effective in such instances. In a severe obsessive-compulsive patient who does not improve with intensive psychotherapy, thyroid hormones may be employed on a trial basis; rarely, such a patient may undergo a lobotomy for the relief of his intense distress.

GENERAL INDICATIONS FOR SOMATIC TREATMENT

The decision to use a somatic method of treatment depends upon the degree of impairment of function which the patient experiences. It is strongly influenced by the dynamic setting of the illness and by the form of psychotherapy selected for the patient's needs. Psychopharmacologic agents are more likely to be employed in acute rather than chronic reactions, and methods are more readily available for the management of anxiety, dissociative, or phobic states than for depressive or obsessive-compulsive forms of psychoneuroses.

Somatic intervention is clearly indicated when pathologic emotions and associated psychopathologic features threaten to interfere with the ability of a patient to fulfill his regular responsibilities. For example, if anxiety so handicaps judgment or concentration that a lawyer cannot prepare important briefs or appear in court when it is required, he will be forced to modify his working situation. Frequently this is not possible, and unless pharmacologic agents are used, the real difficulties which may ensue may undermine any and all psychotherapeutic measures. When pathologic hostility is so intense and continuous that it seriously disrupts the personal relationships of the patient, creating a number of critical situations with his family and colleagues, somatic means may accomplish in days what weeks and months of psychotherapy may be required to achieve. There is little justification for allowing a patient to suffer intensely when it is possible to use appropriate drugs to restore his appetite, sleep, and some degree of well-being, unless his distress is essential to motivate him to participate in therapy and make adjustments necessary for his continued health.

If a psychoneurotic reaction develops suddenly and it is possible to discern well-defined, circumscribed precipitating factors, it is often desirable to terminate the acute episode by somatic means. If, on the other hand, the condition has developed insidiously, the precipitating factors are multiple and complex, and it is apparent that personality factors contribute largely to the patient's reaction, the physician may be wiser to refrain from using somatic agents until the psychodynamic patterns have been elaborated in psychotherapy. The therapist may be inclined to use drugs in the management of a patient whose environmental situation is unsettled in order to promote rapid relief of symptoms, thereby enabling him to utilize his abilities to cope with the external difficulties. For example, if a psychoneurotic patient's intense anxiety and rage are due in part to recent dismissal from his job and he is forced to seek a new position at once, it may be necessary to use somatic methods to relieve these emotions promptly so that he can reestablish himself. If, because of advanced age or serious physical disability, the patient's life expectancy is limited, pharmacologic agents may constitute important timesavers, offering relief from symptoms in patients who are not candidates for extensive analysis. The decision to use medications may be forced on the physician at times by a patient who refuses to accept the presence of psychologic factors in his illness and draws back at the suggestion of discussing even the most superficial personal matters with his family doctor. If a patient who has already undergone psychoanalysis or intensive psychotherapy for his condition experiences a recurrence of symptoms, somatic intervention will frequently be desirable.

When the indications for psychoanalysis or intensive dynamic psychotherapy are present and the patient is willing to pursue such a constructive course of action, it is ordinarily preferable to refrain from the administration of pharmocologic agents. Disturbing emotions often serve as an impetus to drive the patient in his search for self-knowledge and emotional readjustment. They may also facilitate the emergence of important conscious and unconscious dynamic material which frequently would be beyond reach once these emotions have been reduced by medication. On the other hand, during the process of therapy, a patient may develop intense pathologic emotions associated with the discussion of sensitive topics. These features may seriously interfere with his ability to function and may obstruct the progress of therapy. In such a setting, drugs may be most helpful in alleviating the undesirable symptoms and allowing the patient to continue treatment uninterruptedly. For example, in the analysis of a psychoneurotic patient with unconscious sexual conflicts, the removal of resistances and defenses may permit the recognition of disturbing desires and impulses; at times a patient may be temporarily overwhelmed by such an experience. The fear or sexual unrest thus produced may, if unchecked, lead to the development of a panic or excitement, with delusions, paranoid features, hallucinations, and suicidal attempts. The judicious use of the correct pharmacologic agent at the first signs of such a change can prevent very damaging consequences.

The importance of anxiety as a motivation for therapy has been stressed again and again and is offered as a reason for refraining from somatic therapy in patients who are about to enter intensive psychotherapy. There are numerous situations, however, in which it is not possible to begin psychotherapy until pathologic emotions or psychopathologic symptoms have been reduced. Many patients, even though they are aware of the need for therapy and consciously agree to begin this procedure, manifest profound resistance to any kind of analysis. They may force themselves to go to the psychotherapist's office but, once there, are unable to communicate in a meaningful way. Profound hostility may be evident, mounting in intensity, aimed at the physician and the treatment situation, and easily leading to premature termination of the dynamic investigations. The use of a pharmacologic agent may successfully reduce these disturbing emotions, and the resistances, although still present, may assume forms which are considerably less threatening to the treatment situation.

Somatic methods may be used in association with brief or supportive psychotherapy. Here the goals of treatment are limited, and symptomatic relief is of primary importance. Many patients respond excellently to a few psychotherapeutic sessions and never require somatic intervention. Some, however, can discuss their conflicts and obtain intellectual understanding into the dynamic factors without securing symptomatic improvement, and for such patients drugs are frequently of value.

In summary, there appears to be something of an inverse relationship between the indications for intensive psychotherapy or psychoanalysis and those for pharmacologic therapy. The psychoneurotic patient who is able to function, whose anxiety has been manifest for a long period of time, whose environmental situation is relatively stable, and who is motivated and capable of probing extensively into the nature of conscious and unconscious factors contributing to his condition is not as likely a candidate for somatic treatment as the patient who is acutely and intensely ill, unable to carry out his daily routine, whose life is complicated by many real difficulties, and who may reject adamantly any recommendations for intensive analysis. Naturally, there are many exceptions to this generalization, as have already been outlined.

SELECTION OF SPECIFIC SOMATIC METHODS

Once the decision to use a somatic treatment has been made, the particular method of therapy remains to be selected. This decision depends upon the pathologic emotions and associated psychopathologic features prominent in the patient's state and the dynamic setting of the illness, in particular his age and physical health.

Pathologic anxiety is almost universal in psychoneurotic states. This emotion may be manifested directly as a state of general apprehension which is continuous or which recurs episodically. It may be modified by the formation of phobias. Dissociation may foster the development of conversion symptoms, such as paralysis or amnesia. Obsessions or compulsions or depression of mood may represent a more complex management of pathologic anxiety. Anxiety, it will be recalled, is often associated with somatic symptoms, particularly palpitations and tachycardia; gastrointestinal distress, such as anorexia, nausea, vomiting, diarrhea, or constipation; and pain, weakness, dizziness, headaches, fatigue, or excessive perspiration.

The most effective therapeutic agents for the reduction of pathologic anxiety are barbiturates and meprobamate. These drugs are often able to relieve this emotion when it is directly experienced and manifested or when it is handled by the development of phobias. The barbiturate most frequently used for this purpose is phenobarbital, ordinarily administered in doses of 30 to 60 mg repeated several times daily or at critical moments. Meprobamate, in individual doses of 400 to 800 mg, may be used similarly and demonstrates no clear superiority to barbiturates except in situations where definite signs of muscular tension are associated with anxiety. Intravenous Sodium Amytal is valuable in the alleviation of conversion symptoms, facilitating a cathartic release of dissociated emotions during the phase of impaired consciousness, followed by liberation from the disabling symptoms. In some patients in whom pathologic anxiety is associated with depression of mood, the administration of either barbiturates or meprobamate will often lead to marked improvement in the total psychopathologic picture. In other patients with anxiety and depression, these drugs will fail to influence the clinical state. When anxiety leads to the formation of obsessive-compulsive symptoms, neither barbiturates nor meprobamate produces much improvement, although at times they may slightly dull the patient's perception of his distress.

Pathologic hostility is often seen in psychoneurotic patients. When it is directly experienced and manifested as resentment or anger, phenothiazine compounds seem to be most effective in reducing these emotions. These drugs are also the agents of choice when sexual unrest and fear are leading features of a psychoneurotic condition. Current studies indicate that all phenothiazines are capable of reducing these psychopathologic features. However, certain phenothiazines, particularly those with piperazine side chains, such as prochlorperazine or perphenazine, seem to have less of an inhibitory effect on alertness and energy and may be associated with fewer serious side effects, such as jaundice or agranulocytosis, than chlorpromazine and phenothiazines, which more closely resemble them structurally. Hence, they appear to be preferred in the treatment of psychoneurotic conditions.

Rarely, sexual unrest or fear leads to the development of sexual excitements or panics. In such conditions, chlorpromazine is the most reliable and preferred agent, but electroconvulsive therapy may be indicated if immediate relief is necessary or if resistance to phenothiazine treatment has been observed. Pathologic hostility, fear, and sexual unrest are not infrequently associated with depression of mood in psychoneurotic patients, and reduction of these pathologic features often leads to a lifting of the depression. In psychoneuroses, pathologic hostility, fear, or sexual unrest may often be combined with anxiety. In such instances it seems preferable to use the phenothiazine derivatives first and, if, following the reduction of these features, distressing anxiety remains, change to barbiturate or meprobamate therapy.

Mild periods of elation are occasionally seen in psychoneurotic patients but are usually not intense enough to require somatic intervention. Depression of mood, however, may be very severe. Often this mood change occurs in association with anxiety, hostility, sexual unrest, or fear and improves when these pathologic emotions are alleviated. At times, however, depression of mood is the leading manifestation of the illness and may be accompanied by mental and physical retardation, fatigue, or, at times, suicidal inclinations. When somatic measures are indicated in mild depressive states, stimulants such as amphetamine, dextro amphetamine, or methylphenidate may be used effectively. These drugs may be combined with barbiturates to alleviate anxiety occurring in association with the depression or aggravated by the administration of the cerebral stimulants. In more severe conditions these drugs are often ineffectual. In tenacious states of depression, which do not respond satisfactorily to psychotherapy or the use of amphetamines, it seems justifiable to place the patient on a trial of imipramine or monoamine oxidase inhibitors, inasmuch as the role of these compounds in the treatment of psychoneurotic patients has not yet been favorably or unfavorably established.

Pathologic emotions may be associated with the development of tension, sleep disorders, gastrointestinal distress, and over- or underactivity. These symptoms may be treated, directly or indirectly, by somatic methods. For example, when tension is present in association with pathologic hostility, it will frequently be relieved during phenothiazine administration. On the other hand, if it constitutes the leading disturbance and strong emotions are not readily evident, it may be attacked by the use of meprobamate or physical measures, such as warm baths and massage. Insomnia is often the result of anxiety, hostility, sexual unrest, or tension. The reduction of anxiety by barbiturates or of hostility or sexual unrest by phenothiazines will often alleviate the patient's difficulty in falling asleep or his frequent nocturnal interruptions. On the other hand, insomnia may represent the most distressing symptom of the patient's condition, and a more direct method of eliminating this feature may be desired. In such a case, barbiturates, such as pentobarbital or amobarbital in hypnotic doses, or nonbarbiturate soporifics may be utilized. The selection of the particular drug to induce sleep depends on the nature of the sleep disturbance. For example, if only the induction of sleep is required, amobarbital, which has a short duration of activity, may be preferable; if broken sleep, rather than difficulty in falling asleep, is the problem, a longer-acting barbiturate, such as barbital or phenobarbital, may be indicated. Nonbarbiturate hypnotics may be preferable in aging patients, even in the absence of evidence of cerebral organic changes. Variations in physical or mental activity are usually alleviated when the emotions accounting for these changes are reduced. Special drugs, such as propantheline for the relaxation of smooth muscle sphincters and the reduction of peristalsis, gels for the relief of gastric hyperacidity, and cathartics for constipation, are very often prescribed in psychoneurotic patients, but ordinarily these procedures are much less desirable than treating these symptoms indirectly by using methods which will relieve the pathologic emotions and dynamic factors contributing to their existence.

Dynamic Orientation of Combined Therapy

The use of somatic methods in the alleviation of pathologic emotions in psychoneurotic patients carries with it certain definite advantages which have already been discussed. The patient may not only be free of unnecessary and unprofitable distress, but he may also be allowed to carry on in his life routine without undue disability. Frequently, he is better able to use constructively the psychotherapeutic sessions, and a positive attitude toward treatment and the physician is fostered. It is important to recognize, however, that there are certain disadvantages which can accrue from the use of somatic methods in psychoneurotic patients, and appropriate precautions must be considered. The premature elimination of distress can erase the motivation of many patients to pursue an active course of psychotherapy which is essential for their continued well-being. The production of significant dynamic material in sessions may be delayed or entirely prevented in the absence of pathologic emotions. Psychoneurotic patients are often very aware of the slightest side effects of the drugs which are used. They may acutely perceive dizziness, mild retardation, lethargy, and fatigue which can complicate the administration of barbiturates, meprobamate, or phenothiazines, and any interference with concentration, energy, and activity may be quite distressing. Hysterical and hypochondriac patients, in particular, tend to incorporate drug effects, such as motor incoordination produced by phenothiazines, into their pattern of illness, exaggerating the symptoms and using them as resistance to recovery and progress in psychotherapy. Some patients are highly sensitive to these compounds and manifest intellectual bewilderment during their administration. It is not uncommon for the initial improvement associated with prochlorperazine therapy, for example, to be followed by some decrease in spontaneity and cloudiness in thinking, which rapidly disappears when the dose is reduced or the drug is terminated. Such changes do not impress the patient or the therapist when medications have been used to terminate profound psychopathologic reactions, such as paranoid panics or acute schizophrenic excitements. However, they may be as disturbing to the psychoneurotic patient and as disruptive to the progress of psychotherapy as the pathologic emotions which they have replaced. In order to minimize the occurrence of such complications, it is important to use a dose adequate to accomplish the desired goal but no higher than required. The medication should be terminated as soon as the improvement becomes established, usually in a matter of several weeks or less. It may be reinstituted later if required. It seems to be the course of least resistance to allow a patient to continue on medication regularly, long after the indications for it have ceased to be evident.

The conscious and unconscious meaning to the patient of being given a medication is extremely important. To some patients, it is an unspoken denial by the therapist of the importance of the dynamic analysis. Others are threatened by the fear that the use of drugs will stimulate pathologic dependency. It is not uncommon to recommend a definite dose of a drug only to find that the patient has taken only half the amount and therefore has not obtained the desirable effects. This decision may have been based on the patient's desire to demonstrate his independence and overcome his anxiety by sheer power of will. Another patient may fight against his therapist's recommendations by taking more of the drug than prescribed or by obtaining medications from many other sources and using them instead of, or in combination with, the suggested regimen. If a patient possesses unconscious transference hostility directed toward the therapist, he may manifest an antagonistic response to the prescribed drug. If it is a stimulant, he may report lethargy and mental retardation while taking it; if it is a tranquilizer, he may report an intensification of his anxiety, agitation, and insomnia. In such a situation it is usually desirable to terminate the medication and analyze the sources of his resentment and resistance.

When administering a drug to a psychoneurotic patient, it is most important to keep in mind the dynamic structure of his anxiety symptoms. Not only do they cause his distress and impair his function, but they protect him against the awareness of his basic conflicts, reinforce his resistance to working through his difficulties, and secure for him pathologic gain and satisfaction. The premature or abrupt removal of his symptoms, particularly if this is done in the absence of adequate psychotherapy, can easily force him to find some other, more tenacious method of protecting himself from being separated from his illness. For example, the anxious patient receiving meprobamate may lose his apprehensions but gradually manifest depression of mood. The phobic patient may be freed of his inappropriate fears but begin to disrupt his personal relationships through undesirable behavior, creating real life difficulties to distract him from the true, unconscious sources of his psychoneurotic anxiety. Instead of being afraid of heights or closed spaces, he succeeds in alienating his employer or his wife and forcefully insists that his disturbance is the result of these real problems.

In the majority of patients with psychoneurotic illnesses, somatic therapy is not ordinarily indicated. In a select group of such patients, however, pharmacologic agents are very desirable and at times indispensable adjuncts to effective psychotherapy. When the physician has carefully evaluated the dynamic considerations outlined in this chapter and understands the indications for somatic treatment and the meaning of this procedure to the patient, to the doctor-patient relationship, and to the future course of psychotherapy, medications can be employed with a high degree of success.

SUMMARY

Psychodynamic factors are of primary importance in the genesis of psychoneurotic reactions. Therefore, psychotherapy is the fundamental method of treatment for patients with such an illness. Four types of dynamic psychotherapy are available: psychoanalysis, intensive psychotherapy, brief psychotherapy, and supportive psychotherapy. The selection of the particular method of treatment depends to a very great extent upon the dynamic setting of the illness.

Somatic methods of treatment may be valuable as adjunctive measures in the management of certain psychoneurotic patients. The most commonly used agents are barbiturates, meprobamate, phenothiazines, and amphetamine or dextro amphetamine. The decision whether or not to initiate any form of pharmacologic therapy depends largely upon the intensity and complications of pathologic emotions and the dynamic setting of the reaction. The selection of the particular pharmacologic agent is largely determined by the nature of the predominant pathologic emotions, moods, sexual unrest, or associated psychopathologic features.

Table 4   Treatment of Psychoneurotic Reactions

Indications for Psychotherapy

Psychoanalysis or intensive psychotherapy	Brief psychotherapy	Supportive psychotherapy
Long-standing condition	Acute reaction	Chronic unmodifiable condition
Complex precipitating factors	Well-defined, circumscribed precipitating factors	Limited personality assets
Many personality assets	Limited personality assets	Very unsettled environmental situation
Stable environmental situation	Rapid recuperative abilities	Poor physical health, limited life expectancy
Reasonable physical health and life expectancy	Very unsettled environmental situation	Failure of more intensive methods
Good motivation for analysis	Poor physical health, limited life expectancy	
Available resources for treatment	Limited motivation for analysis	
	Limited therapeutic resources	

Indications for Somatic Therapy

All methods	Specific methods
Acute reactions	Barbiturates: Pathologic anxiety, insomnia, dissociative states
Chronic reactions, unresponsive to psychotherapy alone	Meprobamate: Anxiety, particularly in association with muscular tension
Well-defined, circumscribed precipitating factors	Phenothiazines: Pathologic hostility, sexual unrest, fear
Limited personality assets	Amphetamine or dextro amphetamine: Depression, fatigue, retardation
Unsettled environmental situation	Monoamine oxidase inhibitors; imipramine: Trial basis for tenacious depression of mood
Limited life expectancy	ECT (rare): Panic, sexual excitement
Poor motivation for psychotherapy alone	
Limited resources for psychotherapy	
Undue emotional disturbances in the course of psychotherapy	
Significant impairment by symptoms	

16

THE TREATMENT OF SCHIZOPHRENIC
REACTIONS

In the treatment of patients with schizophrenic reactions, the watchword is *specificity*. Whether one deals with a patient who is in the middle of a catatonic excitement or who experiences chronic anxiety in a simple schizophrenic reaction, whether one is attempting to explore historical dynamic material or to guide the patient in obtaining employment, whether one is seeing the patient several times per week or once every 6 months, the content of psychotherapeutic interviews must be specific. Interviews must deal with concrete realities of the environment in which the patient lives and in which he has lived, and they must avoid the use of abstract terms.

The reasons for this need of specificity become clear when the dynamic origin of schizophrenic reactions is considered. Whether they be caused by physiologic or psychologic processes, the schizophrenic reactions have, as their common manifestation, a personalized view of the world. Consequently, when the patient uses abstract terms or associations in describing or evaluating situations, it is likely that he will use them with different meanings and connotations than those which the therapist is accustomed to use. A "bad" situation for the patient might be radically different from what the therapist would describe as "bad"; the patient, for example, might see great danger in a person who wears a red tie, because of his own associations with that color. Similarly, the schizophrenic person may see an employment opportunity as a "good" one because of some objectively peripheral, but personally important, feature; the therapist's more objective view of the opportunity, however, might reveal several aspects of significant danger or disadvantage. It is of extreme importance, therefore, that both the therapist and the patient, as they explore material in interviews, concentrate on describing what has *actually* happened or what is *actually* present in concrete and specific terms; their own value judgments should be eliminated.

In understanding the urgency of this need for specificity, it is profitable to consider analogous situations. Value judgments abound in our everyday life. A $30 watch, for example, may be inordinately expensive for some persons, average in price for others, and dirt-cheap for still others. We are so much aware of these ordinary expressions of personal values that we would be apt to ask for the specific price of the watch, if it were described to us simply as an "expensive" item. By determining the exact price of the article, we are then able to put it into our own personal framework of cheapness or expensiveness. If we do not know the actual price, however, we are left with the need to assess the relationship between our own price framework and the price framework of the person describing the article. The psychotherapy of schizophrenic persons, if it does not deal with specifics, will become mired in the complications of just this kind of juggling, with the two frames of reference being the personalized world of the schizophrenic person and the more objectively oriented world of the therapist.

The need for psychotherapeutic specificity, therefore, must provide the base for all of the treatment programs for schizophrenic patients. So far as possible, the therapist must eliminate his own value judgments from what he says to the patient by making his own words specific. At the same time, he must continually be aware of the fact that the patient's value judgments are not the same as his and must continually question even the most common opinions which the patient expresses. Again and again, he must look for the "price tag," instead of accepting the patient's general assessment. He must be willing to carry this to an extreme degree; if the patient states, "it was a nice day," the therapist must be prepared to ask the nature of the "nice day." When the therapist uses this caution, he will avoid most of the pitfalls which are associated with the treatment of schizophrenic patients. These pitfalls are largely based on misunderstanding, whereby the therapist does not see dangerous areas as they arise or whereby he allows himself to be seen as a misconstrued, threatening person. If all areas are dealt with in a specific fashion, both the therapist and the patient will know where they stand at all times and will be able to carry on psychotherapy, to be described, in a safe and constructive fashion.

ACUTE SCHIZOPHRENIC REACTIONS

In dealing with the treatment of schizophrenic reactions, the acute treatment situations will be considered separately from the chronic treatment situations. In actuality, many of the same principles are followed in the two types of situations, but the emphasis and the techniques are somewhat different. In the acute treatment situations, it is the therapist's major job to obtain relief for the patient. The emphasis in his treatment will be on the amelioration of symptoms.

In attempting to ameliorate major symptoms, several steps are useful. Perhaps the most obvious and most important of these steps is the removal of the patient from the threatening environmental situation in which he finds himself. Almost invariably, the patient with an acute schizophrenic reaction has found himself in an environmental situation with which he cannot cope. The nature of this situation, of course, may be varied. The patient may need removal from a heterosexually stimulating situation, in which he was being led toward a rupture of his moral code. Alternatively, he may require removal from an aggressive, competitive work situation, or from a family setting in which his conflicting feelings are stimulating increasing anxiety and confusion. Whatever the nature of the environmental situation, it is usual to find that the patient with an acute schizophrenic reaction is unable to handle the complicated emotional patterns of everyday living. In consequence, it is usually advisable to have the patient removed to a less stressful and more controlled environmental situation, preferably a psychiatric hospital. In such a situation, he can be allowed an adequate amount of time in quiet and private situations, with a room to himself for sleep and for leisure. Even while the controlled environment provides security and isolation, it fosters limited group activities with other persons. Very frequently, as in military situations and in serious environmental disasters, the simple removal of the patient from the stressful situation can bring the acute schizophrenic episode to a halt.

When the patient has been removed as far as possible from environmental stress, the next step that the therapist must undertake is to relieve the patient's anxiety and fear by psychotherapeutic interviews. The ways in which this may be done are many, and considerable exploration of this material is available in the literature (Fromm-Reichmann, 1950; Hill, 1955). In general, however, the therapist must be understanding and willing to extend himself far beyond the normal limits in order to assure the patient of his protection, understanding, and cooperation. In order to extend himself in this way and yet not harm the patient by distorting the world excessively, the therapist must be keenly aware of his own feelings and able to walk a therapeutic tightrope of sorts. It is probably best for most therapists to extend their sympathy and help in a verbal fashion, emphasizing to the patient the fact that they will listen to his problems and try to understand and deal with them, but, at the same time, they do not necessarily agree with all the reasons and interpretations which the patient uses. The therapist should also emphasize that he lives in the same world as the patient and that this world cannot be changed by the wishes of either patient or therapist. In this fashion, the therapist identifies himself with the patient as a realistic human being, extending to him human sympathy and understanding but avoiding a godlike, messianic sort of protective role.

Certain skilled therapists, with experience, may go further in attempts at relieving major symptoms by actually entering into the delusional and confused world of the schizophrenic patient, in the manner described by Rosen (1947); such ability and technique is, however, beyond the limits of most therapists. The desirability and results of such a method remain to be clarified; clearly, its application is limited (Horwitz, et al., 1958).

In addition to removing the patient from the environmental stresses and relieving anxiety, the third major aim in the treatment of acute schizophrenic reactions is to establish a thorough maximum knowledge and understanding of the patient. The acute schizophrenic episode is a time when the patient is showing his problem in a most florid fashion. His delusions and hallucinations and his distorted behavior are replete with clues to the origin of his conflicts and to the misinterpretations which he uses in judging the world. The very setting of his illness and the things which alleviate or aggravate his symptoms provide the firmest type of evidence for the specific areas in the person's life which are giving him the greatest amount of trouble. The acute schizophrenic episode is the mother lode of dynamic understanding for this individual. Altogether apart from his anxiety-relieving role, therefore, the therapist must spend a great deal of time with the patient in acute schizophrenic episodes in order to prepare for later work in reconstructive therapy. As the acute episode clears and the patient returns to his previous, chronic state, the therapist must be prepared to ensure that the patient does not become reinvolved in the same old conflicts. He can obtain the insight which will allow this by means of careful, repeated, and curious observations of the acutely disturbed patient. Obviously, the same time may be spent in acquiring knowledge and in relieving anxiety. The very interest of the therapist will help to make the patient more secure. It will also serve to cement the patient-physician relationship and ensure that continuing psychotherapy can be carried out when the episode has passed. In using his time with the patient in such a dual fashion, the therapist must keep each purpose clear in his own thinking.

There are, therefore, three general purposes in the treatment of an acute schizophrenic reaction. These are (1) removal of the patient from environmental stress; (2) alleviation of anxiety; (3) establishing the knowledge of the therapist and his firm relationship with the patient. If these three aims are kept in mind, most acute schizophrenic episodes will be brought under control in a fairly rapid fashion and the therapist and the patient will be able to embark on their long-range therapeutic program. As these steps are being carried out, a great amount of help can be provided by various dynamically oriented physical treatments. These may best be considered by listing the various treatments which may be used during acute schizophrenic reactions.

Electroconvulsive Treatment

During acute schizophrenic episodes, electro convulsive treatment may be used to terminate states of excitement or stupor. It may be expected that paranoid and catatonic excitements and paranoid panics will be brought under control with three to five ECTs given at a frequency of one to two times per day. A catatonic stupor may be brought under control with three to five ECTs, which may be administered at any frequency up to two times per day. It is characteristic of the interruption of excitements and stupors by ECT that the patient will have very little recollection of the events which took place during the acute episode after it is terminated by the ECT. It will therefore interfere to some extent with his dynamic understanding of his illness and with the nature of the relationship which he established with his therapist during the acute illness. These reasons are indicative of some disadvantage in the use of ECT during acute schizophrenic reactions. The major advantage which ECT possesses for such reactions is that it works rapidly and effectively. It may be relied on to bring an excitement or stupor under control and thus can be a lifesaving measure.

Phenothiazines

Catatonic excitements and paranoid excitements may also be brought under control by the administration of phenothiazine derivatives, such as chlorpromazine, in the fashion which has been described. Chlorpromazine will not work as rapidly as ECT in bringing excitements under control. Moreover, it will be necessary for the chlorpromazine treatment to continue for a period of about 6 weeks before one can be sure that the danger of immediate occurrence has passed. Chlorpromazine and the related phenothiazine derivatives, however, have a distinct advantage over ECT in allowing for a continuation of psychotherapeutic relationship during the excitement and in the period immediately thereafter. Especially when the excitements are associated with great hostility, the patient is able to recall or be aware of the hostile feelings, the delusions, the hallucinations, and other distortions, while not suffering extreme emotional disturbance because of these experiences. He is therefore able to discuss them in detail with the therapist. By this means, the therapist is frequently able to make great inroads into the patient's distortions of reality, even during the period of acute excitement. When the excitement is over and the chlorpromazine therapy has been discontinued, the patient and the therapist have a considerable head start in approaching the long-term therapeutic problem.

Reserpine

Reserpine, in large doses, can be effective in the treatment of acute schizophrenic reactions which are marked by extreme fear and anxiety. These include those which occur as panics, in settings of simple or paranoid schizophrenic reactions, and can also include the excitements of simple, hebephrenic, and paranoid schizophrenic reactions, *provided* these are associated with primary manifestations of anxiety and fear. If, on the other hand, anger or sexual unrest occurs in such states, reserpine does not possess the effectiveness of chlorpromazine. When reserpine is administered to the excited patient who is fearful, it may be expected that the over-all course will be similar to that which is found with chlorpromazine. The patient's excitement may be expected to be controlled within a period of 2 to 3 weeks from the onset of physical treatment, but his course in therapy will have to be continued for a minimum period of 6 weeks. During this time, once again, the patient and the therapist are able to make considerable inroads into the dynamic understanding of problems which brought the excited state about and to allow the patient to make a head start toward his long-term therapy. Once again, just as with catatonic excitements treated by chlorpromazine, if it is necessary to terminate the excitement or panic more quickly, it is possible to do this by the administration of ECT.

Barbiturates

SEDATION

Barbiturate sedation has little place in the treatment of the acute schizophrenic reactions. Only in those instances of simple schizophrenic reactions associated with moderate amounts of anxiety and fear would it be possible to use barbiturates in order to provide sedation without running the risk of increasing the patient's loss of contact with reality. By and large, the acute schizophrenic reactions are associated with so much confusion and loss of reality testing that the addition of barbiturate sedation would almost always enhance the risk of further disorganization. They are to be avoided until the acute situation has subsided to a marked degree.

Hypnosis

Barbiturates, on the other hand, can be used very effectively to provide sleep during acute schizophrenic reactions. This is of particular importance in dealing with the simple, hebephrenic, and paranoid schizophrenic reactions associated with marked anxiety and accompanying insomnia. In these situations, it is very common to find that sleep is greatly disturbed by homosexual fears and threatening nightmares. Under such circumstances, a wise first step is to have the patient sleeping in a single room. It is then possible to ensure that the patient gets a full night's sleep by using an adequate dosage of barbiturates. It must be remembered, in this connection, that it will usually be necessary to use a minimum dosage of 300 mg barbiturate to insure such sleep and that very frequently it is necessary to increase this dosage to 500 to 700 mg before the effect can be obtained.

SODIUM AMYTAL INTERVIEWS

Sodium Amytal interviews are occasionally of some value in attempting to establish rapport with patients who are in the middle of catatonic stupors. Such patients may continue in a stuporous and uncommunicative state for weeks or months at a time. The execution of a series of Sodium Amytal interviews, however, will almost invariably open up channels of communication by helping the patient to talk while under the influence of the drug. After several such interviews have been carried out, the doctor will have a much better understanding of the patient's dynamic problems and the patient will be better prepared to talk to the physician when he is not under the influence of the medication. Sodium Amytal interviews in this situation can (1) increase therapeutic understanding and (2) facilitate a breakdown of the stuporous resistance. It is unwise to extend the series of Sodium Amytal interviews beyond six interviews in any month, if they prove unsuccessful, because of the dangers of habituation. Sodium Amytal interviews should only be carried out by a therapist who is fully prepared to cope with any material, however delusional, which may be expressed during the interviews.

Meprobamate

Sedation achieved by meprobamate, and other sedative drugs of a like nature, is usually of little avail in the acute schizophrenic reactions. These reactions are usually of too serious and intense a nature to be controlled by the relatively mild effectiveness of the meprobamate group of sedatives. Occasionally, however, just as with the barbiturates, a patient who has a simple schizophrenic reaction and only moderate anxiety may find that symptoms are reduced adequately by this medication.

Antidepressive Drugs

Stimulants and antidepressive drugs have little use during acute schizophrenic episodes. Depression and some retardation may indeed be present during these acute schizophrenic episodes, but the importance of these features in the total psychopathology is very small and therapeutic efforts are more efficiently directed toward the major pathologic elements.

Subcoma and Coma Insulin Treatment

The place of insulin is a secure one in the treatment of acute schizophrenic reactions. As has been indicated in previous chapters, it is particularly useful in the severe schizophrenic reactions which are associated with anxiety and fear. It will apparently promote alleviation of anxiety and enhance the patient's thinking ability. However, it is necessary to recognize that the usual course of insulin treatment will last at least 1 month and frequently 2 or 3 months. The justification for this expenditure of time is that it will allow considerable psychotherapeutic progress to be made, in addition to bringing the acute reaction under control. If it is not likely that this can be done, it is more efficient to utilize ECT to bring about a more rapid termination of the acute episode.

It may be seen that most of the drugs and treatments which have been described in Part Two of this book can be used, according to the nature of the situation, in the therapy of acute schizophrenic reactions. They must be used, however, in such a way that they will forward the major purposes of therapy during the acute reactions: the relief of symptoms, the alleviation of anxiety, and the establishment of a good therapeutic relationship. If they are used in this capacity, they can provide immeasurable help to psychotherapeutic progress.

TREATMENT OF LONG-TERM SCHIZOPHRENIC REACTIONS

In the treatment of long-term schizophrenic reactions, it is still necessary to ensure that the treatment be specific. Once more, it is disastrous if the therapist or the patient becomes involved in imposing his own personal standards on the other; only confusion, hostility, and poor therapeutic results will follow when this takes place. Furthermore, the specific nature of therapy provides a continuing link between the material which has been discussed and utilized during the treatment of the acute episode and that which is utilized as the continuing, long-range treatment progresses.

While the specificity of therapy continues unchanged, there are many aspects of the therapy of long-term schizophrenic reactions which differ from the treatment of acute schizophrenic reactions. First and foremost, perhaps, is the fact that in treatment of long-term schizophrenic reactions therapy is not centered on the restitution of the person to his previous condition. On the contrary, it necessarily involves maintaining the patient in his current state of health or improving his state of health. It is not possible for the therapist dealing with a long-term schizophrenic reaction to remove the patient from stress as he does while treating an acute episode. On the contrary, he must be prepared to help the patient continue to deal with the stresses of life situations and to learn to face new and different stresses as he expands his ability to live. Similarly, it is no longer possible for the therapist to concentrate on relieving anxiety and providing security for the patient; in dealing with a long-term problem, it is necessary for him to stop relieving anxiety and help the patient himself to deal constructively with this anxiety. More and more, as the therapy progresses, it is necessary for the therapist and the patient to devise new techniques whereby the patient can better utilize his assets, better control his emotions, and better face the stresses of the environmental situation.

In order that this growth toward independence may take place, it is usually necessary for the therapist to assume a more realistic role in long-term therapy than that which he assumed during the acute episode. During the acute episode, the therapist frequently goes far out of his way to give the patient the emotional support which he needs and to establish a bond of helpfulness and confidence. Now, however, it is necessary for the therapist to assume a more realistic role; he must be less of a powerful leader and more of an honest and interested guide, helping the patient himself to deal with situations. Naturally, this change in role cannot be made abruptly. Instead, it is necessary for the therapist to interpose himself to varying degrees, according to the nature of specific situations and the amount of emotional stress which the patient is experiencing at any given time. By and large, however, as the long-term therapy progresses, it is more and more necessary for the therapist to reduce his role in the situation to as realistic a one as possible.

Within this framework of continuing specificity and a more realistic therapeutic role, the therapist may then pursue the goals of maintaining and expanding the patient's health and ability to deal with the world. He does this in two ways. The first is by exploring the everyday events which take place in the patient's life. Carefully and repeatedly, the patient and the therapist must examine the finest details of the patient's life. They must explore those areas in which the patient is comfortable and uncomfortable, those areas which he is able to face with confidence and those which he avoids completely. They must explore the social situation, the sexual situation, the religious situation, the food situation, the clothing situation, the home situation, and, indeed, every conceivable aspect of the patient's life. As they do so, they must concentrate on what the situation *actually is* and how the patient deals with it in *actual* terms. The patient must learn what techniques he uses in dealing with these situations and what techniques he might use to deal with them more effectively. As new techniques are discussed and considered, the patient must be supported in experimenting with these new techniques in order to better adjust himself to the environment. As hitherto unrecognized assets are seen, the patient must learn to concentrate his attempts to deal with the world in those areas where his assets work most effectively. When certain situations, e.g., specific kinds of social gatherings, appear especially threatening, the patient may learn that these are to be avoided and that he must obtain his social compensations in other fashions. Whitehorn (1955) has described this method of realignment of assets very well in his description of "evocative therapy."

At the same time as the patient's efforts are rechanneled in his dealings with the daily environment, it behooves both the therapist and the patient to know something of the reasons *why* certain persons are difficult for the patient to deal with while others are easy; *why* some situations are benign and other situations threatening. This may be done, obviously, only by an exploration of past historical dynamic material, which has led to the present situation. In general, it is best for the therapist to take these two steps as two different stages of therapy. In dealing with every schizophrenic patient, it is necessary that the therapist and patient concentrate on day-by-day living. Frequently, because of the patient's anxiety or his limited interest in psychotherapy, it is impossible to do more than concentrate on his pragmatic dealing with the world. When it is possible, however, it is advisable to go to the second stage of therapy, which is to explore the dynamic material which lies behind the day-by-day living. This can only be done, obviously, if the patient is interested and if he can cope with the anxiety which occurs while dynamic explorations are being carried out.

If this second stage of therapy can be carried out, the benefits will be found in understanding and also in the effectiveness of daily operations. When the patient understands better, for example, why he becomes uncomfortable in the presence of aggressive masculine figures, he will be in a far better position to devise new techniques for dealing with this discomfort, which he had previously dealt with by flight. If he recognizes, similarly, his self-defeating tendencies, it will be much easier for him to learn to develop his aesthetic or sympathetic social assets, which he had previously neglected or denied. The pragmatic daily working through of problems and the exploration of historical dynamic material can go hand in hand. The stage that must always be carried out is the examination of the daily activities; the stage that should be carried out whenever possible is the dynamic exploration.

In carrying out this dual kind of therapy, in order to improve the patient's adjustment, it is easily possible to use a number of the somatic treatments which have been discussed previously.

Electroconvulsive Treatment

It frequently happens in the long-range treatment of a schizophrenic reaction that the patient becomes severely depressed as he recognizes more and more clearly the difficulties which he encounters in facing the world. This depression is almost realistic in its nature, being based on the patient's awareness of his own innate difficulties. Such depressions can be manifested by serious symptoms and may easily bring about suicidal attempts. They are found most prominently in patients with simple schizophrenic reactions. In the treatment of such depressions, six to eight ECTs administered at intervals of two times per week will easily terminate the depression itself. Obviously, however, the administration of ECT must be timed in such a way that, when the depression is cleared, the patient will be able to see that he *has* techniques for dealing with the world. If ECT is administered before the proper psychotherapeutic groundwork has been laid, the remission of the depression will be only temporary.

Electroconvulsive therapy may also be used in the long-range treatment of schizophrenic reactions to break long-standing patterns of inadequate defenses. After several years of illness, it is common to find that patients with simple, hebephrenic, and paranoid schizophrenic reactions have developed fixed patterns of thinking and behavior. These may consist of chronic delusions, of antisocial behavior, or of eccentric dress. Whatever the manifestation, it is so firmly entrenched as a habit that no amount of insight or anxiety can change it. Electroconvulsive therapy, however, can break the impasse. It is necessary to administer between 12 and 20 ECTs, given at intervals of two to three times per week. After the twelfth ECT, it is common to find that the patient's patterns of thinking and behavior are greatly broken up and the patient is ready to adopt new modes of thinking and acting. Once more, it is necessary that the proper groundwork be laid for this utilization of ECT. Unless sufficient psychotherapeutic progress has been made, so that the patient is able to adopt new techniques for dealing with the world and knows which techniques to adopt, he will quickly slip back into the previously existing defensive systems and delusional ideation. Thorough psychotherapeutic preparation must be made for this use of ECT. The therapist must be especially certain that hostility has been analyzed and controlled; if it is present to a significant degree, improvement following ECT will be transient in nature.

Lastly, ECT may be used in combination with insulin treatment. This is usually akin to the utilization of ECT for the treatment of depression or for its ability to break up existing patterns. Frequently, after the patient has been on insulin treatment for 1 to 2 months, increasing feelings of depression come to the fore. These can then be terminated by ECT if the psychotherapeutic groundwork has been laid, and the patient can go on successfully in the insulin-facilitated reorganization of personality. It may be similarly used to break up old patterns, while insulin helps the psychotherapeutic construction of new ones.

Phenothiazines

The use of phenothiazine derivatives, in particular chlorpromazine, can be incorporated into the treatment of a long-term schizophrenic problem under specific circumstances. When the patient is facing environmental difficulties which produce emotional turmoil, such as anger or sexual unrest, it is frequently possible to use low dosages of chlorpromazine (300 to 400 mg orally per day) to alleviate the emotional turmoil and allow the patient to handle the problem in his interviews and in the environmental situation. Such a course in therapy may extend as long as the particular problem exists, but it is probably not efficient to utilize the medication for a problem which will last less than 1 week.

A second utilization of chlorpromazine in the long-term treatment of a schizophrenic patient is in dealing with the hostile paranoid patient who has a well-fixed and chronic delusional system. One does not expect the delusional system to be altered under the influence of chlorpromazine, but one hopes that the hostility will be controlled, thereby allowing psychotherapeutic interviews to explore the dynamic background of the paranoid pattern. When sufficient progress has been made in understanding and dealing with the pattern, it may then be possible to break up the pattern by the judicious use of ECT. If sufficient advances have been made psychotherapeutically in advance of the administration of ECT, it should then be possible to resynthesize a more healthful pattern of living.

Reserpine

The administration of reserpine is cumbersome. In its higher dosages, it *can* be used to control intense states of anxiety and fear; in lower dosages, however, its effect is not strong. Consequently, it is rarely indicated for the intermediate types of problems which are found in the long-term treatment of schizophrenic patients. In addition, it must be remembered that the problems of long-term treatment may require that the medication be used over a long period of time. Such chronic administration can frequently lead to serious depression. For these reasons, it is infrequent that reserpine is an efficient agent in the long-term treatment of schizophrenic reactions.

Barbiturates

SEDATION

In long-term treatment of a schizophrenic reaction, the use of barbiturate sedation is frequently of great value. As opposed to chlorpromazine sedation, barbiturate sedation can be used to handle anxiety and fear, especially when these are of relatively short duration, e.g., an acute difficulty in the office, in the home, or in a social situation. If the episode in question can be brought under control within 4 to 5 days, it is easily possible to utilize barbital in doses of 150 mg four times a day to alleviate some of the patient's anxiety and fear while he is dealing with this environmental situation. This approach is most useful for patients with well-organized personalities and can be utilized to advantage in dealing with simple, hebephrenic, and paranoid schizophrenic reactions. It is not effective in dealing with patients whose emotional problems are largely concerned with anger, where it is wiser to use chlorpromazine as sedation. Similarly, it is not effective in problems which involve the continuation of sedation for a period longer than 2 weeks, because of the gradual falling off of medication effect and the danger of habituation. For dealing with anxieties and fears of longer duration, it is probably wiser to utilize meprobamate.

HYPNOSIS

Just as with barbiturate sedation, the production of sleep by means of the administration of barbiturates can frequently be used in crisis situations in the long-term treatment of a schizophrenic reaction. It is most unwise, however, to use barbiturates to produce sleep for a period of time longer than several weeks unless this becomes absolutely necessary. The usual dosage is less than that required in the acute schizophrenic reactions and is commonly about 200 to 400 mg of Sodium Amytal or pentobarbital, given orally at bedtime.

SODIUM AMYTAL INTERVIEWS

Only under extraordinary circumstances, when the patient has a very definitely well-organized personality, when the therapist is skilled at directing Sodium Amytal interviews toward specific problem areas, and when he is prepared to deal with any emergency situation that may arise, should Sodium Amytal interviews be used in patients with long-term schizophrenic reactions. In the rare instances where its use may be indicated, caution should be used.

Meprobamate Sedation

As mentioned previously, the long-term treatment of schizophrenic reactions frequently brings the patient face to face with internal or environmental problems which produce anxiety as they are explored and handled. If the anxiety-producing situations are of moderately long duration, e.g., longer than 1 to 2 weeks, and the anxiety is sufficient to interfere with therapy and adaptation, then the use of meprobamate is indicated to relieve the patient's suffering. Meprobamate will have the advantage in this situation of not dulling the patient's ability to think and deal with the problem realistically and in not slowing his physical activity. In addition, it may be increased to higher dosage levels than may the barbiturates without comparable impairment of the person's operative capacity. Meprobamate is obviously of more utility in dealing with emotional disturbances characterized by anxiety and fear than with those associated with anger or resentment; in the latter instances, phenothiazine derivatives are recommended. The usual dosage of meprobamate for patients with schizophrenic reactions will be 400 to 800 mg orally, four times per day. The lack of organization of the personality of patients with schizophrenic reactions tends to make the utilization of chronic medication outside the hospital difficult. After the first several weeks, it is usual for the patient to begin to "juggle" medication or to use it according to his own plan. It is, therefore, necessary for the physician to exercise great caution and close supervision when he uses meprobamate or any other chronic medication for the treatment of long-term schizophrenic reactions.

Antidepressive Drugs

As has been described previously, it is frequently possible for depression to occur during the long-term treatment of a schizophrenic reaction. In this situation, the antidepressive drugs, in particular imipramine and monoamine oxidase inhibitors, may be effective. It is important, if these medications are utilized, that they be continued until the patient has overcome the difficulties which have brought on the depression. Otherwise, one would be in the same situation as if ECT had been administered prematurely: when the treatment is terminated, the depression will recur. The decision whether to administer ECT to handle the depression or whether to utilize the antidepressive drugs will depend mainly on the severity of the depression. In very severe depressions, where suicidal risk is imminent, ECT will provide a more reliable and rapid method of treatment. In milder depressions, where more time can be taken, the antidepressive drugs may be more easily used and more therapeutically oriented.

Subcoma and Coma Insulin Treatment

Frequently, it becomes apparent in the course of treating a patient with a long-term schizophrenic reaction that it is necessary to relieve anxiety drastically in order to make therapeutic headway. If the situation is sufficiently severe to require hospitalization, it is possible to use subcoma or coma insulin treatment to produce this result. Subcoma insulin treatment can be used to greatest advantage in dealing with chronic simple and hebephrenic schizophrenic reactions which are associated with anxiety and fear. Coma insulin treatment, on the other hand, is more effective in dealing with paranoid schizophrenic reactions, particularly those with chronic and fixed delusional systems. The treatment is exactly the same as for acute schizophrenic reactions, but with a more long-range purpose. If the schizophrenic reactions are associated with marked feelings of depression, it is sometimes necessary to combine the treatment with ECT. Electroconvulsive therapy may also be used in order more efficiently to break up preexisting patterns of operation, while the insulin treatment provides security and fosters a more healthful integration.

Lobotomy

If the chronic schizophrenic illness is of great severity and there appears little likelihood that the patient will respond to any other therapy, it may be valuable to consider a prefrontal lobotomy. This should not be considered until the patient has failed to respond to an adequate course of ECT and has also been exposed to adequate subcoma or coma insulin treatment. Under these circumstances, if the therapist and the patient, as well as the patient's family, are agreed on the fact that the patient will probably require hospitalization for the rest of his life, prefrontal lobotomy may be administered. At the present time, with rapid advances in the treatment of schizophrenic reactions, it would appear that the indications for this treatment are sharply limited.

The various physical treatments may tie in, at one point or another, with the purposes of psychotherapy in the long-term treatment of schizophrenic reactions. By alleviating anxiety, hostility, and other obstacles, by helping to organize thinking processes, by breaking up patterns of depression or delusional ideation, the somatic treatments may smash obstacles to psychotherapy. Exploration of dynamic historical material and experimentation with new techniques of dealing with the environment will be facilitated. The treatment of schizophrenic patients may extend over a period of many months and years; if the therapist remains keenly aware of the many physical methods of treatment which are at his disposal, he will find several of these useful at different stages of his psychotherapeutic course.

SUMMARY

The schizophrenic reactions, with their protean manifestations, provide a complex psychotherapeutic problem. In general, they must be approached on the level of *specificity*. Whenever any activity, idea, or emotion is discussed with a patient, it must be discussed in specific and concrete terms, thereby avoiding the confusion which may arise from the fact that the patient views all these aspects of life from a personalized point of view.

With specificity as the keynote, the treatment of schizophrenic reactions involves the acute schizophrenic reaction and the long-term schizophrenic reaction. During an acute schizophrenic reaction, it is the obligation of the doctor to concentrate his efforts on restoring the person to his usual health by alleviating major symptoms. He may do this by removing environmental stresses, promoting the patient's security, and relieving the patient's anxiety. At the same time, he uses his interviews to obtain more understanding of the patient's problem and to cement his therapeutic relationship. In pursuing all these goals, virtually every kind of physical treatment can provide some help, depending on the diagnostic and psychopathologic situation.

When the acute episode has been terminated, the course of treatment must continue to concentrate on specificity. Now, however, it is possible for the patient and the therapist to attempt to improve the patient's ability to deal with daily environmental problems. They may do this by careful examination of, and experimentation with, the pattern of daily living; this examination and experimentation will be helped by the simultaneous exploration of historical dynamic material. In dealing with the problems on a practical basis and in exploring the anxiety-producing dynamic areas, a great deal of support may be obtained from physical treatments.

It must always be remembered, in both the acute and long-term situations, that the proper utilization of the physical treatments depends on the psychopathologic condition of the patient and the psychotherapeutic stage at which the patient stands. If this is kept in mind, physical methods of treatment provide the physician with a strong and diversified armamentarium in dealing with one of the most serious psychiatric illnesses.

17

THE TREATMENT OF AFFECTIVE
REACTIONS

DEPRESSIVE REACTIONS

The fundamental problem which confronts the physician who treats a patient with a depressive reaction is the need for the patient to reorient his life. This reorientation may be, in some instances, a very minor one; in other instances, it may require a major shift in the patient's fundamental attitudes, beliefs, and values. In all degrees of depression, however, there are psychotherapeutic features which are common.

The first of these is the need for the therapist to be acutely aware of the degree of suicidal drive which is present in the patient at any given time. Only by a keen awareness of the degree of suicidal intent can the therapist adequately protect the patient, while continuing his psychotherapeutic efforts. Many times depressive illnesses display such seemingly minor surface manifestations as hypochondriasis, insomnia, or generalized fatigue. The physician, despite the apparently inconsequential nature of the complaints, must be on the lookout for signs of serious suicidal depression. The paramount signs of suicidal risk may be listed as follows:

1. Marked psychomotor slowing, which includes retardation of speech, retardation of physical movements, constipation, anorexia with eructations, and lack of muscle tone.

2. Severe early morning awakening, with the patient wakening at approximately 3 A.M. and remaining in bed, brooding, until daylight or after.

3. Marked diurnal variation, with the major feelings of depression oc-

curring between 3 and 6 A.M. and the patient feeling relatively well between 6 and 9 P.M.

4. Paranoid ideation, particularly delusions of persecution, nihilism, or world destruction.

5. Overt hostility, particularly toward family members.

6. A history of previous suicidal attempts by the patient or successful suicides carried out by relatives or close associates.

7. The presence of overt suicidal desires, thoughts, or plans on the part of the patient.

If any of these signs are present, the therapist should be sure that his patient is placed in a psychiatric hospital, where the patient can be given adequate supervision and protection while psychotherapy is executed.

With the safety of the patient assured, the therapist must next consider the nature of the patient's daily activities. Depressed patients, by the very nature of their illness, are unable to function efficiently in their environment. It is characteristic of this illness, moreover, that each inadequacy of the patient and each failure which he notes in the course of his day's activities will add to the depression and provide him with additional proof of his own futility and worthlessness. It is, therefore, imperative that the therapist take great pains to provide for the patient an activity program which will minimize the possibility of failure and help the patient to see his own value and ability to succeed. Most frequently, such a program can be constructed by working closely with a skilled occupational therapist in a hospital setting. The occupational therapist can provide the patient with a planned set of work and play activities which are scaled down to such a simple level that the patient cannot do anything but succeed. In the early stages, such work might be as simple as cutting up rags for cleaning purposes. With each success that the patient achieves in such limited activities, the depression will be undermined to that extent and the patient will have that degree of proof that he still possesses value and worth. Gradually, as the depression improves through psychotherapy or other means, the patient becomes more capable. As this progress takes place, the occupational therapy activities are scaled upward, becoming more and more complex. At the same time, the skilled occupational therapist can guide these activities into directions which are expressive of the patient's needs and emotions. The occupational therapy program which started out to provide the patient with proof of his own value can finally shift into helping the patient find better means of expressing his own feelings. In doing so, as will be seen, it will tie in very closely with the psychotherapeutic needs of the situation.

When the patient's safety and daily program have been considered and arranged for, the therapist must plan how he can carry out psychotherapeutic interviews. Most patients with depression have difficulty in spontaneity; even the agitated patient, while he can pour out many words, will show a marked dearth of new ideas. It is therefore a great strain on both therapist and patient to carry out prolonged interviews. For all therapists except those who are most skilled, therefore, it is wise to limit psychotherapeutic interviews to 15 to 25 minutes, held three to five times per week. The therapist should enter these interviews prepared to listen to the spontaneous productions of the patient and to explore dynamic material in a nondirective fashion. He should also, however, be sufficiently cognizant of the nature of depressive reactions to know that very frequently the patient will be unable to produce such material voluntarily. When no spontaneous material is produced, he should be prepared to explore with neutral questioning the dynamic areas which would seem important in the patient's illness. If the therapist is unprepared to explore a number of avenues in this active way, the therapeutic interview, like other activities in which the patient engages, will be but one more proof of the patient's failure. Later, as the depression clears under the influence of therapy, the patient will become more productive, and there will be less need for the therapist to assume such a directive role in therapy. In the early stages of the treatment of most patients with depression, however, such a gently directive role is imperative.

A corollary to the need for the therapist to assume a directive role in early interviews is his need to obtain a clear understanding of his patient's personality. For many therapists, this is a difficult task. When they deal with patients with schizophrenic or psychoneurotic reactions, they are dealing with persons who are going through the kind of problems which the therapists themselves have faced during their own adolescence and early adulthood. In dealing with the older depressed patient, however, there is a tendency to lose sympathy with the patient and to fail to recognize his emotional needs. To compensate for this difficulty, it is wiser for the therapist to demand of himself that he have a full understanding of how the patient actually lives in extreme detail. The extent of the detail is important here. The therapist must find out how the patient rises in the morning, how he feels when he gets out of bed, how he selects his clothes, how he feels at breakfast, how he goes about reading his daily newspaper; he must follow the patient's footsteps minute by minute and hour by hour through day after day of his usual life. Only in this way, usually, is it possible for the therapist to get a full appreciation of his patient as a human being. In addition to such exploration with the patient, there is also the obligation of the therapist to have extensive interviews with the patient's spouse and other relatives in order to get a full picture of the personality of his patient.

These are the common denominators which should guide psychotherapy of any depressed patient. They are (1) protection of the patient; (2) provision of an adequate daily program of activities, emphasizing occupational therapy; (3) brief interviews, with the therapist prepared to assume a leading role, if necessary; (4) the therapist's keen awareness of his patient's personality and life situation, as a necessary preliminary to all other steps. With these thoughts in mind, we may now go on to consider the specific aims and techniques which may be used in achieving specific psychotherapeutic goals.

In following the four general principles described, the therapist has in mind achieving some reorientation of the patient's life. To some extent, the degree of indicated reorientation will depend on the severity of the depressive reaction. Even more, however, it will depend on the nature of the problems which brought about the depression. It is this etiologic difference which really indicates the course of the psychotherapy and which determines how physical treatments can be useful adjuncts to the therapy.

There are many possible approaches to an understanding of the problems which contributed to the development of a depression. For purposes of the present volume, these may best be considered in three classes: (1) depressions resulting from the need to alter behavioral patterns; (2) depressions resulting from distorted personality structure; (3) depressions resulting from chronic psychoneurotic disability. Each of these types will now be examined in its psychotherapeutic aspects.

DEPRESSIONS RESULTING FROM THE NEED TO ALTER BEHAVIORAL PATTERNS

Depressions brought about by a need to alter behavioral patterns are most commonly the retarded depressions in the fifties and the agitated depressions in the sixties. Very frequently, these depressions are precipitated by discrete events in the environment, such as success in business, the departure of children to college, or serious physical illness. They may also be precipitated by the onset of aging with its limitations on the intellectual and physical capacities of the patient; for this reason, many of the cases of so-called involutional melancholia fall into this category.

Most of these depressions constitute a relatively simple psychotherapeutic process. The therapist finds that he deals with a patient with a well-organized personality who has relatively good insight into his own needs and desires but who has adhered to an excessively rigid pattern of living. As a consequence, the person is unable to adapt to his new situation and becomes ill. Usually, the simple stress of the illness and the fact that the illness itself will alter the person's pattern of living will ensure that recovery will be accompanied by sufficient alteration in the patient's living patterns that he will not have future depressions. The psychotherapist's main job in such a situation is to speed the process of recovery and adaptation as much as possible and to help to reorient the patient's life in the healthiest possible fashion.

Sometimes the problem of recovery and adaptation is not so simple. A successful executive, for example, may be suffering from the early signs of arteriosclerotic cardiovascular disease, with shortened attention, diminished memory, and markedly impaired imagination and initiative. When this executive enters a depression, it constitutes a more serious psychotherapeutic problem because the extent of the required adaptation is well-nigh heroic. The treatment of such a problem provides a model for the way in which the problems of altered behavioral adaptation may be handled. In such an instance, the therapist needs to explore, in detail, the nature of the patient's personality: his drives, motivations, and ambitions, as they have existed throughout his life. He must recognize, in doing so, that the same needs for prestige, accomplishment, love, respect, and integrity which existed prior to the onset of the arteriosclerosis still remain in the individual. Now, however, the individual is no longer able to utilize or even to approximate the same behavioral mechanisms to satisfy these needs. The therapist's work then becomes twofold: he must first demonstrate clearly to the patient that the previous modes of adaptation are no longer effective; in doing so, he must recognize the fact that such an awareness will temporarily increase the severity of the patient's depression. At the same time, as he leads the patient to face the problem, he must help the patient to work out new modes of adaptation, which satisfy his needs and do so in accordance with the capabilities which he currently possesses. Such new modes, very frequently, involve using assets which the patient has not drawn on in the past. The executive, for example, will no longer have his old imagination and initiative; he now needs to draw on experience, the wisdom of past accomplishments, and the memory of previous details, which are not available to his younger and more energetic colleagues. By the adequate use of these hitherto neglected assets, he will usually be able to maintain all the position which he had before. He will do so, however, in a different way.

In the same fashion, one may treat the housewife who can no longer devote herself to raising her children but can channel her activities into church work or cultural organizations. One can help the physically active person who has had a myocardial infarction to direct his energies toward virile accomplishments which do not place the same burden on his physical system. One can help the lady who has lost her youthful beauty to recognize the esteem in which she is held and the love which she receives from others on the basis of her warmth and sincerity, rather than because of her complexion. In all these instances, and many more, the technique is basically the same. The therapist cannot alter the facts of reality; it is necessary for him to help the patient recognize the inescapable truth of his situation, whether this be loss of intellectual capacity, loss of physical ability, or whatever. Once having accomplished this recognition, he helps the patient to find a better way of satisfying his need, in accordance with the reality which has been clarified. The extent of the behavioral change may be great or small, and the difficulty of psychotherapy will vary accordingly. In some instances, adaptation may be virtually spontaneous, if symptoms are relieved. In other instances, months of psychotherapy may be required. In all cases, however, the new adaptation must be sufficiently good to prevent recurrence.

In carrying out this psychotherapeutic program, much help can be received from a variety of somatic treatments.

Electroconvulsive Treatment

A series of six to eight ECTs, administered at a frequency of two to three times per week, will almost invariably terminate depressions which are brought about by the need to alter behavioral adaptation. Occasionally, ECT is not necessary once the psychotherapeutic aims as described above have been accomplished. More frequently, however, the inertia which is inherent in depressive reactions does not permit recovery in less time than several months. When the patient has recognized the reality of the situation, therefore, and is ready to move into new adaptational patterns, it is usually worthwhile to bring about this movement by clearing up the depression with a course of ECT. When the illness is mild and the amount of needed behavioral change is minimal, such a course of ECT may be given early and may indeed constitute the major element in the psychotherapeutic program. It should always be timed, however, in accordance with the psychotherapeutic needs of the situation. The ECT will be most effective, naturally, in the setting of marked anxiety and fear, such as is seen in agitated depressions, or in the presence of paranoid ideation, provided that this is not associated with excessive hostility. The ECT will often not be effective, and there will be a great likelihood of recurrence, if the depression is associated with marked hostility.

Phenothiazines

In the depressions which we are considering, it is not common to find marked hostility and resentment as a pertinent factor in the illness. If these symptoms occur, however, they argue against the utilization of ECT. In such a situation, it is wise to utilize phenothiazine derivatives, such as chlorpromazine in an oral dosage of 300 to 500 mg per day, and to continue psychotherapeutic exploration of the hostility until the hostility is alleviated. At such a time, one resumes the regular psychotherapeutic course of these depressions, utilizing ECT if necessary.

Barbiturates

SEDATION

Barbiturate sedation is frequently helpful in dealing with patients with milder depressions of this sort, provided that they do not have any marked organic brain disease. For patients who show mild agitation in the late fifties, doses of barbital in the range of 150 mg three to four times a day will frequently diminish the agitation and make the patient's life less full of suffering. Barbiturate sedation is not very effective in the treatment of paranoid or very severe depressions. Retarded depressions are usually made worse by the administration of barbiturate sedation.

HYPNOSIS

Nighttime sedation is of great value in the treatment of patients who have depressions. Since the major problem for most patients with depression is early morning awakening, to which may be added difficulty in going to sleep in the case of agitated depression, the optimal medication for such persons is a combined dosage. This involves the oral administration of 300 mg Sodium Amytal and 200 mg barbital at bedtime. Such a dosage will usually provide 7 or 8 hours of continuous, dream-free sleep.

Antidepressive Drugs

Antidepressive drugs may be useful in the treatment of these depressions, and pharmacologic agents may eventually supplant the use of ECT. They can be administered at any time in the psychotherapeutic course, but it is necessary that the patient be able to achieve a readjustment of his life orientation before the medications are terminated. Otherwise, just as with ECT, depression will occur with the cessation of the drug. A current drawback, of course, is the fact that the antidepressive drugs work slowly; in the case of serious suicidal risk, therefore, the antidepressant drug should not be substituted for rapid hospitalization or the use of ECT.

DEPRESSIONS RESULTING FROM DISTORTED PERSONALITY STRUCTURE

Depressions associated with the need to change basic personality patterns are those which are associated with manic-depressive illnesses. One deals with a personality constellation of a fixed and permanent nature, probably associated with equally fixed genetic components. The therapeutic problem is a serious one. It is one which has been explored in some detail by a few workers, but definitive treatment remains uncertain and in an investigative stage (Cohen, et al., 1954; Kohl, et al., 1954).

In its broad outline, however, the definitive treatment of patients with manic-depressive depressions depends on 1 to 2 years of intensive exploratory psychotherapy, aimed at providing the patient with an extensive understanding of his personality drives and motivations. In the course of treatment, great emphasis is placed on his emotional needs and his previous inability to recognize or satisfy these needs. The paradoxical aspect of therapy, of course, is the fact that these patients have led behaviorally satisfactory lives and have produced in other persons great emotional warmth, love, and devotion toward themselves. It is because they have not recognized their own emotional needs and do not know how to communicate these needs that they are unable to reap the rewards of this behavior. It therefore becomes the obligation of the therapist to help the patient see the feelings which exist within him and to open his eyes to the fact that he can satisfy these emotional needs simply by breaking down the barriers which exist within himself. When it is expressed so briefly, this goal of psychotherapy seems ultrasimple. When it is recognized, however, that the breaking down of such emotional barriers is opposed to the very principles of the person's life, it becomes obvious that a therapeutic problem is a complicated and serious one.

In achieving the psychotherapeutic goal of personality reorganization, the therapist must be prepared to guide the patient through recurring depressions which go on during the course of therapy. Therapy may also be marked by one or more outbursts of manic excitement. The patient, therefore, must be prepared to endure therapy inside and outside the psychiatric hospital, as his condition varies. The therapist must be ever on the alert for increased signs of suicidal drive or elation and must have no compunction about giving his patient protection during increased depression or excitement.

If it is not possible for the therapist to approach the manic-depressive patient in this definitive intensive psychotherapeutic fashion, he must then fall back on the classical treatment of manic-depressive illnesses. This treatment is mainly watchful waiting, associated with as much prophylaxis as possible. Basically, it involves the establishment of a close, warm, mutually trusting relationship with the patient, with the patient seeing the therapist repeatedly, whether he be in good health or poor health. When the patient, in the course of routine visits, displays any evidences of increasing psychopathology, the therapist has to prevent this psychopathology from interfering with the welfare of the patient or his family by hospitalization and symptomatic treatment.

Both the reorganizing and the symptomatic types of psychotherapeutic approach to the treatment of depressions resulting from distorted personality structure can be helped by the use of somatic treatments.

Electroconvulsive Treatment

In the intensive psychotherapeutic treatment of manic-depressive depressions, ECT plays only a small role. When sufficient progress has been made psychotherapeutically, it is sometimes observed that the patient who is otherwise prepared to become well and remain well stays in a state of chronic depression. In such a situation, it is frequently possible to terminate the depression artificially, by means of six to eight ECTs administered two to three times per week. Such treatment does not differ in any way from the use of ECT in depressions associated with the need for behavioral adaptation. It must be used very sparingly, however, in the course of treating manic-depressive depressions. In such instances, the lack of sufficient psychotherapeutic progress will almost inevitably result in a recurrence of depression, and ECT becomes less and less effective with each repetition.

In the more symptomatic type of treatment of manic-depressive depressions, ECT may also play a role. It is here that ECT may be used on a long-term, chronic basis. After a patient's depression is terminated by the administration of six to eight ECTs, he then may receive ECT once a month, or once every 2 or 3 months, for the remainder of his life. The frequency with which prophylactic ECT may be given depends on the condition of the patient and on the frequency necessary to prevent recurring depressions. In the hands of several therapists, such prophylactic use of ECT has proved useful. With an interval of more than 1 month between treatments, there is little danger of serious organic damage to the brain.

Phenothiazines

It will be recognized that the treatment of patients with manic-depressive depressions by intensive psychotherapy is a treatment which requires that the patient remain in depressed states for months at a time, while the therapist and the patient explore dynamic material vigorously, regardless of the patient's suffering. In these instances, patients can undergo excruciating torture from their suicidal ideation and the emotional turmoil which accompanies the psychotherapeutic exploration. Very frequently, it is possible to alleviate some of this suffering while psychotherapy is being carried on by the administration of phenothiazine derivatives, such as chlorpromazine in low doses (200 to 300 mg orally per day). Chlorpromazine administration does not alter the behavioral patterns of the patient significantly, nor does it offer any specific psychotherapeutic advantage. Its main purpose is a humane one, to lessen the patient's discomfort while the needed but painful course of psychotherapy is being undertaken.

In addition, of course, there are times in the treatment of a manic-depressive illness, both from a supportive and prophylactic point of view and from a psychotherapeutic point of view, when the depression is associated with marked anger and resentment. In such instances ECT is frequently ineffective, and chlorpromazine will facilitate psychotherapeutic exploration of the anger and resentment before ECT is employed.

Barbiturate Sedation and Hypnosis

Barbiturates may be used in these depressions in a fashion similar to that used in depressions associated with need for behavioral adaptation.

Antidepressive Drugs

Antidepressive drugs may be used in the course of prophylactic treatment of manic-depressive depressions, but they are associated with a high incidence of physical complications. Hence it is unclear whether they can be used with safety in their present forms over the many years that it is necessary to continue such prophylactic treatment. They appear to have little place in the intensive psychotherapeutic management of manic-depressive depressions.

Lobotomy

As has been noted, lobotomy has been recommended for the treatment of chronic recurrent manic-depressive depressions. Its use should be restricted, however, to those patients who are suffering intensely and for whom there is no alternative hope.

DEPRESSIONS RESULTING FROM CHRONIC PSYCHONEUROTIC DISABILITY

In many instances, it is not the personality of the patient or external environmental situations which bring the patient to grief but, instead, the existence of a long-standing, moderately severe psychoneurotic condition. The existence of such a psychoneurotic reaction, over the course of the years, can gradually drain away the satisfactions a person obtains from his life to such an extent that he eventually enters into a depression. Most typically, such depressions begin in the fifth decade of life and are very frequently associated with paranoid features. They have a gradual, insidious onset and do not usually have classical psychomotor manifestations in as straightforward a fashion as do the two previous types of depression.

When these depressions are observed, the clinical picture is an easy one to delineate. The patient will reveal the history of some kind of psychoneurotic reaction which has existed since his early twenties. Such manifestations, commonly, are marked anxiety with phobias and obsessive-compulsive patterns and behavior, very frequently associated with impotence, sexually perverse activities, and chronic dissatisfaction with life. Occasionally, there have been brief episodes of depression of a psychoneurotic nature in the early or middle thirties.

The therapeutic problem with depressions of this nature is a complicated one. In essence, the therapist must deal with two separate illness processes. The first is the psychoneurotic illness which has contributed to the onset of the depression. The second illness is the depression itself, which comes on because of dissatisfaction with the way of life created by the psychoneurosis. Obviously, the treatment of the depression involves altering the behavioral pattern of the patient. In this instance, however, altering the behavioral pattern of the patient requires alteration of the psychoneurotic behavioral pattern. It is this duality of treatment purposes which makes the treatment of these illnesses difficult.

In this complicated situation, usually it is wise to adopt the straightforward principles of treatment for a depressive reaction as the first step. This will mean that the patient is placed in the hospital, given an adequate daily program of activities, and guided into psychotherapeutic interviews in the manner described in the introduction to this chapter. When this has been accomplished, however, there is then a great emphasis placed on the exploration of the psychoneurotic personality mechanisms which exist in the patient. This will be a far more intensive exploratory emphasis than is usually placed on defense mechanisms in the treatment of depressions. The exploration is done, moreover, with the knowledge that by the time a patient reaches the age of 40, there is little likelihood that psychotherapy can obtain a complete eradication of psychoneurotic mechanisms. The mechanisms must be explored, however, because they *must* be altered in some way, sufficient to allow the patient to obtain satisfaction in life, if his depression is to be terminated. Usually, one needs to focus on the sources of anxiety, particularly aggressiveness and sexuality, and help the patient learn means of controlling and tolerating this anxiety. This is done in the fashion which has previously been described for the psychotherapy for psychoneurotic reactions. When this has been accomplished, usually over the course of several months, one can return to the classical treatment of depressive reactions. When the patient has been shown that he can obtain new satisfactions in other ways, he is urged to reenter life activities, with intensive support from the therapist.

In the treatment of depressions resulting from chronic psychoneurotic disability, somatic treatment may be helpful.

Electroconvulsive Treatment

Electroconvulsive therapy may occasionally be of value in the treatment of depressive reactions associated with chronic psychoneuroses. It must be recognized, however, that a series of six to eight ECTs, administered two to three times per week, can only be effective *after* the basic psychoneurotic defense mechanisms have been dealt with. If, at this time, the patient is ready to move ahead into new methods of adaptation, ECT will reliably clear up the depression and allow this movement to take place.

Phenothiazines

It is a frequent finding that depressions associated with chronic psychoneurotic reactions are also associated with marked anger and resentment. These are not usually immediately apparent, however, being masked by psychoneurotic symptoms of an obsessive-compulsive or phobic nature. Instead, the hostility and resentment become obvious in the course of psychotherapy. If they do, they may be alleviated to some extent and psychotherapy facilitated by the administration of phenothiazine derivatives in low oral doses, for example, chlorpromazine in doses ranging from 200 to 400 mg per day.

Barbiturate Sedation and Hypnosis

Barbiturate sedation and hypnosis may be used in the manner described for the treatment of depressions associated with the need to alter behavioral patterns. The only modification arises from the fact that one deals here with a psychoneurotic problem and must guard more strongly against the formation of excessive dependency on drugs.

Antidepressive Drugs

These may be utilized in order to terminate the depression, when the psychoneurotic condition has already been dealt with. At this time, the patient is usually in the hospital, and there is no urgency about the administration of ECT. Consequently, these drugs may afford a satisfactory way of terminating psychotherapy in this type of depression.

MANIC EXCITEMENTS

A manic excitement is, characteristically, a short-lived episode. Within a matter of weeks, the patient enters a state of increasing excitement, achieves the peak level of activity, and returns to his preexcitement state. During this time, the psychotherapeutic responsibilities of the physician are fairly straightforward. In the first place, of course, it is necessary for the physician to minimize danger to the patient in the course of the excitement. This can usually best be done by hospitalizing the patient in a psychiatric hospital, where he will be kept from injuring himself or others and from destroying his financial and social position.

Secondly, it is the responsibility of the physician dealing with the manic excitement to bring the symptoms under control in the shortest possible period of time without harm to the patient. This usually requires the use of some somatic therapy. If somatic therapy is not used, indeed, there is serious danger to the patient's life from physical overactivity.

The third obligation of the physician in treating a manic excitement is to utilize this episode in the patient's illness in as therapeutic a fashion as possible. To accomplish this task is a difficult and delicate feat. The patient in a manic excitement is hostile and abusive and becomes extremely paranoid when his wishes are frustrated. His speech and thinking are often rambling and incoherent, and it is frequently difficult to make any sense out of his behavior.

In the face of these difficulties, the physician should follow a relatively steadfast psychotherapeutic line. He should see his patient at least daily for brief intervals. These intervals should be no longer than 15 minutes in duration. When they are together, the therapist should listen carefully to the patient's requests, demands, and comments. He should carefully avoid contradicting the patient or seeking points of argument. Instead, he should make it clear to the patient that he is seeking to help him in every way possible and that he is keenly aware of the emotional turmoil which the patient is undergoing. It is this last point which is of major importance in the psychotherapeutic approach to patients with manic excitements. Only a short distance beneath the surface, in every patient with manic excitement, lies an awareness of psychologic pain, which the elation is resisting and concealing. By changes of facial expression and by simple, nondirective questions, the physician can focus the patient's attention on this awareness. He can thereby make it clear to the patient that he recognizes the suffering and is prepared to do anything he can about it. The physician must not expect the patient to agree wholeheartedly to this or to be overtly grateful. Instead, the patient may spend 3 to 4 minutes discussing the indicated topic and immediately shift back to some grandiose ideation. In the course of time, however, such a psychotherapeutic technique will allow the physician to become intimately aware of the emotional conflicts which the patient faces. At the same time, it will give the patient a feeling of trust and confidence in the physician. By these two means, it will be possible for the patient and physician to continue the useful psychotherapeutic relationship while the patient is recovering and after he has reached a normal state. Since the likelihood for manic excitements is that the illness will recur unless long-term psychotherapeutic treatment is carried out, the establishment of such a liaison is of crucial psychotherapeutic importance.

Within this framework, somatic treatments can be used in several ways.

Electroconvulsive Treatment

Once a manic excitement has reached its peak, five ECTs, administered on a daily or every-other-day basis, will usually bring the excitement under control. If ECT is administered prior to the peak of the excitement, increasing excitement will usually reappear once the treatment has been terminated. When ECT is given and achieves a successful result, the patient is promptly restored to a normal behavioral state, usually with amnesia for the time of his illness and denial of the illness as a serious factor in his life. Under such circumstances, it is frequently difficult to persuade the patient to agree to any further psychotherapeutic efforts. This "antipsychotherapeutic" aspect of ECT must be regarded as a severe drawback to its use in the treatment of manic excitements.

Phenothiazines

Phenothiazine derivatives have proved to be a very valuable addition to the treatment of manic excitements. If chlorpromazine is used, a typical schedule may be as follows: On the first day, 100 mg is administered. On subsequent days, the intramuscular total dosage is increased to 200, 300, 400, and 500 mg, with the progressive increase being halted when the symptoms are brought under control. Usually such control appears when the dosage of intramuscular chlorpromazine has reached the level of 300 to 400 mg daily. The intramuscular dosage is stabilized for 2 to 3 days and then gradually shifted to twice the total dosage, given orally. By such means, one can bring the manic excitement under control within 3 to 4 days. Chlorpromazine is the best established of the phenothiazine derivatives in the management of manic excitements. The entire group, however, has a marked advantage over the use of ECT in the treatment of these states. This advantage springs from the fact that the patient, while his behavior becomes slowed and his emotional turmoil decreases, does not completely lose the thinking pattern that exists during the manic excitement. On the contrary, his ideas subside only gradually. The physician is therefore given the opportunity to establish a clear liaison with the patient, which he is denied when he uses ECT. Using this liaison, he obtains far more understanding of the patient and is in a far better position to keep therapy going when the manic episode is over.

Barbiturates

SEDATION

Barbiturate sedation is definitely contraindicated in manic excitements. The barbiturates usually are ineffective. If they *do* become effective, they impose a feeling of restraint on the manic patient, which will only increase his efforts to rid himself of all controls. Finally, if the sedation reaches the point of clouding the patient's consciousness, then one will have confusion added to the basic behavioral problem of the excitement. Usually, therefore, barbiturate sedation should not be attempted with a patient in a manic excitement.

HYPNOSIS

Sleep may be brought about by the use of barbiturates in manic excitements under special circumstances. Usually this is done in conjunction with the administration of chlorpromazine. In some instances, it is necessary to use barbiturates without chlorpromazine. In such instances, very large doses of barbiturates need to be administered in order to put the patient to sleep. These may range anywhere from 500 to 1,200 mg Sodium Amytal, given intravenously. Such heroic measures, which carry with them a risk to the patient, can only be justified by the urgent necessity to provide the patient with rest in the face of serious and prolonged hyperactivity which threatens the patient's life.

SUMMARY

In the treatment of affective reactions, one deals with a situation where physical treatments have clear-cut, effective roles. Depressions may reliably be terminated by the use of ECT and antidepressant drugs. Similarly, manic excitements can be brought under control by the use of phenothiazine derivatives or ECT. In all affective reactions, therefore, the physician can readily draw on specific measures which will terminate the symptoms of the illness.

The very availability of specific treatments for these affective symptoms serves only to emphasize how necessary it is to use such specific treatments in accordance with an over-all psychotherapeutic plan. If depression is relieved prematurely by ECT, it may recur. If a patient with a depression associated with a psychoneurotic reaction is not given adequate psychotherapy, he can receive course after course after course of ECT or be continually on antidepressant drugs, with no significant or permanent relief from his basic problem.

On the other hand, the dependence of psychotherapy on the use of somatic treatments is also clearly illustrated in the treatment of affective illnesses. After months of psychotherapy with a patient suffering from a depression resulting from chronic psychoneurotic disability or after years of psychotherapy with a patient in a manic-depressive depression, one may have achieved one's psychotherapeutic goals. The patient's personality will have been explored and new patterns of behavior devised in an absolutely satisfactory fashion—yet the patient will remain depressed. Depressive illnesses have a peculiar tendency to remain intact, even when the psychotherapeutic work has supposedly been done. In this situation, ECT or antidepressant drugs may be used to terminate the depression at the optimal time in the optimal way. By this means, psychotherapy has produced remedial effects which will help the patient for the rest of his life, and physical treatments have helped by terminating the acute episode without any wasted time or motion.

The affective illnesses, therefore, provide a working model of the relationship between physical treatments and psychotherapy. Only by the judicious combination of both can the over-all treatment achieve maximum efficiency.

18

THE TREATMENT OF PARANOID
REACTIONS

The treatment of paranoid reactions follows rather clearly from an understanding of the nature of this illness. When the physician deals with a patient with a paranoid reaction, he is entitled to assume that, beneath the rigidity and the delusions which the patient displays, there exists a large reservoir of emotions, most of which cannot be expressed directly. The therapist's work, therefore, is to help the individual better to recognize these emotions and to obtain satisfaction for them in an acceptable fashion. If this general aim is kept in mind, the course of treatment of a paranoid reaction will follow logically from it.

With these thoughts in mind, the treatment of paranoid reactions may be divided into three phases: Phase 1 involves exploration and the reduction of the delusional material; phase 2 is focused on a study of daily living, in order that the patient can achieve a better recognition of his own feelings; phase 3 is devoted to helping the patient learn better means of dealing with these same feelings. As will be seen, the three phases will overlap to a certain extent. They do, however, involve different techniques and intermediate goals, and it is convenient to consider them as separate entities.

PHASE 1

The first and foremost obligation which the physician undertakes, when he begins the treatment of a patient with a paranoid reaction, is the reduction of the delusional symptomatology which the patient manifests.

This can usually be accomplished rapidly when the patient is removed from the environmental stresses in which the delusions developed. If the illness is mild, such a liberation from stress can be obtained by manipulation of the environment, e.g., by having the patient take several months away from work or by allowing a housewife to take a vacation from household chores. Usually, however, the impracticality of such a move and the severity of the illness contraindicate this type of manipulation. In the great majority of paranoid reactions, it is wiser to have the patient shielded from environmental stresses by placing him in a psychiatric hospital. Within the psychiatric hospital, the patient will find freedom from the external stresses and strains which are causing him to develop a delusional system. Within a matter of 3 to 4 weeks, delusions will frequently have subsided, as the patient becomes integrated into the community life of the hospital.

It is a common misconception that paranoid patients constitute "escape risks" and that they show marked resistance to being hospitalized. The fact of the matter is that resistance and hostility toward hospitalization are functions of the amount of coercion and force which is used to effect hospitalization. The committed patient, particularly the patient who finds himself locked in the psychiatric hospital or placed in seclusion or restraints, will fight hospitalization vigorously and clamor for early release from the hospital. Paradoxically, when the hospitalization is a voluntary one and it is quite clear that the patient will remain only so long as he wishes, the paranoid patient will usually cling to the security of the hospital with might and main. Within the hospital, he finds himself an accepted part of a social group and does not find himself exposed to many of the stresses of everyday life; as long as the hospitalization is noncoercive, he will do everything in his power to stay in this secure setting.

At the same time that symptoms are being reduced by environmental manipulation, the therapist must achieve a clear and detailed understanding of his patient. In a minimum of two to three interviews per week, he must spend large amounts of time in exploring the patient's personal and family history and acquiring an understanding of the origins of the patient's insecurity and anxiety. The paranoid patient is usually quite cooperative in this but tends to use the anamnestic period of history development as a means for blaming his illness and his insecurity, which he recognizes, on other persons, especially family members. The therapist must use the early rapport, which is established as he and the patient seek for the origins of insecurity, in order to help the patient find that it was not only the *other* persons but also *himself* who contributed to the development of patterns which have led to anxiety and insecurity. At the earliest possible moment, the patient should be helped to see how he *and* the environment combined to produce the difficulties which have led to this illness.

During this time of relief of symptoms and exploration of the origin of defensive patterns, a number of physical treatments may provide help in achieving the therapeutic goals.

Electroconvulsive Treatment

Only rarely is ECT an efficient tool in the early stages of treating a patient with a paranoid reaction. It can sometimes be useful in terminating an excitement which may mark the early treatment of the paranoid reaction, however. In such treatment, ECT should be administered on a daily basis, with a total of three to five treatments. Since the phenothiazines are available, such a use of ECT is limited to situations in which there is danger to the life or health of the patient should the excitement continue. The great danger in using ECT early in the treatment of a patient with a paranoid reaction lies in the specious improvement which follows the treatment. The disruptive effect of ECT will temporarily relieve the delusions. All too frequently treatment is terminated, and the patient suffers a recurrence within several months.

Phenothiazines

It is sometimes possible to relieve the symptoms of a paranoid patient by the administration of phenothiazine derivatives, for example, chlorpromazine, while the patient is outside the psychiatric hospital. Treatment can be carried on far more inexpensively, although such an outpatient treatment loses the benefits of the controlled therapeutic environment within the psychiatric hospital. Usually, it is wiser to begin treatment in a hospital, thereby minimizing risks and speeding eventual recovery. In both outpatient and inpatient usage, the chlorpromazine is used to control the hostility which is associated with the paranoid delusions and to facilitate the patient's cooperation in the exploratory stage of psychotherapy. The usual dosage required is between 300 and 500 mg chlorpromazine per day, orally. It should be continued for a period of 2 months or more, until the therapist is quite sure that he has established a strong and understanding relationship with the patient and that his patient sees clearly the need for further and continuing psychotherapy when the drug is terminated.

Reserpine

Occasionally one may see a patient with a paranoid reaction who enters a panic. If such a panic interrupts the early course of the treatment of a paranoid reaction, it may be controlled with the use of reserpine or the related rauwolfia derivatives. Usually, however, the development of a panic may be prevented by close observation of the patient, avoidance of stress and excessively fast exploration, and early psychotherapeutic reassurance. Phenothiazines are usually preferred.

Barbiturates

SEDATION

Barbiturate sedation is contraindicated in the early stages of the treatment of paranoid reactions. The retarding effect which barbiturates have on the cerebral cortex increases the paranoid patient's fears and hostilities, in the same fashion as locks on the doors and other restraining measures. In consequence, the use of such sedation is to be avoided whenever possible.

HYPNOSIS

Barbiturate hypnosis, in order to produce a regular sleep pattern, is frequently a valuable aid in the treatment of a paranoid reaction. Like those with severe schizophrenic reactions, patients with paranoid reactions require large doses of nighttime barbiturates, and the dose required to produce adequate sleep is usually between 300 and 500 mg per night, orally. The shorter-acting barbiturates are preferred, to lessen the likelihood of residual barbiturate effect the next day.

SODIUM AMYTAL INTERVIEWS

Sodium Amytal interviews are usually not useful in the early stages of treating a patient with a paranoid reaction. Until the first month or two of treatment has elapsed, the patient is usually productive in interviews and is actively exploring the background of his illness. During this same period, the threat of the therapist's intervention, through the force of the drug, is also much more likely to produce panic or hostile resistance. It is in the later stages of treatment that Sodium Amytal interviews become more useful.

Meprobamate

If anxiety is as prominent a part of the clinical picture as hostility, it is sometimes possible to use meprobamate, instead of chlorpromazine, to relieve the patient's emotional turmoil. Usually, however, this is possible only if the illness is a mild one. In instances where the anxiety is of intense proportions and causes pronounced disorganization of thinking and loss of concentration, it is far more valuable to utilize insulin or rarely reserpine for control of the anxiety.

Subcoma Insulin Treatment

If the anxiety reaches such proportions that the person's total life pattern becomes disorganized, then it may be valuable to use a course of 30 to 45 subcoma insulin treatments to facilitate organized thinking and psychotherapeutic progress. The same course, shortened to 30 treatments, can also be used to handle panics which interrupt the regular treatment in a paranoid reaction.

PHASE 2

In phase 2 of the treatment of paranoid reactions, the work to be accomplished by the patient and the therapist is an exploration of the feelings, emotions, and attitudes which the patient experiences deep within himself about the events of his daily life. In order to accomplish this end, it is necessary for the patient and the therapist to explore the small events of daily living in extreme detail. They must find out how the patient *actually* feels when he misses his favorite television program, when he receives a compliment or a rebuff, when he succeeds at a difficult task, or when he fails. These events, and the reaction to them, can seem insignificant to the patient, at first; their significance will gradually become clear, however. It must be remembered that the patient with a paranoid reaction is having emotional responses to such "small" events continually and is denying their existence to himself. He is therefore constantly accumulating a store of emotional frustration; with his personality structure, such suppressed emotions can only be expressed by delusions and withdrawal. It is necessary for the patient and the therapist, therefore, to explore instance after instance after instance of such denial and frustration. Finally the patient will become keenly aware of the nature of his actual feelings, without such detailed and guided examinations.

As this current-event exploration takes place, the patient will experience great concern, and frequently considerable guilt, as he recognizes the feelings which he has previously denied to himself. He will feel guilt especially as he comes to recognize feelings of resentment and both heterosexual and homosexual desires. At this point, it is of crucial importance that the therapist be able to take a directive and reassuring role. The physician must be able to interpose himself as an authority and to give the patient definite reassurance that the feelings which he recognizes are not, in themselves, dangerous or "bad." He does this in a common-sense way, indicating that the feelings might be dangerous if they were unbridled or if they led to criminal activities but that their mere existence is far from being bad, and is actually the common experience that the patient shares with other persons. To the paranoid patient, the revelation that other persons have the same feelings is astounding. It is the greatest reassurance that he can have at this stage in therapy and can only come from a secure therapist with whom the patient has a sound relationship.

Naturally, phase 1 of the treatment of a paranoid patient does not end on a certain day and phase 2 begin thereafter. On the contrary, daily events should be examined as soon as possible in the course of the exploratory interviews during phase 1. In general, however, more than 90 per cent of the interview time for the first couple of months of therapy is devoted to past historical material. During this time, references to the present are used only as illustrations of how the patterns which developed in the past still show up at the present time. After several months, the balance between the two poles gradually shifts. When phase 2 has begun, most of the time in interview is spent in understanding current everyday reactions and some time in each interview is spent in reviewing how a particular pattern, a particular denial, or a particular defense originated in the past. Throughout the interviews in both phases of treatment, there is a constant interplay between the past and the present. In phase 1, the emphasis is on the past; in phase 2, the emphasis is on the present.

Usually the third and fourth months in the treatment of a patient with a paranoid reaction are occupied in this exploration of present-day emotional responsiveness. Phenothiazine and meprobamate sedation are not useful in this stage of therapy. Both these forms of sedation have as their basic characteristic the blunting of emotional responses. It is the very aim of therapy during this phase in the treatment of a paranoid reaction that the patient become more keenly aware of his emotional responses. Therefore, if progress is to be made toward the intermediate goal of phase 2 of treatment, chlorpromazine, meprobamate, and other sedative drugs are to be avoided. There are, however, some somatic treatments which are useful in this phase of treatment.

Barbiturates

HYPNOSIS

The paranoid patient should not be on regular nightly medication by the time he is reaching the end of phase 2 of treatment. Occasionally, however, the emotional turmoil which is associated with recognition of feelings during phase 2 can produce marked anxiety and insomnia which interfere with the patient's progress. Moreover, the insomnia sometimes aggravates the heterosexual or homosexual fears which the patient experiences. Therefore, it is thoroughly legitimate to use a regular dose of nighttime sedation with barbiturates during the early stages of phase 2.

The dose required will be between 200 and 400 mg, orally; intermediate- and short-acting barbiturates are preferred.

SODIUM AMYTAL INTERVIEWS

At this stage in the treatment of paranoid reactions, Sodium Amytal interviews may be of invaluable aid. Patients with this illness usually have great difficulty in recognizing feelings and emotions, and a series of three to six Sodium Amytal interviews, given over a period of 2 weeks, can help them to see the many different emotions, feelings, and opinions they experience in dealing with daily life. Once the block has been removed through Sodium Amytal interviews, the patient can usually continue to see new aspects of his responsiveness without the aid of the interviews. Very frequently, all progress will stop if such aid is not provided.

PHASE 3

Once again, it is not possible to draw a distinct line between phase 2 and phase 3 in the treatment of paranoid reactions, since the activities of the two phases must merge to some extent. In general, however, phase 3 occupies the fifth and sixth months in the treatment of a patient with a paranoid reaction. It consists in the patient's using his previously acquired understanding of his personality formation and his recognition of the actual feelings which he has in daily situations to develop new methods for dealing with himself and his environment. It is, therefore, a phase of exploring new techniques and of learning how to obtain better satisfaction from the world. In order to achieve the goal of this phase in the treatment of a paranoid reaction, it is necessary for the environment to provide a wide scope of activities for the patient to engage in. Most frequently, the psychiatric hospital cannot provide a sufficiently wide scope in itself. It is usual, therefore, that hospitalized patients visit out of the hospital to participate in work or home life. These visits are scattered at first but gradually occur at daily intervals. In this transitional way, the hospitalized patient finds an adequate scope of living in which to do his psychotherapeutic work. With patients who have been treated outside of the psychiatric hospital, phase 3 is the time during which they should gradually be resuming their full-time activity program.

A word of caution must be entered at this point. As the scope of the patient's activities is increased, the physician must remember that the patient is expected to experiment with new techniques of dealing with the environment. It would be an extremely unusual patient, or an extremely unusual human being, who could even experiment with new modes of behavior without sometimes making a mistake. It is wise, therefore, that the patient's experiments be guided and that he be protected from making serious mistakes in dealing with critical aspects of his environment during this phase of his treatment. This can be done both inside and outside a hospital, but obviously the possibility of protecting the patient is somewhat easier when he is using a hospital as a base of operation.

In learning the new techniques of dealing with the environment, it is of crucial importance that the patient do this as independently as possible. Therefore, it is unwise to use physical treatments during phase 3 in the treatment of paranoid reactions, with one exception.

Electroconvulsive Treatment

Occasionally, one sees the patient with a paranoid reaction associated with marked elements of depression. These elements of depression do not usually hinder therapy during the first or second phase but will markedly diminish the patient's willingness to accept, and capability for, exploration of new methods of dealing with the environment. Therefore, it is sometimes wise to use four to eight ECTs, administered at intervals of two times per week, in order to clear up depression in the early days of phase 3. It must be noted that this ECT must be administered at a time when the patient is ready to move ahead in trying out new methods for dealing with the world.

SUMMARY

In the treatment of a patient with a paranoid reaction, the organization of a treatment program usually covers a period of 6 months. During phase 1 of the treatment, in the first 2 months, the patient's symptoms are relieved, and dynamic historical material is explored. During this phase, somatic treatments can be utilized in order to speed the disappearance of symptoms. The phenothiazine compounds, especially, can help to relieve the hostility of the paranoid patient. They may also be used to control intervening excitements and panics.

During phase 2 of treatment, in the third and fourth months, the emphasis should be on the exploration of the patient's emotional responses to daily living. It is of crucial importance that this work be achieved in as independent a fashion as possible; therefore somatic treatments are not of much use, with several notable exceptions. The first is the use of barbiturates to produce sleep during stormy periods of treatment, and the second is the Sodium Amytal interview, which may overcome the inherent difficulties which the patient faces in recognizing his own feelings.

During phase 3 of treatment, in the fifth and sixth months, the patient needs to learn new methods for dealing with his newly discovered feelings, emotions, and opinions. During this phase, somatic treatments should be held to a minimum. It is occasionally necessary, however, to overcome a residual depression by the use of a brief course of electroconvulsive treatment, in order that this phase of treatment may be carried on actively.

Following the plan which has been outlined, good success can be expected in the treatment of patients with paranoid reactions. The over-all psychotherapeutic program can be greatly aided, at each step, by the appropriate use of proper somatic treatment.

19

THE TREATMENT OF PERSONALITY DISORDERS

It is unusual for somatic treatment to be important in the therapy of the patients with personality disorders (psychopathic personalities). This is understandable, because personality disorders are illnesses which involve the total personality structure of the individual. Unlike the psychoneurotic, schizophrenic, and affective reactions, these illnesses do not manifest themselves primarily through internal discomfort and symptoms. On the contrary, their basic manifestations is a behavioral one which is not usually amenable to biological treatment. There are, however, a few exceptions to this, and these will be detailed in later paragraphs.

At our present stage of psychotherapeutic knowledge, the treatment of personality disorders must follow one of two lines. The first and classical line is one which accepts the disability of the patient with a personality disorder as a relatively unchangeable feature of his life and attempts merely to control the disability. This approach concentrates on the fact that the primary manifestations of the personality disorder consist of the patient's need for immediate gratification and failure to profit from experience, while the patient views his actions as egosyntonic. The entire course of therapy is guided by a recognition of these characteristics and pursues a course which is intended to control them. This is a psychotherapeutic method which may be followed by almost any physician, but it is a frequently discouraging method and requires great patience.

In detail, this classical method for the psychotherapeutic treatment of patients with personality disorders involves the establishment of a regular relationship with the patient, in which he is seen at least weekly, in order to discuss the pattern of his activities. So far as possible, interviews attempt to elucidate the background of the patient and the dynamic factors which have contributed to his personality development. The work of therapy, however, is concentrated on the discussion of the immediate present. In these discussions, great emphasis is placed, repeatedly, upon the results which come about when the patient fails to utilize rational thinking in satisfying his immediate needs. Again and again, in discussion of minute details of behavior, the consequences of immediate gratification of needs are made clear to the patient. The loss of prestige, money, personal relationships, and security, which results from the patient's use of alcohol or from other behavioral manifestations, is repeatedly emphasized to the patient. In effect, the therapist is pursuing a consistent rational course, emphasizing the greater gains which the patient will achieve by controlling his impulses. He holds these gains out as a stimulus to the patient, at the same time emphasizing the suffering which the patient undergoes by succumbing to his need for immediate gratification. When the therapist assumes this role, it is obvious that he is attempting to fulfill the stabilizing and organizing influence which was not present in the patient's childhood. His success, therefore, depends on the success with which he can achieve a satisfactory relationship with the patient. If his relationship becomes a punitive or threatening one, the patient will desert therapy. If he maintains an excessively permissive or evasive attitude, the patient will not adhere to any of the injunctions of the therapist. The therapist must achieve an intermediate role, therefore, in which he is an admired and respected teacher, a parent surrogate on whom the patient can lean when it is necessary for him to undergo the hardship of delayed gratification.

As has been indicated, this course of treatment is an arduous and frequently disappointing one. Only if the patient's personality disorder is a mild one can the therapist expect to achieve success by this means. Any success is a result of his own patience, restraint, and adroitness in avoiding the twin dangers of overindulgence and overpunitiveness. While success is not frequent with this method, it can achieve some modification of the headlong course which is followed by the patient with a personality disorder and thereby minimize the disastrous consequences of the patient's behavior on himself, his family, and his associates. Such therapy must include close cooperation between the physician and the patient's relatives and associates in order that they may make positive contributions to treatment and be in a position of security in dealing with the dangers which the patient's manipulativeness may create.

In this guiding and didactic type of psychotherapy, some somatic treatments may be of occasional use in fostering the psychotherapeutic efforts.

Disulfiram

In the treatment of certain patients with alcoholism who demonstrate passive and dependent personalities, the use of disulfiram can frequently prove helpful. These patients, by virtue of their personality structure, need outward signs of dependency on the therapist and also need a continuing bond with the therapist. Both of these are provided by the continuing administration of disulfiram. At the same time, the medication provides a strong and constant prohibition of the alcohol and a constant symbol of the therapist's interest and concern. The use of disulfiram in patients who do not have passive and dependent personalities is less impressive. Those with personality disorders associated with rebelliousness against authority will simply discard the use of disulfiram in anticipation of drinking, and psychoneurotic persons will similarly avoid the conflict.

Anticonvulsants

In those personality disorders which are associated with electroencephalographic abnormalities, it is sometimes possible to control the impulsiveness and unpredictable behavior by attempts to regulate central nervous activity through the medium of anticonvulsants. Such a utilization of these drugs depends on clear-cut indications of impulsiveness in the behavioral patterns of the individual and on verification by equally clear-cut electroencephalographic findings.

The second course of psychotherapy available to the physician who is treating the patient with personality disorders is one which aims at the analysis and reconstruction of the entire personality structure. In this therapy, it is necessary to analyze the origins of the personality in detail, with intensive exploratory psychotherapy. This requires a minimum of two interviews a week, the more usual number being four or five; therapy may continue for a number of years. In the course of therapy, the therapist adheres as closely as possible to the classical, nonintervening, nonjudgmental, analytic role. He will attempt to analyze the origins of the patterns and feelings which the patient has and the significance of the needs which the patient attempts to gratify. Such a therapeutic course depends, naturally, on the motivation of the patient, as well as on his intelligence and environmental situation. Experience with this form of therapy is limited, and it must currently be regarded as an experimental approach. One needs extensive experience and training before one is prepared to enter into this type of psychotherapy with patients with personality disorders. If successful, the results can be outstandingly good, but the difficulties are prominent. Somatic treatment has little place or value in this psychotherapeutic regimen.

20

THE TREATMENT OF ORGANIC
REACTIONS

The crucial factor in the treatment of patients with organic reactions is the physician's recognition that the organic lesion exists in a total personality setting. The organic lesion is an added factor which is superimposed on the basic personality of the patient and upon any other psychiatric illness which the patient has. Arteriosclerotic cardiovascular disease may be found in rigid persons with an obsessive-compulsive psychoneurosis, brain tumors may be found in schizophrenic persons, and delirium tremens may be found in a patient with a severe personality disorder. If the fact that the organic illness co-exists with a personality structure and with other possible psychiatric symptoms is kept in mind, then it is clear that the therapist must divide his attention. He must consider both the treatment of the organic lesion itself and the proper psychotherapeutic handling of the associated personality and symptom structure. Naturally, the physician must concentrate the maximal curative efforts on the organic lesion. He must guide the patient into such efforts, however, in the light of the patient's psychologic status. His instructions, medications, and rehabilitation programs will be radically different for two patients with a similar brain tumor, one of whom has a rigid personality structure and one of whom has a poorly organized personality structure.

If it is kept in mind that the personal variation of the patient will control the details of how the therapeutic program is executed and that this personalization of the therapy is the keynote in directing a program to treat a person with an organic reaction, it is possible to describe several general measures which may be taken in such reactions. Within the framework of this book, it has been necessary to limit examples to three

275

major fields, which are found frequently in the practice of most physicians. These fields are the delirious reactions, the reactions of aging, and the problems which follow brain tumors and injuries.

DELIRIOUS REACTIONS

On the following pages delirious reactions will be considered from a general point of view. Such reactions may occur as a result of a number of disordered metabolic states. Delirious reactions may be found following the administration of excessive quantities of barbiturates, bromides, or other agents which inhibit central nervous system activity. They may also follow the excessive ingestion of stimulants; they may be the result of vitamin deficiency, diminished oxygen supply to the brain, and some hormone imbalances. A delirium is a frequent occurrence in the immediate postoperative period, as well as in states of serious infection, both within and without the central nervous system. In all these conditions, the fundamental pathology is the same: because of the addition of toxic substances or the absence of necessary nutrition, the metabolism of the central nervous system has been impaired. With this impaired cellular function, the patient is less able to think and to understand in a rational and coherent fashion. The groundwork is laid for a delirious reaction.

Once this metabolic groundwork has been established, the pattern of a delirious reaction is a relatively standard one. It may be considered in three separate stages. During the first, or introductory, stage of a delirious reaction, the patient shows mild impairment and retardation in thinking. He manifests anxiety through repetitious questions and pleas for reassurance. He shows some restlessness and mild insomnia. Pulse and respiration are usually slightly increased. This stage of a delirious reaction is not, obviously, one of great severity. It is frequently seen in patients postoperatively and is usually handled excellently by the psychotherapeutic measures employed by most physicians. These measures include the administration of reassurance in a simple, understanding, attentive fashion and minimizing confusing elements in the patient's treatment by limitation of visitors, noise, and confusion.

Stage 2 of a delirious reaction is marked by an exaggeration of stage 1. The patient's difficulty in comprehension is noticeable. Frequently he distorts his perceptions of the environment by illusions: shadows become strangers in his room; meaningless noises become words and conversation. There are temporary losses of orientation, and anxiety now reaches the point of obvious fear. The patient's requests for reassurance and explanation are almost incessant, and he shows very marked motor restlessness. Sleep diminishes to 1 to 2 hours during a 24-hour period, and pulse and respirations are increased markedly. Altogether too frequently psychotherapeutic efforts at this stage of the delirious reaction are ineffective. If a delirium has reached this point, it is necessary to use strong environmental and individual measures. The patient should be placed in a single room, with continual lighting throughout the day and night. Sharp objects and suicidal opportunities should be removed, lest the patient injure himself in a sudden panic. All nursing care should be given by a selected team of nurses, and only one physician should visit the patient, making sure that all explanations and reassurances are given in consistent and very simple fashion. Outside visitors should be limited to the immediate family, and all conversation should be kept simple and reassuring.

Stage 3 in the delirious reaction is the culminating stage. At this point, the patient's fear and impaired understanding have caused him to lose contact with reality. Fear has mounted to the point of panic, and the patient is disoriented, with fearsome delusions and hallucinations, e.g., a railroad train running across the end of his bed, bats flying around the room, and animals crawling over his skin. The patient does not understand what is going on, does not know where he is, does not recognize the persons who surround him, and does not know what is going to be done to him. In this extreme state of fear, he may succeed in killing himself in desperate attempts to avoid threatening situations. At this point in the delirious reaction, the psychotherapeutic program should be similar to that which is carried on in stage 2, and the patient should have constant companionship of kind, understanding persons.

In the over-all treatment of delirious reactions, the major somatic treatments which have proved useful are sedatives, hypnotics, and hormones.

Phenothiazines

With their rapid effectiveness and the control which they exert over activity, phenothiazine derivatives such as chlorpromazine have proved very valuable in treating the third stage of delirious reactions. Within a matter of hours, the administration of repeated doses of 25 mg chlorpromazine intramuscularly can bring profoundly excited, delirious patients under control. This is especially true in the case of delirium tremens. The use of chlorpromazine is contraindicated in the presence of delirious reactions which are associated with seriously disordered metabolism of liver or kidneys.

Barbiturates

SEDATION

It is a frequent occurrence for the psychiatric consultant to find that a patient in a delirious reaction has been receiving barbiturate sedation.

Clearly, the delirious reaction is based on a functional deficiency of the cerebral cortex. In such a situation, the addition of barbiturate sedation can only be expected to increase the intellectual impairment of the patient, thereby making the likelihood of an increase in the delirious reaction greater. It is true that in some instances the barbiturate sedation will sufficiently relieve anxiety and that this good effect will counteract the harmful increased impairment of thinking. On the whole, however, the dangers of administering barbiturates for sedation to anybody with impaired cerebral functioning far outweigh the chance of benefit, and barbiturate sedation should clearly be contraindicated in any such condition.

HYPNOSIS

On the other hand, the use of barbiturates to put the delirious patient to sleep is *not* contraindicated. In this respect, the use of barbiturates in delirium follows an all-or-nothing rule. Either none should be given, or enough should be given so that the patient is placed into deep sleep. In stage 1 of the delirious reaction, 300 to 500 mg barbiturates, taken orally, will allow the patient 6 or 7 hours of sleep; on awakening, his anxiety will be diminished, and he will be less likely to proceed further into the delirium. In stage 2, a similar response is found. In stage 3, it is frequently advisable to use 300 to 700 mg Sodium Amytal intravenously to produce deep sleep. On awakening, the patient may have only 15 to 30 minutes of clear thinking before the delirium gradually develops again. In such a situation, if 6 hours have elapsed since the previous dose, it is possible once again to administer intravenous Sodium Amytal and several hours of sleep will follow. After three to four repetitions of these measures, the period of lucidity that follows sleep will have been increased to the point of several hours, and the treatment of the delirium can resume the pattern which may be followed in stages 1 and 2.

Analgesics

It is worthy of note, at this time, that the analgesics have a definite role to play in the treatment of delirious reactions. Frequently, the physician, aware of the danger of barbiturates and other sedatives, leans over backward and also eliminates analgesics from his treatment program. In doing so, he may subject the patient with impaired ability to think to additional stress, in the form of pain. This pain may be due to postoperative or traumatic conditions or to disturbing painful influences of toxic illness. In any event, the additional stress may only serve to increase the likelihood of serious delirious developments. Therefore, it is wise to use any analgesics which are legitimately necessary for the relief of pain during the course of the delirium. Such analgesics as morphine and Demerol have a slight sedative effect; the benefits of the analgesic effect are usually far greater than the detrimental effects of the sedation.

Anticonvulsants

In delirium tremens, which follows the withdrawal of alcohol after a prolonged period of heavy drinking, there is frequently a danger of repeated convulsions. These may lead to status epilepticus, with great risk to the patient's life. It is therefore imperative that the patient be given adequate anticonvulsive therapy. A minimum dosage of 400 mg Dilantin per day is indicated in most deliriums which follow the withdrawal of alcohol.

Hormone Therapy

In the treatment of delirious reactions which are the result of metabolic imbalances, the use of cortisone, thyroid, or adrenal hormones is sometimes indicated. In the case of delirium tremens, both adrenal cortical extract and cortisone have proved helpful in modifying delirious symptoms. The use of these hormones is complicated, however, and the utilization of chlorpromazine and other measures is probably simpler and just as effective.

REACTIONS OF AGING

The major reactions of aging are those associated with senile degenerative changes in the brain and arteriosclerotic cardiovascular disease. The former presents a pathologic picture of interstitial fibrosis, with a gradually developing, evenly progressive course which is not associated with neurologic impairment. Arteriosclerotic changes, on the other hand, are associated with a progressive but intermittent course, associated with sudden increases in thinking disability and with demonstrable neurologic impairment; these progressive changes occur as cerebral vessels are occluded by spasm, thrombosis, or hemorrhage. In brief, the course of senility is a smoothly progressive one, with mainly central symptoms; the course of arteriosclerosis is an unevenly progressive one, with both central and peripheral symptoms. It is rare, however, that one sees senility without arteriosclerosis, or vice versa. Almost invariably, the condition is a mixed one, and the differentiation is not important clinically, except for the prophylactic measures which may be taken to combat the extension of arteriosclerosis.

The typical behavioral pattern of these illnesses begins in the early or middle sixties. A previously well individual shows gradually failing intellectual function, first manifest in recent memory, as he becomes unsure of immediate past events, commitments, and appointments. As cerebral damage increases, immediate and recent memory impairment becomes profound and the patient gradually loses his orientation to time, place, and person. With further impairment, the patient's contact with his environment decreases, and he gradually withdraws into a confused and helpless state. Partly as a result of the lack of orientation and contact with surrounding reality and partly as a result of neurologic impairment, the patient becomes unable to care for himself. Initially, this is manifest only in terms of outgoing activities, but gradually the disability increases and involves personal care, hygiene, eating, and sleeping. Eventually, the patient is reduced to an invalid status, requiring constant nursing attention.

The psychotherapeutic management of the problems of aging requires a recognition of the unalterable physical changes which have taken place. The elderly person has the impairment of comprehension and orientation which has been indicated, and the psychotherapeutic problem of the physician is to mobilize other assets within the individual and within the environmental situation to combat the unchangeable disability. The environmental measures which may be taken are relatively clear. It is necessary for the elderly person to live in a simple, well-organized environment. Within such an environmental setting, there should be a sufficient amount of activity which satisfies his personal needs; the activity should include social contact, work, and recreation. All these should be scaled to the physical and intellectual capacity of the individual. In addition, the personality and background of the individual must be considered. A nursing home may be an ideal for one individual but absolutely contraindicated for another. Great care must be taken to individualize the environmental arrangements.

Coupled with this environmental manipulation, the therapist and the patient should evaluate carefully and realistically the patient's disability. Frequently physicians attempt to reassure elderly patients about their disabilities, minimizing the real drawbacks which the patient is experiencing. In doing so, they sometimes urge the patient to disregard crippling difficulties; such a disregard can only result in increased confusion, discomfort, and withdrawal. Overoptimism and unrealistic encouragement are contraindicated. On the contrary, the physician should help the patient to recognize and discuss the intellectual impairment which he is facing. With such recognition and discussion, it becomes much easier for the patient to take compensatory measures, e.g., writing appointments and events down in a notebook, simplifying work schedules, and not undertaking jobs which require imagination and active recent memory but pursuing employment which depends more on past memory, experience, and prestige. With a realistic view of himself, the elderly person is frequently able to function at far higher levels than he can achieve when he pretends that he has *not* lost some of his faculties. The amputee who tries to pretend that he has not lost a leg will repeatedly fall on his face; the amputee who recognizes his difficulties can control them.

At the same time that these environmental and personal psychotherapeutic measures are undertaken, the physician needs to consider certain psychopathologic and emotional features which are very common during this age period. Anxiety and depression are the most prominent characteristic emotions to appear, as the elderly person faces his disability and the constriction of his life. These emotions are apt to occur whether the patient grapples with his problems overtly or attempts to avoid them by denial; in either event, he experiences considerable fear and depression. Characteristically, the emotions will heap more coals on the fire; they will increase the patient's retardation and concentration difficulty, thereby greatly exaggerating the intellectual deficits which his organic situation imposes on him. The manifestations of these emotions are frequently tremulousness, insomnia, tearfulness, early morning awakening, diurnal variation, and fleeting suicidal ideation. When the alert physician recognizes these features, he can deal with them psychotherapeutically, using the measures that have been described for the treatment of affective reactions and psychoneurotic reactions. Even if they have not reached the proportions of the major diagnostic entities, they are frequently present as sidelights to the otherwise straightforward organic picture and need specific treatment.

In the treatment of the disorders of aging, most of the somatic treatment which is available is concentrated on the emotional difficulties which accompany the major organic deficit.

Hypnotic Medication

Producing sleep by means of barbiturates is sometimes acceptable in older persons. Frequently, however, barbiturates appear to have a prolonged impairing effect on the elderly person's thinking, thereby exaggerating the organic defects. The use of 1 to 2 Gm of chloral hydrate, administered at bedtime, is a preferable method of producing sleep. By the production of such adequate sleep, there will frequently be a marked diminution of anxiety, and the patient's alertness during his waking hours will be increased.

Phenothiazines

Phenothiazine derivatives, for example, chlorpromazine, in a daily dosage ranging from 200 to 400 mg orally, can frequently aid in controlling agitation and resentment in older persons. At this age level, the incidence of parkinsonlike side effects is high, and the use of anti-Parkinson drugs is usually recommended.

Meprobamate Sedation

For elderly persons whose functions are impaired by anxiety, meprobamate sedation is often useful. The daily oral dosage seldom need exceed 1,600 mg. The sedative effect can be achieved, furthermore, without the impairment of intellectual functioning which is so commonly a side effect of barbiturate sedation in the elderly.

Antidepressive Drugs

Because of the frequent presence of borderline depression associated with the organic changes, the use of antidepressive drugs is frequently valuable in the treatment of organic reactions in elderly persons. Metrazol has also been used, in small intravenous doses, as an alerting device at this time of life.

REACTIONS FOLLOWING BRAIN TUMORS AND BRAIN INJURIES

In the treatment of patients who have organic disease which follows the removal of brain tumors or have sustained injuries or accidents, the same principles of psychotherapy hold that were described in the treatment of aging patients. In this instance, once again, it is necessary to help the patient recognize the deficit which he has. Whether this deficit be an aphasia, a memory difficulty, a visual loss, or an emotional impairment, it is necessary for the patient to spend the first period of therapy in a painstaking, patient, and systematic analysis of the exact nature of his impairment. When the impairment has been clarified for the patient in his own terms and at his own level of understanding, it is then possible for the physician and patient to make further plans for the adjustment of the patient's life. At the same time, the physician can help the patient to adjust to this difficulty and ease the emotional blow which impairment presents. Just as in the problems of aging, the use of medications and treatments in this condition may be guided by the need to relieve anxiety and depression which the patient experiences as a result of his impairments. The use of chloral hydrate to produce sleep, the use of stimulants to relieve depression, and the use of anticonvulsants to relieve impulsiveness and seizure episodes may all be indicated, at different times, in the treatment of reactions which follow brain injury. Similarly, phenothiazines and meprobamate may be used to control excessively strong emotions and to lessen excitement and overactivity.

I

Drug names	Trade names
alseroxylon	Rauwiloid
amobarbital	Amytal
amphetamine	Benzedrine, Amphetamine, Raphetamine
azacyclonol	Frenquel
barbital	Veronal
benactyzine	Suavitil, Phobex
benztropine methanesulfonate	Cogentin
β-phenylisopropylhydrazine	Catron
butabarbital	Butisol, Butabarbital
chlorpromazine	Thorazine, Largactil
deanol	Deaner
deserpidine	Harmonyl
dextro amphetamine	Dexedrine, Dextro Amphetamine, d-Amfetasul
diphenhydramine	Benadryl
diphenylhydantoin sodium	Dilantin, Diphenylhydantoin
disulfiram	Antabuse
heptabarbital	Medomin
hexobarbital	Evipal
hydroxyzine	Atarax
imipramine	Tofranil
iproniazid	Marsilid
isocarboxazid	Marplan
mepazine	Pacatal
mephobarbital	Mebara
meprobamate	Equanil, Miltown, Meprospan
methabital	Gemonil
methaminodiazepoxide	Librium
methamphetamine	Methedrine, Desoxyephedrine, Desoxyn
methantoin	Mesantoin
methitural	Neraval
methoxypromazine	Tentone
methylphenidate	Ritalin
nialamide	Niamid
paramethadione	Paradione
pentobarbital	Nembutal
perphenazine	Trilafon
phenacemide	Phenurone

Drug names	Trade names
phenelzine	Nardil
phenobarbital	Luminal
phensuximide	Milontin
primidone	Mysoline
prochlorperazine	Compazine
promazine	Sparine
promethazine	Phenergan
propantheline bromide	Pro-Banthine Bromide
rescinnamine	Moderil
reserpine	Rauloydin, Raurine, Rau-Sed, Reserpine, Reserpoid, Sandril, Serfin, Serpasil, Serpate
secobarbital	Secobarbital, Seconal, Evronal
thiamylal	Surital
thiopental	Pentothal
thiopropazate	Dartal
thioridazine	Mellaril
trifluoperazine	Stelazine
triflupromazine	Vesprin
trihexyphenidyl	Artane
trimethadione	Tridione
vinbarbital	Delvinal

GLOSSARY OF DRUGS

II

Trade names	Drug names
Amphetamine	amphetamine
Amytal	amobarbital
Antabuse	disulfiram
Artane	trihexyphenidyl
Atarax	hydroxyzine
Benadryl	diphenhydramine
Benzedrine	amphetamine
Butabarbital	butabarbital
Butisol	butabarbital
Catron	β-phenylisopropylhydrazine
Cogentin	benztropine methanesulfonate
Compazine	prochlorperazine
d-Amfetasul	dextro amphetamine
Dartal	thiopropazate
Deaner	deanol
Delvinal	vinbarbital
Desoxyephedrine	methamphetamine

Trade names	*Drug names*
Desoxyn	methamphetamine
Dexedrine	dextro amphetamine
Dextro Amphetamine	dextro amphetamine
Dilantin	diphenylhydantoin
Diphenylhydantoin	diphenylhydantoin
Equanil	meprobamate
Evipal	hexobarbital
Evronal	secobarbital
Frenquel	azacyclonol
Gemonil	methabital
Harmonyl	deserpidine
Largactil	chlorpromazine
Librium	methaminodiazepoxide
Luminal	phenobarbital
Marplan	isocarboxazid
Marsilid	iproniazid
Mebaral	mephobarbital
Medomin	heptabarbital
Mellaril	thioridazine
Meprospan	meprobamate
Mesantoin	methantoin
Methedrine	methamphetamine
Milontin	phensuximide
Miltown	meprobamate
Moderil	rescinnamine
Mysoline	primidone
Nardil	phenelzine
Nembutal	pentobarbital
Neraval	methitural
Niamid	nialamide
Pacatal	mepazine
Paradione	paramethadione
Pentothal	thiopental
Phenergan	promethazine
Phenurone	phenacemide
Phobex	benactyzine
Pro-Banthine Bromide	propantheline bromide
Raphetamine	amphetamine
Rauloydin	reserpine
Raurine	reserpine
Rau-Sed	reserpine
Rauwiloid	alseroxylon
Reserpine	reserpine
Reserpoid	reserpine
Ritalin	methylphenidate
Sandril	reserpine

Trade names	*Drug names*
Secobarbital	secobarbital
Seconal	secobarbital
Serfin	reserpine
Serpasil	reserpine
Serpate	reserpine
Sparine	promazine
Stelazine	trifluoperazine
Suavitil	benactyzine
Surital	thiamylal
Tentone	methoxypromazine
Thorazine	chlorpromazine
Tofranil	imipramine
Tridione	trimethadione
Trilafon	perphenazine
Veronal	barbital
Vesprin	triflupromazine

BIBLIOGRAPHY

This bibliography is not meant to be comprehensive. It represents those important books and articles which seem pertinent to the text and which may be of interest to the reader.

General

PARTS ONE AND THREE

Basowitz, H.; Persky, H.; Korchin, S. J., and Grinker, R. R.: Anxiety and Stress, McGraw-Hill Book Company, Inc., Blakiston Division, New York, 1955.

Bowlby, J.: Maternal Care and Mental Health, World Health Organization, Geneva, 1952.

Cohen, M. B.; Baker, G.; Cohen, R. A.; Fromm-Reichmann, F., and Weigert, E. V.: An Intensive Study of Twelve Cases of Manic-Depressive Psychosis, Psychiatry 17:103, 1954.

Cole, J. O., and Gerard, R. W.: Psychopharmacology, in Proceedings of the National Academy of Science–National Research Council, Washington, 1959.

Diethelm, O.: Treatment in Psychiatry, 3d ed., Charles C Thomas, Publisher, Springfield, Ill., 1955.

Drill, V. A.: Pharmacology in Medicine—A Collaborative Textbook, McGraw-Hill Book Company, Inc., New York, 1958.

Flach, F. F.; Celian, C. I.; Stokes, P. E., and Rawson, R. W.: The Influence of Thyroid Hormones on Metabolism in Psychiatric Disorders, J. Clin. Endocrinol. 19:454, 1959.

Flach, F. F.; Liang, E., and Stokes, P. E.: The Effects of Electric Convulsive Treatments on Nitrogen, Calcium, and Phosphorus Metabolism in Psychiatric Patients, J. Ment. Sc. 106, 1960.

Freud, S.: Standard Edition of the Complete Psychological Works of Sigmund Freud (J. Strachey, Ed.), Hogarth Press, Ltd., London, 1958.

Fromm-Reichmann, F.: Principles of Intensive Psychotherapy, University of Chicago Press, Chicago, 1950.

Goodman, L. S., and Gilman, A.: The Pharmacological Basis of Therapeutics, 2d ed., The Macmillan Company, New York, 1955.

Hill, L. B.: Psychotherapeutic Intervention in Schizophrenia, University of Chicago Press, Chicago, 1955.

Hoch, P.: Drugs and Psychotherapy, Am. J. Psychiat. 116:305, 1959.

Hoch, P., and Polatin, P.: Pseudoneurotic Forms of Schizophrenia, Psychiat. Quart. 23:248, 1949.

Hollingshead, A. B., and Redlich, F. C.: Social Class and Mental Illness: A Community Study, John Wiley & Sons, Inc., New York, 1958.

Horney, K.: Neurosis and Human Growth, W. W. Norton & Company, Inc., New York, 1950.

Horwitz, W. A.; Polatin, P.; Kolb, L. C., and Hoch, P. H.: A Study of Cases of Schizophrenia Treated by "Direct Analysis," Am. J. Psychiat. 114:780, 1958.

Jasper, H. H.; Proctor, L. D.; Knighton, R. S.; Noshay, W. C., and Castello R. D. (Eds.): Reticular Formation of the Brain, Little, Brown & Company, Boston, 1958.

Kalinowsky, L. B.: Appraisal of the "Tranquilizers" and Their Influence on Other Somatic Treatments in Psychiatry, Am. J. Psychiat. 115:294, 1958.

Kalinowsky, L. B., and Hoch, P.: Shock Treatments, Psychosurgery and Other Somatic Treatments in Psychiatry, 2d ed., Grune & Stratton, Inc., New York, 1952.

Kohl, R. N., and Flach, F. F.: Intensive Dynamic Psychotherapy of Depressions, A. M. A. Arch. Neurol. & Psychiat. 72:383, 1954.

Leighton, A. H.; Clausen, J. A., and Wilson, R. N.: Explorations in Social Psychiatry, Basic Books, Inc., New York, 1957.

McIlwain, H.: Chemotherapy and the Central Nervous System, Little, Brown & Company, Boston, 1957.

New and Nonofficial Drugs, A. M. A. Council on Drugs, J. B. Lippincott Company, Philadelphia, 1959.

Opler, M. K., and Singer, J. L.: Ethnic Differences in Behavior and Psychopathology: Italian and Irish, Internat. J. Soc. Psychiat. 2:11, 1956.

Rennie, T. A. C.; Srole, L.; Opler, M. K., and Langner, T. S.: Urban Life and Mental Health, Am. J. Psychiat. 113:831, 1957.

Ripley, H. S., and Wolf, S.: Long-term Study of Combat Area Schizophrenic Reactions, Am. J. Psychiat. 108:409, 1951.

Rosen, J.: The Treatment of Schizophrenic Psychosis by Direct Analytic Therapy, Psychiat. Quart. 21:117, 1947.

Rosenthal, D.: Some Factors Associated with Concordance and Discordance with Respect to Schizophrenia in Monozygotic Twins, J. Nerv. & Ment. Dis. 129:1, 1959.

Sargent, W., and Slater, E.: An Introduction to Physical Methods of Treatment in Psychiatry, The Williams & Wilkins Company, Baltimore, 1948.

Sullivan, H. S.: The Interpersonal Theory of Psychiatry, W. W. Norton & Company, Inc., New York, 1953.

Whitehorn, J. C.: Understanding Psychotherapy, Am. J. Psychiat. 112:328, 1955.

Somatic Therapies

PART TWO

The Phenothiazines

Ayd, F. J., Jr.: A Clinical Appraisal of Trilafon, Am. J. Psychiat. 114:554, 1957.

Ayd, F. J., Jr.: Fatal Agranulocytosis Due to Triflupromazine Hydrochloride, Am. J. Psychiat. 114:940, 1958.

Azima, H.: Vesprin and Mopazine: Two New Phenotropic Substances, Am. J. Psychiat. 114:747, 1958.

Azima, H.: Sleep Treatment in Mental Disorders—Results of Four Years Trial, Dis. Nerv. System 19:523, 1958.

Azima, H.; Durost, H., and Arthurs, D.: The Effect of Thioridazine (Mellaril) on Mental Syndromes, Canad. M. A. J. 81:549, 1959.

Barsa, J. A.; Saunders, J. C., and Kline, N. S.: Trifluoperazine in the Treatment of Chronic Schizophrenics, Am. J. Psychiat. 115:812, 1959.

Berg, S.; Gabriel, A. R., and Impastato, D. J.: Comparative Evaluation of the Safety of Chlorpromazine and Reserpine Used in Conjunction with ECT, J. Neuropsychiat. 1:104, 1959.

Bonafede, V.: Chlorpromazine Treatment of Disturbed Epileptic Patients, A. M. A. Arch. Neurol. & Psychiat. 77:243, 1957.

Cahn, C. H., and Lehmann, H. E.: Perphenazine—Observations on the Clinical Effects of a New Tranquilizing Agent in Psychotic Conditions, Canad. Psychiat. A. J. 2:104, 1957.

Cohen, S.: TP-21, A New Phenothiazine, Am. J. Psychiat. 115:358, 1958.

Delay, J.; Deniker, P., and Harl, J. M.: Utilisation en thérapeutique psychiatrique d'une phenothiazine d'action centrale elective (4560 R. P.), Ann. méd.-psychologiques 2:112, 1952.

Delay, J.; Deniker, P., and Harl, J. M.: Traitement des états d'excitation et d'agitation par une méthode médicamenteuse dérivée de l'hibernothérapie, Ann. méd.-psychologiques 2:267, 1952.

Denber, H. C. B., and Bird, E. G.: Chlorpromazine in the Treatment of Mental Illness: IV. Final Results with Analysis of Data on 1,523 Patients, Am. J. Psychiat. 113:972, 1957.

Dransfield, G. A.: A Clinical Trial Comparing Prochlorperazine ("Stemetil") with Chlorpromazine ("Largactil") in the Treatment of Chronic Psychotic Patients, J. Ment. Sc. 104:1183, 1958.

Edisen, C. B., and Samuels, A. S.: Thiopropazate Hydrochloride (Dartal) Chemotherapy for Emotional Disorders, A. M. A. Arch. Neurol. & Psychiat. 80:481, 1958.

Erwin, H. J.: Clinical Observations on the Use of Promethazine Hydrochloride in Psychiatric Disorders, Am. J. Psychiat. 113:783, 1957.

Feldman, P. E.: A Comparative Study of Various Ataractic Drugs, Am. J. Psychiat. 113:589, 1957.

Feldman, P. E.: Clinical Evaluation of Pacatal, Am. J. Psychiat. 114:143, 1957.

Feldman, P. E.: Two-year Fate Study of Pacatal-treated Patients, Am. J. Psychiat. 115:736, 1959.

Fink, L., and Vlavianos, G.: Clinical Impressions of the Response to Promazine Therapy, Am. J. Psychiat. 114:1031, 1958.

Flach, F.: The Use of Chlorpromazine to Facilitate Intensive Dynamic Psychotherapy in Depression, Psychiat. et neurol. 134:21, 1957.

Flach, F., and Regan, P. E., III: The Influence of Chlorpromazine on Pathologic Emotions and Sexual Unrest, J. Nerv. & Ment. Dis. 129:171, 1959.

Freyhan, F. A.: Therapeutic Implications of Differential Effects of New Phenothiazine Compounds, Am. J. Psychiat. 115:577, 1959.

Gosline, E.; Walters, C. J., and Saunders, J. C.: Clinical Report on Methoxypromazine: A New Phenothiazine, Am. J. Psychiat. 115:939, 1959.

Hegarty, J. G.: MC4703, A New Phenothiazine Derivative, J. Ment. Sc. 104: 870, 1958.

Himwich, H. E.; Rinaldi, F., and Willis, D.: Examination of Phenothiazine Derivatives with Comparisons of Their Effects on the Alerting Reaction, Chemical Structure, and Therapeutic Efficacy, J. Nerv. & Ment. Dis. 124: 53, 1956.

Ilem, P. G., and Sainz, A.: The Psychiatric Application of Vesprin, Psychiat. Quart. 33:9, 1959.

Kinross-Wright, V. J.: The Evaluation of a New Tranquilizing Drug, Thioridazine, Scientific Exhibit, Clinical Meeting of the American Medical Association, Minneapolis, Dec. 2–5, 1958.

Kruse, W.: Experience with Trifluoperazine in 110 Female Schizophrenics, Am. J. Psychiat. 115:1031, 1959.

290 *Bibliography*

Lehman, H. E., and Hanrahan, G. E.: Chlorpromazine, A. M. A. Arch. Neurol. & Psychiat. 71:227, 1954.

Lesse, S.: An Evaluation of Promazine Hydrochloride in Psychiatric Practice, Am. J. Psychiat. 113:984, 1957.

Malitz, S.; Hoch, P. H., and Lesse, S.: A Two-year Evaluation of Chlorpromazine in Clinical Research and Practice, Am. J. Psychiat. 113:540, 1956.

Mathews, F. P.: Dartal: A Clinical Appraisal, Am. J. Psychiat. 114:1034, 1958.

Mendel, W. M.: Observations on the Comparative Effects of Tranquilizers on Patients Previously Treated with Prochlorperazine, Am. J. Psychiat. 115: 466, 1958.

Pennington, V. M.: Clinical Results of Triflupromazine (Vesprin) in 132 Psychotic Patients, Am. J. Psychiat. 115:749, 1959.

Psychiatric Research Reports, American Psychiatric Association, No. 8, 1957.

Riesenman, F. R., and Pettit, M. B.: Clinical Efficacy of Prochlorperazine (Compazine) in Mental Illness, Am. J. Psychiat. 115:1032, 1959.

Roebuck, B. E.; Chambers, J. L., and Williams, E.: An Evaluation of the Therapeutic Use of Triflupromazine in Mental Disease, J. Nerv. & Ment. Dis. 129:184, 1959.

Rudy, L. H.; Himwich, H. E., and Tasher, D. C.: Clinical Evaluation of Two Phenothiazine Compounds—Promazine and Mepazine, Am. J. Psychiat. 113:979, 1957.

Rudy, L. H.; Rinaldi, F.; Costa, E.; Himwich, H. E.; Tuteur, W., and Glotzer, J.: Triflupromazine and Trifluoperazine: Two New Tranquilizers, Am. J. Psychiat. 114:747, 1958.

Samuels, A. S.: Phenergan in Treatment of Psychiatric Patients, Dis. Nerv. System 28:183, 1957.

Sibilio, J. P.; Andrew, G.; Dart, D.; Moore, K. B., and Stehman, V. A.: Treatment of Chronic Schizophrenia with Promazine Hydrochloride, A. M. A. Arch. Neurol. & Psychiat. 78:419, 1957.

Simpson, R. W.: The Effects of Pacatal on Chronic Mental Illness, J. Ment. Sc. 103:610, 1957.

Smith, J. A.; Christian, D.; Rutherford, A., and Mansfield, E.: A Comparison of Triflupromazine (Vesprin), Chlorpromazine, and Placebo in 85 Chronic Patients, Am. J. Psychiat. 115:253, 1958.

Sundby, P., and Lien, J. B.: Prochlorperazine and Chlorpromazine: A Comparative Clinical Trial, Acta psychiat. et neurol. scandinav. (Supp. 136) 34:82, 1959.

Thimann, J., and Gauthier, J. W.: Control of Acute Alcoholism with Prochlorperazine, New England J. Med. 260:915, 1959.

Tolan, E. J., and Peppel, H. H.: Preliminary Observations on Trifluoperazine in Schizophrenia, Am. J. Psychiat. 115:935, 1959.

Trifluoperazine—Clinical and Pharmacological Aspects, Lea & Febiger, Philadelphia, 1958.

Weiss, I. I.; Rubinger, J. H.; Sorin, M., and Ryzen, N.: Trilafon Treatment in Psychotics, Am. J. Psychiat. 114:1118, 1958.

Winkelman, N. W.: An Appraisal of Chlorpromazine, Am. J. Psychiat. 113:961, 1957.

Reserpine

Barsa, J., and Kline, N. S.: Use of Reserpine in Disturbed Psychotic Patients, Am. J. Psychiat. 112:684, 1956.

Cutler, R. P.; Monroe, J. J., and Anderson, T. E.: Effects of "Tranquilizers" upon Pathological Activity in Psychotic Patients: II. Reserpine, A. M. A. Arch. Neurol. & Psychiat. **78**:61, 1957.

Ferguson, R. S.: A Clinical Trial of Reserpine in the Treatment of Anxiety, J. Ment. Sc. **102**:30, 1956.

Hes, J., and Bracha, S.: The Influence of Reserpine on a Disturbed Male Ward and a Method for Assessing This, J. Ment. Sc. **102**:546, 1956.

Malamud, W.; Barton, W.; Fleming, A. M.; Middleton, P. McK.; Friedman, T. T., and Schleifer, M. J.: The Evaluation of the Effects of Derivatives of Rauwolfia in the Treatment of Schizophrenia, Am. J. Psychiat. **114**:193, 1957.

Reserpine (Serpasil) and Other Alkaloids of Rauwolfia Serpentina: Chemistry, Pharmacology, and Clinical Applications, Ann. New York Acad. Sc. **59**:1, 1954.

Reserpine in the Treatment of Neuropsychiatric, Neurological, and Related Clinical Problems, Ann. New York Acad. Sc. **61**:1, 1955.

Savage, C., and Day, J.: Effects of a Tranquilizer (Reserpine) on Psychodynamic and Social Processes, A. M. A. Arch. Neurol. & Psychiat. **79**:590, 1958.

Wing, L.: The Use of Reserpine in Chronic Psychotic Patients: A Controlled Trial, J. Ment. Sc. **102**:530, 1956.

Meprobamate

Barsa, J.: Use of Meprobamate in the Treatment of Psychotic Patients, Am. J. Psychiat. **112**:1023, 1956.

Folkson, A.: Use of Meprobamate in Tension States, J. Ment. Sc. **103**:860, 1957.

Gardner, A.: Meprobamate—A Clinical Study, Am. J. Psychiat. **114**:524, 1957.

Heller, G. C.; Walton, D., and Black, D. A.: Meprobamate in the Treatment of Tension States, J. Ment. Sc. **103**:581, 1957.

Lemere, F.: Habit-forming Properties of Meprobamate, A. M. A. Arch. Neurol. & Psychiat. **76**:205, 1956.

Meprobamate and Other Agents Used in Mental Disturbances, Ann. New York Acad. Sc. **67**:671, 1957.

Tucker, K., and Wilensky, H.: A Clinical Evaluation of Meprobamate Therapy in a Chronic Schizophrenic Population, Am. J. Psychiat. **113**:698, 1957.

Uhlenhuth, E. H.; Canter, A.; Neustadt, J. O., and Payson, H. E.: The Symptomatic Relief of Anxiety with Meprobamate, Phenobarbital, and Placebo, Am. J. Psychiat. **115**:905, 1957.

Electroconvulsive Treatment

Funkenstein, D. H.; King, S. H., and Drolette, M. E.: Mastery of Stress, Harvard University Press, Cambridge, Mass., 1957.

Kalinowsky, L. B., and Hoch, P. H.: Shock Treatments, Psychosurgery, and Other Somatic Treatments in Psychiatry, 2d ed., Grune & Stratton, Inc., New York, 1952.

Regan, P. F.: Effective Utilization of Electric Convulsive Treatment, Am. J. Psychiat. **114**:351, 1957.

Shagass, C.; Naiman, J., and Mihalik, J.: An Objective Test Which Differentiates between Neurotic and Psychotic Depression, A. M. A. Arch. Neurol. & Psychiat. **75**:461, 1956.

292 Bibliography

Bibliography

Stimulants and Antidepressive Agents

Amine Oxidase Inhibitors, Ann. New York Acad. Sc. **80**:551, 1959.

Ayd, F. J., Jr.: A Preliminary Report on Marsilid, Am. J. Psychiat. **114**:459, 1957.

Azima, H., and Vispo, R. H.: Effects of Imipramine (Tofranil) on Depressive States, A. M. A. Arch. Neurol. & Psychiat. **81**:658, 1959.

Breitner, C.: Marsilid in Catatonic Schizophrenia, Am. J. Psychiat. **114**:941, 1958.

Carey, B.; Weber, M., and Smith, J. A.: Methyl-phenidylacetate Hydrochloride (Ritalin) in the Treatment of Chronic Schizophrenic Patients, Am. J. Psychiat. **113**:546, 1956.

Cole, C. E.; Patterson, R. M.; Craig, J. B.; Thomas, W. E.; Ristine, L. P.; Stahly, M., and Pasamanick, B.: A Controlled Study of Efficacy of Iproniazid in the Treatment of Depression, A. M. A. Arch. Gen. Psychiat. **1**:513, 1959.

Davidoff, E.; Best, J. L., and McPheeters, H. L.: The Effect of Ritalin (Methylphenidylacetate Hydrochloride) on Mildly Depressed Ambulatory Patients, New York J. Med. **57**:1753, 1957.

Davidoff, E., and Reifenstein, E. C., Jr.: The Results of Eighteen Months of Benzedrine Sulfate Therapy in Psychiatry, Am. J. Psychiat. **95**:945, 1939.

Feldman, P. E.: Preliminary Report on Imipramine (Tofranil), Am. J. Psychiat. **115**:1117, 1959.

Ferguson, J. T., and Funderburk, W. H.: Improving Senile Behavior with Reserpine and Ritalin, J. A. M. A. **160**:259, 1956.

Ferreira, A. DeL., and Freeman, H.: A Clinical Trial of Marsilid in Psychotic Depressed Patients, Am. J. Psychiat. **114**:933, 1958.

Hoshino, A., and Cease, E.: Iproniazid Phosphate in the Treatment of the Chronic Hospitalized Schizophrenic, Am. J. Psychiat. **114**:1111, 1958.

Houston, F.: A Preliminary Investigation into Abreaction Comparing Methedrine and Sodium Amytal with Other Methods, J. Ment. Sc. **98**:707, 1952.

Kuhn, R.: The Treatment of Depressive States with G22355 (Imipramine Hydrochloride), Am. J. Psychiat. **115**:459, 1958.

Pleasure, H.: Psychiatric and Neurological Side-effects of Isoniazid and Iproniazid, A. M. A. Arch. Neurol. & Psychiat. **72**:313, 1954.

Scanlon, W. G., and White, W. M.: Iproniazid (Marsilid): Its Use in Office Treatment of Depression, Am. J. Psychiat. **114**:1036, 1958.

Special Supplement on the McGill University Conference on Depression and Allied States held in Montreal, March, 1959, Canad. Psychiat. A. J. **4**:1, 1959.

Zimmerman, F. T., and Burgemeister, B. B.: Action of Methyl-phenidylacetate (Ritalin) and Reserpine in Behavior Disorders in Children and Adults, Am. J. Psychiat. **115**:323, 1958.

Insulin Treatment and Lobotomy

Greaves, D. C.; Regan, P. F., and West, L. J.: An Evaluation of Subcoma Insulin Therapy, Am. J. Psychiat. **112**:135, 1955.

Kalinowsky, L. B., and Hoch, P. H.: Shock Treatments, Psychosurgery, and Other Somatic Treatments in Psychiatry, 2d ed., Grune & Stratton, Inc., New York, 1952.

Regan, P. F., and Browne-Mayers, A. N.: Electroencephalography, Frequency Analysis, and Consciousness, J. Nerv. & Ment. Dis. **124**:142, 1956.

Slocum, L.; Bennett, C. L., and Pool, J. L.: The Role of Prefrontal Lobe Surgery as a Means of Eradicating Intractable Anxiety, Am. J. Psychiat. **116**:222, 1959.

Whitehorn, J. C., and Betz, B. J.: A Comparison of Psychotherapeutic Relationships between Physicians and Schizophrenic Patients When Insulin Is Combined with Psychotherapy and When Psychotherapy Is Used Alone, Am. J. Psychiat. **113**:901, 1957.

Endocrine Therapy

Bower, W. H., and Altschule, M. D.: Use of Progesterone in Treatment of Postpartum Psychosis, New England J. Med. **254**:157, 1956.

Chance, J.; Lotsof, E. J.; Pine, I.; Patterson, R. M., and Craig, J.: Effects of Cortisone on Psychiatric Patients, Psychosom. Med. **16**:516, 1954.

Cohn, J. B.; Karnosh, L. J., and Stecher, R. M.: Clinical Trials with Cortisone in the Treatment of Chronic Schizophrenia, Dis. Nerv. System **12**:291, 1951.

Danziger, L., and Kindwall, J. A.: Thyroid Therapy in Some Mental Disorders, Dis. Nerv. System **14**:3, 1953.

Dunn, C. W.: Stilbestrol Induced Testicular Degeneration in Hypersexual Males, J. Clin. Endocrinol. **1**:643, 1941.

Flach, F. F.; Celian, C. I., and Rawson, R. W.: Treatment of Psychiatric Disorders with Triiodothyronine, Am. J. Psychiat. **114**:841, 1958.

Flach, F. F.; Celian, C. I.; Stokes, P. E., and Rawson, R. W.: The Influence of Thyroid Hormones on Metabolism in Psychiatric Disorders: I. The Effect of 3:5:3'-Triiodothyronine on Calcium and Phosphorus Metabolism in Psychiatric Patients, J. Clin. Endocrinol. **19**:454, 1959.

Gallagher, W. J.; Schroeppel, A. B., and Pfeiffer, C. C.: Effects of Reserpine, Iproniazid (Marsilid), and Triiodothyronine (Trionine) and of Reserpine Alone, A. M. A. Arch. Gen. Psychiat. **1**:215, 1959.

Gjessing, R.: Disturbances of Somatic Functions in Catatonia with a Periodic Course, and Their Compensations, J. Ment. Sc. **84**:608, 1938.

Gornall, A. G.; Eglitis, B.; Miller, A.; Stokes, A. B., and Dewan, J. G.: Long-term Clinical and Metabolic Observations in Periodic Catatonia, Am. J. Psychiat. **109**:584, 1953.

Hardwick, S. W.; Pearse, J. J., and Petrow, V.: 6 Beta-hydroxy-3:5-cyclopregnan-20-one in Mental States, J. Ment. Sc. **103**:835, 1957.

Hoagland, H. (Ed.): Hormones, Brain Function, and Behavior, Academic Press, Inc., New York, 1957.

Hoskins, R. G.: The Biology of Schizophrenia, W. W. Norton & Company, New York, 1946.

Polatin, P.; Lesse, S., and Harris, M. M.: Use of Large Doses of Cortisone in Schizophrenia, A. M. A. Arch. Neurol. & Psychiat. **73**:485, 1955.

Rees, L., and King, G. M.: Intensive Cortisone Therapy in Schizophrenia, J. Ment. Sc. **102**:155, 1956.

Reiss, M. (Ed.): Psychoendocrinology, Grune & Stratton, Inc., New York, 1958.

Reiss, M.; Hemphill, R. E.; Gordon, J. J., and Cook, E. R.: Regulation of Urinary Steroid Excretion: I. Effects of Dehydroisoandrosterone and of Anterior Pituitary Extract on the Pattern of Daily Excretion in Man, Biochem. J. **44**:632, 1949.

Ripley, H. S.; Shorr, E., and Papanicolaou, G. N.: The Effect of Treatment of

Depression in the Menopause with Estrogenic Hormone, Am. J. Psychiat. 96:905, 1940.

Sands, D. E., and Chamberlain, G. H. A.: Treatment of Inadequate Personality in Juveniles by Dehydroisoandrosterone, Brit. M. J. 2:66, 1952.

Strauss, E. B.; Sands, D. E.; Robinson, A. M.; Tindall, W. J., and Stevenson, W. A. H.: Use of Dehydroisoandrosterone in Psychiatric Treatment, Brit. M. J. 2:64, 1952.

Vlavianos, G., and Fink, L.: The Clinical Effect of Nor-eth-androlone on Incontinent Mental Patients, Am. J. Psychiat. 115:164, 1958.

Wiedorn, W. S., Jr.: Psychological Effects of Cortisone in Acute Catatonic Excitement, Am. J. Psychiat. 112:457, 1955.

Miscellaneous Drugs

Alexander, L.: Chemotherapy of Depression—Use of Meprobamate Combined with Benactyzine (2-Diethylaminoethyl Benzilate) Hydrochloride, J. A. M. A. 166:1019, 1958.

Barsa, J. A.: Azacyclonol (Frenquel) in the Treatment of Chronic Schizophrenics, Am. J. Psychiat. 113:255, 1956.

Bonafede, V.: Chlorpromazine Treatment of Disturbed Epileptic Patients, A. M. A. Arch. Neurol. & Psychiat. 77:243, 1957.

Bowes, H. A.: The Ataractic Drugs: The Present Position of Chlorpromazine, Frenquel, Pacatal, and Reserpine in the Psychiatric Hospital, Am. J. Psychiat. 113:530, 1956.

Brooks, C.: The Use of Reserpine (Serpasil) in Mentally Ill Epileptics, Dis. Nerv. System. 18:275, 1957.

Feldman, D. J.: Drug Therapy of Chronic Alcoholism, M. Clin. North America, March, 1957.

Forster, F. M. (Ed.): Modern Therapy in Neurology, The C. V. Mosby Company, St. Louis, 1957.

Green, J. R., and Steelman, H. F. (Eds.): Epileptic Seizures, The Williams & Wilkins Company, Baltimore, 1956.

Jacobsen, E.; Kehlet, H.; Larsen, V.; Munkvad, I., and Skinhøj, K.: The Autonomic Reaction of Psycho-neurotics to a New Sedative: Benactyzine NFN, Suavitil (R) (Benzilic Acid Diethylaminoethylester Hydrochloride), Acta psychiat. et neurol. scandinav. 30:627, 1955.

Kinross-Wright, V., and Moyer, J. H.: Observations upon the Therapeutic Use of Benactyzine Suavitil, Am. J. Psychiat. 114:73, 1957.

Lemere, F.: Failure of Azacyclonol (Frenquel) to Relieve Non-experimental Mental Confusion and Hallucinations, Am. J. Psychiat. 113:840, 1957.

Lemere, F., and Lasater, J. H.: Deanol (Deaner), a New Cerebral Stimulant for the Treatment of Neurasthenia and Mild Depression: A Preliminary Report, Am. J. Psychiat. 114:655, 1958.

Martensen-Larsen, O.: Five Years' Experience with Disulfiram in the Treatment of Alcoholics, Quart. J. Studies Alcohol 14:406, 1953.

Moriarity, J. D., and Mebane, J. C.: Clinical Uses of Deanol (Deaner): A New Type of Psychotropic Drug, Am. J. Psychiat. 115:941, 1959.

Munkvad, I.: Treatment of Psychoses and Psychoneuroses with a New Sedative (Suavitil), Acta psychiat. et neurol. scandinav. 30:729, 1955.

Pfeiffer, C. C.; Jenney, E. H.; Gallagher, W.; Smith, R. P., and Bevan, W., Jr.: Stimulant Effect of 2-Dimethylaminoethanol—Possible Precursor of Brain Acetylcholine, Science 126:610, 1957.

Rathod, N. H.: Toxic Effects of Disulfiram Therapy, Quart. J. Studies Alcohol 19:418, 1958.

Rinaldi, F.; Rudy, L. H., and Himwich, H. E.: The Use of Frenquel in the Treatment of Disturbed Patients with Psychoses of Long Duration, Am. J. Psychiat. 112:343, 1955.

Sherfey, M. J., and Diethelm, O.: Evaluation of Drugs in the Treatment of Alcoholism, in Psychiatric Treatment, Proceedings of the Association for Research in Nervous and Mental Disease 31:287, 1953.

Simms, L. M.: Use of Hydroxyzine in Neuropsychiatric States, Dis. Nerv. System 19:225, 1958.

Symposium on Newer Antidepressant and Other Psychotherapeutic Drugs, Supplement, Dis. Nerv. System 21:3, March, 1960.

Toll, N.: Deaner, an Adjunct for Treatment of Schizoid and Schizophrenic Patients, Am. J. Psychiat. 115:366, 1958.

Winkelman, N., Jr.: Evaluation of Two Ataractic Agents—Experience of One Year with Prochlorperazine and of Seven Months with Benactyzine, Dis. Nerv. System 20:27, 1959.